THE WISDOM OF
MILTON H. ERICKSON

THE WISDOM OF MILTON H. ERICKSON

By
Ronald A. Havens

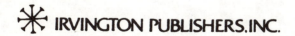

IRVINGTON PUBLISHERS, INC.

Library of Congress Cataloging in Publication Data

Erickson, Milton H.
    The wisdom of Milton H. Erickson.

    Bibliography: p.
    Includes index.
    1. Hypnotism—Therapeutic use—Addresses, essays,
lectures.   2. Psychotherapy—Addresses, essays, lectures.
3. Psychology—Addresses, essays, lectures.   I. Havens,
Ronald A.   II. Title.   [DNLM: 1. Hypnosis.   2. Psychotherapy.   WM 415 H385W]
RC495.E74   1984   616.89′162   82-21377
ISBN 0-8290-0963-9

Printed in the United States of America

TABLE OF CONTENTS

ACKNOWLEDGEMENT

Many thanks are due to my friend and colleague, Dr. Richard Dimond, for his encouragement and contributory ideas and for his assistance in copying many of the quotations eventually used in this book. Thanks also to Sandy McGuire and Maryanna McCall for their patience and skill in typing from the original handwritten manuscript which was a genuine nightmare of inserts, corrections, and bibliographic details. My wife, Marie, deserves special mention and thanks for her warmth, sacrifice, support, and editorial review of my work.

Finally, the author wishes to acknowledge the following journals, publishers, and individuals who generously provided permission to use quotations from sources copyrighted by them:

American Medical Association (*Archives of Neurology and Psychiatry*), American Psychiatric Association (*American Journal of Psychiatry*), American Psychological Association

(*Journal of Abnormal and Social Psychology and Journal of Experimental Psychology*), American Society of Clinical Hypnosis (*American Journal of Clinical Hypnosis*), American Society of Psychosomatic Dentistry and Medicine (*Journal of the American Society of Psychosomatic Dentistry and Medicine*), British Psychological Society (*British Journal of Medical Psychology*), Brunner/Mazel, Elsevier Publishing Co. (*Psychosomatic Medicine*), Encyclopaedia Britannica, *Family Process*, Grune & Stratton, Jay Haley, Harper & Row Publishers, Irvington Publishers, Journal Press (*Journal of General Psychology* and *Journal of Genetic Psychology*), Herbert S. Lustig, M.D., Macmillan Company, Merck, Sharp & Dohme (*Trends in Psychiatry*), Physicians Postgraduate Press (*Diseases of the Nervous System*), Psychoanalytic Quarterly Inc., Plenum Publishing Corporation (for Appleton-Century-Crofts), Science & Behavior Books (for Meta Publications), Society for Clinical and Experimental Hypnosis (*Journal of Clinical and Experimental Hypnosis*), Springer Verlag New York, W. B. Saunders (*Medical Clinics of North America*), William Alanson White Psychiatric Foundation (*Psychiatry*), Jeffrey K. Zeig, Ph.D.

In accordance with the procedures requested or required by the relevant parties, acknowledgement is hereby provided that portions of the copyrighted material specified below have been reprinted by permission of the copyright holders:

Abridged sections from "Basic Psychological Problems in Hypnotic Research" by Milton H. Erickson, M.D. in *HYPNOSIS: Current Problems*, edited by G. H. Estabrooks. Copyright © 1962 by George H. Estabrooks. Reprinted by permission of Harper & Row Publishers, Inc.

Bandler, Richard & John Grinder. *Patterns of the Hypnotic Techniques of Milton H. Erickson, M.D. Volume I*, Science & Behavior Books, Inc. Palo Alto, California, copyright © 1975 by Meta Publications.

Erickson, M.H. Development of apparent unconsciousness during hypnotic reliving of a traumatic experience. *Archives of Neurology and Psychiatry*, 1973, *38*, 1282–1288, Copyright © 1937 by American Medical Association.

Erickson, M.H. Negation or reversal of legal testimony. *Archives of Neurology and Psychiatry*, 1938, *40*, 549–555. Copyright © 1938 by American Medical Association.

Erickson, M.H. Demonstration of mental mechanisms by hypnosis. *Archives of Neurology and Psychiatry*, 1939, *42*, 367–370, Copyright © 1939, American Medical Association.

Erickson, M.H. Hypnotic investigation of psychosomatic phenomema: Psychosomatic interrelationships studies by experimental hypnosis. *Psychosomatic Medicine*, 1943, *5*, 51–58, Copyright © 1943 by the American Psychosomatic Society, Inc.

Erickson, M.H. The therapy of a psychosomatic headache. *Journal of Clinical and Experimental Hypnosis*, October, 1953, 2–6, Copyright © by The Society for Clinical and Experimental Hypnosis, October, 1953.

Erickson, M.H. A clinical note on indirect hypnotic therapy. *Journal of Clinical and Experimental Hypnosis*, July, 1954, 171–174. Copyright © by The Society of Clinical and Experimental Hypnosis, July 1954.

PREFACE

The material in this book was compiled in an attempt to clarify the concepts and attitudes necessary for an effective application of the Ericksonian forms of therapy and hypnosis. It is not a compilation of Ericksonian techniques nor is it a theoretical analysis of Dr. Erickson's work. It is, instead, simply a collection of the observations and ideas that Dr. Erickson himself presented in numerous publications and lectures in an effort to communicate the wisdom that guided his interventions. It is an effort to capture and to convey the essential ingredients of his solution to the most fundamental problem facing us all, i.e., how to enjoy and use life to its fullest and how to enable those around us to do the same. Some people spend more time than others grappling with this problem and many, such as psychotherapists, earn their living doing so. Ultimately, however, this issue forms a common denominator between us all in our universal search for insights, understandings, and truths about ourselves.

Rarely in this search are we presented with straightforward observations about how people operate or about what factors influence human behavior. Information about people typically is so tightly embedded within a specific theoretical framework that it is impossible to determine fact from fancy. As we read various texts on personality theory, hypnosis, and psychotherapy, we are confronted by the contradictory theoretical assumptions of either the Freudians, the Jungians, the Adlerians, the Rogerians, the Skinnerians, or some other prominent school of thought. Each of these theoretical systems views people in an entirely different light and each leads to entirely different dogmatic observations and recommendations about what to do and when. As a result, human nature and human behavior continue to be confusing mysteries for most psychotherapists; a phenomenon we participate in without real understanding and attempt to influence in ourselves and others without much effect.

It would be especially significant, therefore, if someone came along who had taken the time and effort simply to observe what people actually do and what variables actually influence their behavior. It would be even more significant if this person had translated these observations and had demonstrated how to apply them for the benefit of oneself and others. Anyone could certainly benefit from such accumulated wisdom.

Milton H. Erickson did just that! He observed, he noticed every detail, and he applied his observations in his practice of hypnotherapy. He devoted his life to careful observation of himself and others and, as a result, he became more familiar with the nature of people than perhaps anyone else before or since. As a consequence, he learned how to enable others to utilize potentials they did not know they had and he helped them resolve personal and interpersonal problems that no other professional had been able to touch.

And he tried to teach others the wisdom he had accumulated by those years of observation. He wrote and he lectured and he taught throughout his entire professional career. He taught, in fact, until several days before his death on March 25, 1980 at the age of 78.

This book is a distilled synopsis of what this remarkable man observed and what he taught throughout his lifetime. Naturally, the wisdom contained in these pages should be of tremendous value for anyone seriously interested in becoming an effective hypnotist or psychotherapist. Erickson was a master of both and his comments on these endeavors may represent the best advice and instruction available.

On the other hand, his general knowledge about people represents such a unique perspective of such proven value that it deserves serious consideration even by social scientists who believe that both hypnosis and psychotherapy are useless or irrelevant to their interests. Every psychologist, sociologist, anthropologist, or other professional involved in the study of people should find it worthwhile to learn what Erickson had to say because his observations have significant implications for an understanding of all aspects of human functioning.

What Erickson noticed about people provides a perspective on ourselves which seems to be descriptively accurate, objectively valid, conceptually challenging, and totally beyond the boundaries of any existing paradigmatic perspective. Here, at last, is a person who told us simply what people are and what they do without imposing a set of biased and limiting assumptions or theoretical constraints between his perceptions and the world around him. All theoreticians, researchers, and clinicians owe it to themselves to take a fresh look at people through Erickson's perspective. What they see may or may not strike them as useful, but it is guaranteed to give them something to wonder about and it is likely to open their awareness to aspects of human behavior that they had previously ignored.

A similar comment could be made about people interested in becoming more aware and more effective, no matter what their age, vocation, role, or status. Erickson's wisdom is universal in its application and impact and, as such, it deserves to be deciphered and shared with everyone. The basic perspective Erickson taught in the lecture hall was identical to what he taught to his patients in his office. In both instances he was simply attempting to teach others a way of being and perceiving that would motivate and enable them to use their inherent capacities and previous learnings to cope most effectively with the realistic demands of their lives. It is hoped that this book will facilitate that process in some small way for students of psychology and psychiatry, for practitioners of therapy, counseling, and hypnosis and even for nonprofessionals interested in learning about themselves and others.

AN INTRODUCTION TO MILTON H. ERICKSON, M.D.

Milton H. Erickson was probably the most creative, dynamic, and effective hypnotherapist the world has ever seen. Not only could he hypnotize the most difficult and resistant patients imaginable, he could even do so without their conscious awareness that they were being or had been hypnotized. He hypnotized people by talking about tomato plants in a certain way, by describing the objects in his office in a certain way, and even by shaking hands in a certain way. There were, in fact, several colleagues who refused to shake hands with him after he had successfully demonstrated his handshake induction upon them. During a lecture in Mexico City in 1959 he hypnotized a nurse in front of a large audience using only pantomime gestures, a feat made even more impressive by the fact that this Spanish-speaking nurse had no idea when she volunteered that she was to be a subject in a demonstration of hypnosis. In a sense, the variety and effectiveness of

Erickson's hypnotic inductions defies imagination, though none seems less likely to be effective than his "Shut up, sit in that chair there and go into a deep trance!", an induction technique that he made work.

As a psychotherapist he was equally creative and effective. It is doubtful that many therapists would conclude that effective intervention should involve teaching patients how to squirt water between their teeth, stepping on patient's feet, sending them out to climb mountains, having them strip naked in the office and point to each part of their bodies, or having them eat a ham sandwich. Yet these are some of the strange strategies that Erickson employed with outstanding success, and with each patient he seemed to generate another unique and almost outlandish intervention. His psychotherapy style was so completely innovative and his success rate was so high that many of his patients were people referred to him by other psychotherapists or were those other psychotherapists themselves.

It should come as no surprise, therefore, that Milton H. Erickson has been described by other hypnotherapists in some of the most laudatory terms imaginable. At various times he has been referred to as a master hypnotist, as a psychotherapeutic wizard, and as the world's foremost authority on hypnotherapy and brief strategic psychotherapy. In 1976 he became the first recipient of the only award presented by the International Society of Hypnosis: the Benjamin Franklin Gold Medal. This medal was inscribed *"To Milton H. Erickson, M.D. — innovator, outstanding clinician, and distinguished investigator whose ideas have not only helped create the modern view of hypnosis but have profoundly influenced the practice of all psychotherapy throughout the world."*

In December of 1980 several thousand professionals descended upon Phoenix, Arizona to pay posthumous tribute to him and to participate in workshops and presentations on his hypnotherapeutic techniques. This *International Congress of Ericksonian Approaches to Hypnosis and Psychotherapy* had been preceded for years by a constant stream of professionals to training sessions in his office in Phoenix. Elsewhere throughout the country and throughout the world workshops on Ericksonian techniques have become almost mandatory inclusions in the programs of professional conferences in psychotherapy and hypnosis. Books by and about him have become bestsellers almost overnight and Dr. Ernest L. Rossi has even edited a four-volume collection of almost all of his numerous published and unpublished articles. In short, it probably would not be an exaggeration to state that Erickson has had a greater impact upon the human services professions than any other single individual since Freud.

It is somewhat ironic that the peak of his public recognition should have occurred only after he reached the age of seventy. Prior to that time the value of his work was acknowledged only by a relatively small group of devoted followers. His therapeutic techniques were rarely mentioned in textbooks on psychotherapy and even books and articles on hypnosis by some of the most prominent scientific investigators in the field often gave no more than a brief mention of his techniques or research contributions. In fact, it is easy to get the impression that Erickson was intentionally ignored by many of his contemporaries. Whether or not this was the case, the fact remains that he was a maverick to a large extent, a unique person with strong and unusual convictions, and an unselfconscious person who was not afraid of confrontations. His background and professional activities both explain and demonstrate this quite clearly.

Erickson was born on December 5, 1901, in the now defunct town of Aurum, Nevada. His pioneer parents eventually moved "east" in a covered wagon and settled on a farm in a rural section of Wisconsin. Even as a child he experienced the world in ways that were quite different from those of his friends and relatives. Aside from an intense curiosity and a general reluctance simply to accept the beliefs and superstitions of his rural community, Erickson's world was different from others for physiological reasons as well. For example, he had an unusual form of color blindness that enabled him to perceive and enjoy the color purple but little else. As a result, he surrounded himself with this color in later life and eventually became quite interested in the hypnotic induction of color blindness. He was also arrhythmic and tone deaf, phenomena that led to his intense interest in the effects of alterations in breathing patterns associated with the "yelling" that others called singing. In addition, he experienced dyslexia. The various difficulties created by that anomaly actually intensified his familiarity with and interest in the meanings and implications of words. It is especially intriguing that a person who would eventually become one of the world's experts on the use of language did not learn to talk until the age of four and even then, because of his arrhythmia and tone deafness, spoke in a rhythm totally unlike most Americans. Various experts have compared his speech pattern to that of a Central African tribe, that of a Brazilian tribe, and that of a Peruvian tribe.

Finally, Erickson experienced a lifetime of physical ailments beginning with a life threatening bout of polio at age 17 and culminating in a second case of polio in 1952. Although he was able to recover almost completely from the total paralysis of his first bout with polio, the unusual second case took a more severe toll. For most of his later years he was confined to a wheelchair with no real use of his legs, little or no use of his right arm, and restricted use of his left arm. Eventually, he was able to use only half of his diaphragm to speak and his mouth had become partially paralyzed as well. In addition he suffered from chronic intense pain which he moderated with autohypnosis.

In spite of his many physical discomforts and handicaps he remained active and therapeutically effective until his death on March 25, 1980. Throughout his lifetime he was forced to overcome an incredible variety of adversities, but he had a way of turning all of his difficulties into advantages and valuable opportunities for learning. He was fond of saying that life's difficulties were merely necessary roughage. Few other people have ever made more effective use of so much roughage.

Perhaps because he was so atypical physiologically, Erickson began observing and influencing the behavior of others while still a small child. For example, he enjoyed walking to school early through the new fallen snow, leaving behind him a crooked path. His journey home that afternoon was then made more interesting by observing how many other children had walked to school following his crooked path instead of creating a straighter one of their own. Similarly, as he slowly recovered from the total paralysis of polio he spent many days simply observing the behavior of those around him and gradually, as a result, he became remarkably sensitive to body language and developed methods to elicit needed help from others without asking for it directly.

He used his skills at influencing the behavior of others during a one-man canoe trip of over 1200 miles that he undertook as physical therapy in the summer of 1921 following his first year as an undergraduate. When he began this summer trip he was so weak from the aftereffects of polio that he could swim only a few yards at a time and could not even lift his canoe out of the water. He had some beans, some rice, and slightly more than two dollars with him to purchase additional supplies. Yet without ever directly asking for assistance he managed to elicit enough fish from curious fishermen, money from odd jobs along the river, and help in getting his canoe over dams to manage quite well. In fact, by the time he returned to Wisconsin he could swim a mile, could carry his own canoe, and was more than ready to begin his second year of classes at the University of Wisconsin.

During the first semester of his sophomore year at the University of Wisconsin, Erickson experienced one of his many spontaneous autohypnotic phenomena. This experience seems to have had a profound effect upon his thinking and may have set the stage for his subsequent introduction to hypnosis by Clark Hull. Erickson had decided that he wanted to earn some extra money by writing editorials for the local newspaper and he had planned to write them by using an ability he had discovered when he was younger. This ability consisted simply of sometimes being able to dream the correct solutions to arithmetic problems. Accordingly, he planned to study until 10:30 P.M. at which time he would go to bed and awaken at 1:00 A.M. to write the editorial he hoped he would have created in his dreams in the meantime. He awoke the next morning with no memory of having written the editorial, yet there it was, carefully placed under his typewriter. He decided not to read that editorial or any of the others he produced in the same mysterious manner and submitted to the newspaper that week, but each day he looked in the paper to see if he could find one he thought he might have written. He discovered that he was unable to recognize his own editorials, each of which had been published, and concluded that "there was a lot more in my head than I realized." That experience also led him to conclude that he should begin to trust his own understandings and not allow them to be distorted "by somebody else's imperfect knowledge."

In spite of these and other similar experiences, Erickson did not begin to think in terms of hypnosis until the end of his sophomore year when he observed a demonstration of hypnosis by Clark L. Hull. Erickson was so excited by this demonstration that he subsequently managed to get Hull's subject to allow Erickson to hypnotize him and he spent the following summer hypnotizing anyone who would cooperate with him.

He reported on the various experiences and conclusions accumulated over that summer during a graduate seminar on hypnosis conducted by Clark Hull the following fall. Erickson's conclusions conflicted sharply with those of Hull, who approached hypnosis from an experimentalist and learning theorist point of view. Hull's emphasis upon a standardized approach and de-emphasis of the importance of any inner processes of the subject were directly contrary to Erickson's own observations and this difference of opinion led to considerable acrimony and estrangement between the two men. According to Erickson, Hull regarded his views as "unappreciative disloyalty and willfull oversight" (Erickson, 1967). Erickson, in turn, has since labeled Hull's standardized approach an "absurd" and "futile" endeavor that disregards "...the subject as a person, putting him on a par with inanimate laboratory apparatus..." (Erickson, 1952).

Needless to say, Erickson was unable to convince Hull that he was wrong. Instead, Hull formalized his views further, conducted a series of experiments based upon them and published this material in his book, *Hypnosis and Suggestibility: An Experimental Approach*, in 1933. The conceptual and experimental assumptions underlying this landmark book formed the foundation for the modern scientific view of hypnosis, a view that continues to reject or to conflict with Erickson's perspectives.

Hull was also unable to convince Erickson that Erickson was wrong. Undaunted by Hull's rejection of his perspective, Erickson continued to utilize and to do research in hypnosis. He consulted with others at the university including Dr.

William Blackwen of the Psychiatric Department and Dr. Hans Rees, a professor of neurology, regarding the design of a research project to determine the inherent or basic differences between hypnotized and non-hypnotized subjects. This and other research projects on hypnosis were begun and conducted on an extracurricular basis throughout the remainder of his academic career. Thus, by the time he had completed his B.A. in 1927 and his M.A. in psychology and M.D. degrees in 1928 at the University of Wisconsin, he had developed an extensive background and high level of expertise in this area.

Along the way, he found it necessary to solicit the help of a psychiatrist-lawyer to prevent his dismissal from graduate school for dealing with the black art of hypnosis. When he began his internship at the Colorado General Hospital (1928–1929) he emphatically was forbidden even to mention the topic of hypnosis under the threat of dismissal and refusal of his state licensing application. Characteristically, however, Erickson was able to continue his work in hypnosis by associating with the Colorado State Psychopathic Hospital where he eventually received a special residency in psychiatry following his internship and licensure.

During the year following his special residency in psychiatry (1929–1930) he was an Assistant Physician at the Rhode Island State Hospital for Mental Diseases after which he joined the Research Service of Worcester State Hospital in Massachusetts. When he left, four years later, he had become chief psychiatrist on the Research Service.

From 1934 to 1939, he was Director of Psychiatric Research at the Eloise Hospital and Infirmary in Eloise, Michigan where he subsequently was promoted to Director of Research and Psychiatric Training, a position he held until 1949. While in Michigan, Erickson was a prolific writer and researcher in the field of hypnosis. The productivity of this period is even more remarkable given his joint appointment in psychiatry at Wayne University College of Medicine from 1938 to 1948 and his joint appointment as a professor in the Graduate School of Wayne State University from 1943 to 1948. He also was a Visiting Professor of Clinical Psychology at Michigan State University in East Lansing, Michigan for a brief time.

Erickson met his second wife, Elizabeth, while teaching at Wayne State University where she was a psychology student and graduate assistant. His first marriage had ended in divorce and when he married Elizabeth in 1936 he brought three children with him from that marriage. Subsequently they had five additional children, which may partially explain why Erickson was so familiar with and referred so often to the process of human development and early learning in his lectures.

In 1948, primarily for health reasons, the Ericksons moved to Phoenix, Arizona where, after working briefly in a local institution, Erickson established a private practice. The remainder of his life was spent in Phoenix where he continued to practice in an unpretentious office at his home. Eventually, his cramped office became cluttered with various mementos and presents from patients who had flown from as far away as New York or Mexico City to be treated by him. In his later years he would meet with eight or more people at a time in his small office to teach and to conduct hypnotherapy. These people came to Phoenix to learn from the master, though a number of them reportedly ended up learning more about themselves and less about hypnotherapy *per se* than they had originally expected.

Erickson himself was unconcerned that his cramped and cluttered office did not accurately reflect his growing stature and prestige in the field. In fact, his first office had held only a card table and two chairs, but he had defended his decor by stating *"I* was there." He may have been unpretentious but he was not unconvinced of his own prowess and competency! As quoted in Zeig (1980), Erickson states, "As for my dignity ... the hell with my dignity. (Laughs) I will get along all right in this world. I don't have to be dignified, professional." He also says, "And I am very confident. I look confident. I act confident. I speak in a confident way ..." These two comments are a remarkable summary of Erickson's life and style and provide some insight into the man who was so convinced that he was right and so unconcerned with what others thought of him that he was able to challenge the traditional assumptions and techniques of the scientific and professional community and to blaze his own unique path.

During the early 1950's Erickson undertook a series of teaching seminars in hypnosis throughout the United States and other countries. As a result of his presentations before a group of professionals in Chicago, the Seminars on Hypnosis Foundation was established. Many of the members of this teaching group, of which Erickson was the senior member, had participated in his early seminars in Chicago. Subsequently, the Seminars on Hypnosis Foundation evolved into the American Society of Clinical Hypnosis — Education and Research Foundation.

In 1957 Erickson became the founding president of the American Society of Clinical Hypnosis. This society provided a more clinically oriented alternative to the previously formed Society for Clinical and Experimental Hypnosis. SCEH had been established in 1949 within a Hullian scientific tradition and it had maintained that experimental tradition quite emphatically. As a determined opponent of the theories and hypnotic techniques of this tradition and as a dedicated clinician, Erickson founded ASCH and served as its president from 1957 to 1959. In 1958 he became founding editor of the *American Journal of Clinical Hypnosis* and served in this capacity until 1968, during which time he was able to provide a forum for authors whose interests and theoretical assumptions may not have been appropriate for SCEH's *Journal of Clinical and Experimental Psychology.*

From 1967 on, Erickson received an increasing amount of recognition for his psychotherapeutic skills in addition to his hypnotic abilities. Although his publications during that period continued to focus upon the techniques and considerations underlying hypnosis, various books about him began to appear that focused instead upon his therapeutic interventions (cf. Bandler & Grinder, 1975; Haley, 1967; 1973). These publications brought him to the attention of a much broader audience and ensured an ever-increasing following.

Prior to his death Erickson had received numerous honors and awards. He was a Life Fellow of the American Psychiatric Association, the American Psychological Association, and the American Association for the Advancement of Science. He had received a diplomate from the American Board of Psychiatry and had been a member of the American Psychopathological Association. The July, 1977 issue of the *American Journal of Clinical Hypnosis* was dedicated solely to his work in honor of his 75th birthday. The list of achievements and honors could go on, but the point simply is that Milton H. Erickson was a person worthy of our careful study and attention; a unique, effective, and influential hypnotherapist who evidently knew something very special about people and translated that knowledge into effective hypnotic and therapeutic strategies.

HOW AND WHY THIS BOOK WAS CREATED

Unfortunately, Erickson never translated his unique body of knowledge and learning into an organized, detailed account of his conceptual framework. Although he was a prolific author (over 140 scholarly articles and co-author of several books) and lecturer, he rarely provided more than brief, general glimpses of his underlying system of thought. Erickson once stated, "If I started teaching by precision I'd bore them." (Zeig, 1980) and it is safe to say that his audiences were rarely bored. As a result, however, there is no single publication of his that offers the interested and motivated reader a genuine or complete sense of the wisdom that guided him throughout his hypnotherapeutic career. The observations and conceptual perspective underlying his strategies have remained remarkably elusive and it seems safe to assert that there are few hypnotists or therapists in the world who could rightly claim to understand Erickson's approaches thoroughly or to be able to utilize them as effectively and creatively as he did.

As a consequence of the conceptual void left by his reluctance to do more than hint at the underlying observations or
concepts that guided his work, Erickson's traditionally trained
colleagues often tended to view his interventions as illogical,
confusing, mysterious, magical, irrelevant, or even irreverant.
Apparently it was easier for many to dismiss him as a show-
off, a charlatan, or a lunatic than to undergo the perspective
shift and careful observation necessary to appreciate what he
had to offer.

On the other hand, even among his followers there often
seemed to be much confusion as to whether his effectiveness
should be attributed to him as a person, to his unique perspective and wisdom, or to the specific techniques he developed
and described. Those who held fast to the first view formed
little more than a cult following and the third view was held
primarily by those who had become particularly effective at
imitating his physical and verbal mannerisms and in training
others to do likewise.

Although it is obvious that Erickson was a powerful personality and that imitation of his mannerisms may be effective
under some circumstances, it also seems apparent that only by
learning the fundamental concepts and information that guided him, and thus adopting his underlying perspective, can we
hope to understand the logic of his actions or to create similar
interventions on our own. Erickson may not have presented a
direct or complete explanation of his work, but fortunately he
did attempt to communicate bits and pieces of it to others.
Comments pregnant with meaning and implications are scattered throughout his lectures, case histories, and research sum-
maries like the parts of a complex jigsaw puzzle.

Unfortunately, the actual meaning and implication of each
of these jigsaw statements are apparent only within the context
of the entire pattern of his knowledge. Each of his general

comments seems to be meaningful alone, but that meaning shifts and changes slightly as other statements of his are read or heard. The problem with understanding what Erickson was trying to tell us is that each of his comments is almost invariably interpreted within our own framework of understanding because his was so unique and, thus, difficult to comprehend. The meaning we tend to impose upon his comments is not necessarily the meaning he intended to communicate and, paradoxically, it is probably impossible to comprehend the meaning he was trying to communicate until we can comprehend it *in toto* from within the framework of his specific perspective.

The limitations generated by this natural distorting and misunderstanding process were very familiar to Erickson. He typically admonished his students in the following manner: "So, I warn all of you, don't ever when you are listening to a patient, think you understand the patient, because you're listening with your ears and thinking with your vocabulary. The patient's vocabulary is something entirely different." (Zeig, 1980, p. 58). Later on he adds the comment that "We always translate the other person's language into our own language." (Zeig, 1980, p. 64). Even Dr. Ernest Rossi, who spent many years studying with Erickson, was subject to this error for which he received the following admonition: "You were placing *your* meaning on my words. But what was *my* meaning?" (Erickson & Rossi, 1981, p. 211). This may be the ultimate question facing all students or practitioners interested in becoming proficient in an Ericksonian approach or anyone interested in learning what this man knew about people. What was *his* meaning?

· The idiosyncratic meanings of Erickson's conceptual comments and their presentation in a diversity of sources are major obstacles to a widespread appreciation and utilization of his wisdom. Furthermore, the amount of time involved in a thorough review and reorganization of his work to isolate and organize his more pertinent comments regarding the nature of people, the purpose of psychotherapy, etc. is not available to everyone who might be interested in doing so. By a lucky coincidence, however, my fascination with the work of Erickson and the granting of a sabbatical leave from my teaching responsibilities at Sangamon State University provided me with both the motivation and the opportunity to conduct such a review.

I began this project solely to satisfy my own personal need to understand once and for all what this incredible clinician had to offer. I had a purely selfish and admittedly grandiose desire to comprehend what Erickson knew, a desire that had not been satisfied by the numerous analyses of his work which I had read previously or by my relatively unorganized and cursory exposure to his numerous articles and books. Whenever I began to feel that I understood what he was saying, I would run into another quotation that confused me, added some new twist, or directly contradicted my original notions. Finally my patience ran out and I decided to use the time available to me to read everything of his that I could get my hands on and to consolidate in an organized fashion all of his comments that seemed to be direct expressions of his accumulated knowledge and basic observations. In essence, I hoped to create a concordance of Erickson's concepts and knowledge that would guide and direct my own thoughts, observations, and clinical activities.

The initial stage of this project consisted of a thorough and careful reading of Erickson's published works. At first it was necessary to rely upon the bibliography of his writings compiled by Gravitz and Gravitz (1977) to find these materials. However, the publication of his collected works by Rossi

(Erickson, 1980) facilitated this process considerably. Additional books, transcripts, and audio tapes contributed further insights and notable quotations. Eventually it was possible to review almost every publication by or about him prior to 1981.

As these books, transcripts, and articles were read, statements that expressed his general observations, basic concepts or underlying assumptions in any way were carefully noted. Such statements were rarely lengthy and usually were scattered rather widely through his writings, inductions, and speeches. In addition, I eventually decided to use only comments that were directly attributable to Erickson himself, a decision that eliminated much of the material in most co-authored works. Accordingly, what began as several thousand pages eventually was reduced to several thousand "significant" quotations of varying length and complexity.

Each isolated quotation was assigned to a general category on the basis of its predominant content. Those dealing with hypnosis were placed in one category, those dealing with therapy were placed in another, and those providing broad generalizations about people were placed in the third. All quotations in each category were reviewed and subdivided further into smaller groups in accordance with their primary topics. Eventually, all comments about the conscious mind were in the same file, all of those about the unconscious in another, etc.

Next, all of the quotations from each subcategory were spread around several large tables and small clusters of highly related or similar statements were created. It was quite startling to realize how frequently Erickson had discussed the same points over the years. Apparently he had referred over and over again to a fairly limited number of issues, sometimes repeating previous statements almost verbatim, typically adding new details or insights. It was somewhat comforting to learn that he had not undergone any dramatic changes in his perspective during his professional career. It simplified my task and seemed to emphasize the significance of his position.

As the statements assigned to each cluster were reviewed and organized, it became apparent that the material contained an inherent organization. In spite of their original separation in time, the statements within each category almost had to be organized in a specific hierarchical arrangement if they were to be understood. Some comments simply could not be appreciated until others were read. Similarly, there seemed to be a necessary hierarchy of importance to many of the topics covered. An understanding of what was conveyed in some categories seemed to form the foundation for what was said in others.

It is difficult to convey the impact created by my first thoughtful reading of the resultant condensed and organized collection of Erickson's words. What had emerged from my efforts was more than I could have anticipated or had any reason to expect. As I read through those organized quotations, an entirely new conceptual reality began to take form before me. When I had finished, the clarity, coherence, implications and seemingly unchallengeable validity of what I had read was overwhelming. Throughout the years Erickson had developed a view of reality, of people, of hypnosis, and of therapy that was simple, direct, and yet remarkably insightful. The how and why of his effectiveness as a hypnotist and psychotherapist suddenly became blatantly obvious and had an immediate effect upon me. As the scattered shards of wisdom organized themselves into meaningful gestalts, the truth and beauty of the final form became genuinely compelling.

Other readers may not experience the same opening up of new worlds of observation and understanding or feel the same impact upon their personal and interpersonal patterns of thought and interaction as I did. They may not even find anything new in these collections of quotations. After all, everything in them has been said before by Erickson and much of it has been summarized effectively or alluded to by others in their reviews of his work. At least for me, however, once the actual words of this man had been allowed to organize themselves in a fashion that enabled them to speak their whole message at once, they seemed to speak with a clarity and a directness that I had been unable to experience when reading them separately or as interpreted by someone else. Because of this, I quickly concluded that I had a responsibility to share what I had discovered in order to provide Erickson with a final forum before *his* words faded into the background and those of his well-meaning followers and interpreters began to replace them. The result is this book.

My first impulse was to publish only the set of organized quotations thereby providing readers with nothing more or less than Erickson in his pure form. However, it soon became apparent that this would be inadequate. A context needed to be provided for some sections, connections needed to be established between others, and the entire collection required an ongoing process of introduction and summary. I have not endeavored to present a theoretical analysis of Erickson's work nor to relate his work to other theories or research. I have merely attempted to facilitate the reader's comprehension of the material quoted.

An effort has been made to eliminate irrelevancies and to organize the quotations in such a manner that each section holds together as a coherent whole and does not read as a jumbled array of disconnected comments. No doubt there are instances where the original or intended meaning has been distorted by the decision to place a statement in a particular context. Every effort was made to avoid this and I believe that any instance where this occurs is rare and relatively inconsequential. In the interests of space, clarity, and the avoidance of undue repetition, not all of the quotations originally isolated and placed in each category have been presented here. As mentioned earlier, Erickson reiterated most of his fundamental points on a number of different occasions, and only those comments which capture the essence of his perspective most effectively were incorporated into this final product.

This is not a book to be read quickly and effortlessly. Every quotation requires careful consideration and integration with previous comments. Erickson knew what he was talking about. I hope I have succeeded in allowing his words to speak to you.

SECTION I
HUMAN BEHAVIOR

SECTION I

HUMAN BEHAVIOR

The material contained in this section is the essence of Milton Erickson's success. All of his hypnotic techniques and psychotherapeutic strategies were derived from a perspective or approach to life that led to careful objective observations and understandings of people. Although an understanding of his perspective will not turn anyone into a master hypnotist or therapist, it should provide the framework or foundation and motivation necessary to learn how to be one. More importantly, perhaps, it may provide an attitude toward oneself and others that can generate a clarity of vision, a sense of purpose, and a philosophy of life that is genuinely liberating and that can initiate a new focus for the conduct of one's life and work.

CHAPTER ONE

OBJECTIVE OBSERVATION YIELDS WISDOM

Erickson maintained one fundamental orientation toward life that will be emphasized numerous times in this book. This orientation may have grown out of his heroic battles with life-threatening and crippling effects of polio as a teenager or, as I strongly suspect, may have emerged much earlier as an expression of his family's pioneer spirit. Whatever its time of origin or source, it runs as a connecting thread throughout his work, emerging over and over again in various contexts in one form or another. It provided his definition of normal versus pathological functioning, specified his goal of hypnotherapy, and guided the style of his hypnotherapeutic work. The significance of this fundamental orientation to life within the context of the present chapter, however, is that it generated his awareness of the necessity for careful, objective observation as opposed to theoretical constructs.

Erickson's fundamental orientation toward life, perhaps the central theme of his work, was that people must learn to recognize, to accept, and to utilize what actually is in order to meet their needs, accomplish their goals, and satisfy their purposes. Rather than lamenting, distorting, or denying the unpleasant facts of life or fantasizing about an easier, more ideal reality, Erickson proposed that people must experience and acknowledge the realities of their situation and apply whatever capacities they have in order to cope as effectively or purposefully as possible with those realities. He recognized that this often is a difficult or confusing task, but argued that to do otherwise is to create artificial restrictions, unnecessary handicaps, and unrealistic perspectives.

Erickson entered the fields of psychology, psychotherapy, and hypnosis with this orientation and applied it unerringly in those fields. As a consequence, he rapidly concluded that no single theory could explain or describe adequately the incredible variety and unique complexity of individual functioning. From his perspective, the use of theoretical constructs and generalizations about people was a lazy and inadequate method of describing individuals and a useless exercise in fantasy, as well. Accordingly, he did not subscribe to any particular theoretical perspective nor did he develop one of his own. Those who would search for the theory underlying his strategies are doomed to frustration and failure and those who would impose a theoretical model upon his techniques merely demonstrate that they have missed his major point altogether. The fact is that he did not have a theory of human behavior to guide him nor did he use a theory to develop his intervention strategies.

Erickson may not have used a theory to guide his interventions, but what he did during his therapy sessions was neither arbitrary nor magic. He often spent hours considering the structure and content of his interventions and rarely, if ever, relied upon intuitive hunches or trial and error, even though these sometimes seem to be the easiest explanations for his sometimes bizarre, always unique, strategies. Somehow, without depending upon a carefully constructed theoretical model of human behavior, Erickson was able to decipher the complexities of people and to elicit curative responses from his patients. The question is, of course, what secret wisdom or knowledge did he use to plan and accomplish these therapeutic breakthroughs.

Erickson's secret was an incredibly simple and yet audaciously revolutionary concept. He developed his remarkable understandings of how people behave purely by observing them very, very closely, open-mindedly, and almost naively. He did not sit in his office reading or thinking about how people operate — he watched them. He did not become immersed in theories which he then tried to apply to various patients — he noticed what his patients did and modified his thinking in response. Erickson's spectacular success was based upon his willingness to let people teach him what was real or true about themselves and not upon unique theoretical constructs. The marvelousness of his concepts is that they are descriptively accurate truisms about people and not mere speculations about imaginary dynamics. He learned how to intervene in and how to influence human thought and behavior in the same way that most people learn how to ride a bicycle as children. He paid close attention, he experimented, and he made notes of what happened. As a result, he had no more use for theoretical constructs than a child has for the notions of momentum or velocity when learning to ride a bike.

But Erickson observed in a manner and with an intensity not typical of most people. First of all, he observed himself in incredible detail internally and externally. Secondly, he observed others with an intensity that surpassed even the most self-conscious analysis. Finally, he unashamedly observed people other than patients. Almost everyone was fair game to

7

satisfy his curiosity and to fill in the gaps in his understanding. He hypnotized his sisters and told them to undress in preparation for a complete physical examination just to see what they would do (they refused). Similarly, he attempted to induce other subjects to play practical jokes on their friends, to destroy prized possessions, to lie, to verbally abuse others, and even to steal. All of these "experiments" were carried out under carefully controlled conditions, but they indicate the lengths to which he was willing to go to obtain information. Even strangers in train stations and airports or members of his audiences became opportunities to note how people responded under various circumstances and in response to various stimuli.

Erickson's emphasis upon careful observation pervaded his teachings and lectures. Over and over again he emphasized the necessity of observing subjects with an open-mindedness and precision that most people can only approximate. It may seem odd to us that simply looking at what people do under various circumstances gave this man such a unique understanding of others that he became one of the most effective hypnotists and psychotherapists of all time and developed one of the most innovative and powerful conceptions of human behavior of the century. But, as Erickson often demonstrated, most of us are so *unobservant* that we would be lucky to notice a car careening toward us in broad daylight. As an example Erickson mentions the case of a woman wearing sandals who walked into his office with her husband (Zeig, 1980). Erickson noticed that the second and third toes of both feet of the woman were partially webbed, but both the husband and *the woman herself* were ignorant of that simple fact. On another occasion (ASCH, 1980) he described an incident wherein he had instructed a group of interns to observe silently an elderly woman lying under the covers in a hospital bed until they noticed something unusual that would suggest a diagnosis to them. After three hours of supposedly careful observation, none of them had taken notice of the seemingly obvious fact that both of her legs had been amputated in mid-thigh.

As mentioned in the brief biographical sketch in the beginning of this book, Erickson suffered from a series of perceptual and physical defects. It is apparent that his childhood dyslexia, tone deafness, arrhythmia, color blindness and his eventual bouts with polio caused him to pay closer attention than others do both as a form of compensation and because he did not automatically perceive or respond in the same way as others. For this reason, Erickson had a life-long ability to observe the details of human behavior and to notice things that others missed. This childhood ability eventually became a professional pastime or obsession that resulted in a general description and utilization of human functioning *par excellence*.

Before we move on to a review of his general observations regarding the nature of human consciousness, however, it may be informative and useful to examine briefly the details of the observations upon which these more general conclusions were based or from which they were derived.

Observations Regarding the Influence of Breathing Patterns

Possibly the clearest examples of perceptual deficits that led Erickson to notice things that most of us miss were his tone deafness and arrhythmia. As a result of these "deficiencies" Erickson became puzzled and curious in grade school about the behavior of his classmates and sisters whenever they listened to music or singing (cf. Erickson, 1980, Vol. 1, Chapter 16). For some inexplicable reason they began to move their hands and feet and bodies in regular patterns whenever music was played and what confused him most was that their breathing patterns all shifted in unison when one song ended and another began, even though none was actually singing ("yelling" to Erickson) at the time. Erickson felt no urge to move about in this manner and was unaware of any shift in his own breathing pattern. But he became intensely aware that his classmates consistently began humming the songs sung by soloists after awhile. Thus, what is commonplace, expected, and generally ignored by most of us became a source of considerable concern and interest to him because he did not naturally respond in the same way.

After some experimentation he found that when he mimicked the pattern of breathing associated with a particular song, those around him would begin humming or even singing that song and assume it was a tune that had just come to them out of the blue. (His questions about this phenomenon were met with rebuffs and disapproval, a response he later indicated merely stimulated his interest and observations further.)

Erickson's observations eventually revealed to him that a particular pattern of breathing could initiate not only humming or singing but even yawns, a discovery that he employed surreptitiously to interrupt recitations by classmates, to initiate yawning in an entire classroom, or even to disrupt the lecture of a boring professor. Eventually he became convinced that breathing patterns could be used to communicate a variety of messages in an unobtrusive and unrecognized fashion, a recognition that he often employed when inducing a hypnotic trance.

It is worth noting that young children were able to notice the intentional shifts in his breathing pattern and the effects of these changes even when adults could not. One two and one-half year old told Erickson that "you breathe me to sweep" and other children observed that he just breathes differently to get someone to go to sleep or to wake up. This and other demonstrations of the relative perceptiveness of children eventually had a profound influence upon his general descriptions and understandings of adult behavior, as will become apparent later.

Observations Regarding Learning About One's Body

When Erickson went through the process of re-learning how to move following the total paralysis created by his first bout with polio, he naturally was forced to pay close attention to a learning process most of us have long since forgotten. What he observed in himself he also noticed later in his children as they developed. These various observations eventually coalesced into an understanding of the essential characteristics or basic pattern of human functioning. Aspects of human development that most of us take for granted, rarely consider, or even ignore totally became of central concern for him at that time and what he observed eventually was incorporated into his basic model of human behavior and into his hypnotherapeutic strategies.

Location of Body Parts: One of the first things Erickson had to re-learn as he recovered from polio was how to locate and recognize the signals from the various parts of his body. His nurse would touch his hand or his toes or his face and he would try to guess where the sensation had originated. It took him a long time simply to recognize what each sensation meant in terms of location and intensity of pressure.

The difficulty of reconstructing an understanding of one's body parts, the relationship between them, and the location of stimuli from them gave Erickson a profound sympathy for the immense amount of learning confronting a developing child. He carefully watched his children go through this learning process and noticed the manner in which they gradually discovered their physical identity. He noticed their puzzlement when they first tried to grasp their right hand *with* their right hand, something that children apparently do before they learn that the object *is* their right hand. Then he watched them discover and explore their right hand with their left hand and vice versa. He observed the details of their examination of the location, movement and sensation of each finger, of each arm and of each leg. He noticed how they determined the location of one ear by feeling it with one hand and then with the other. All parts, he concluded, had to be located in relationship to all others.

Later he noticed that children became awkward and confused as they grow because the relative distances between these various body parts changes. The head gets smaller relative to the rest of the body and the arms and legs move farther and farther away from their original anchor points. New patterns of response in relationship to oneself and the environment have to be learned continuously. Suddenly, one day it is no longer possible to walk under the kitchen table; the child has grown too tall.

He watched children learn these and many other things about their bodies and about the relationship of their bodies to the world around them and he became increasingly aware of how many things people learn, know, and use every day but do not remember learning and do not know that they know. His appreciation for this aspect of human functioning eventually formed a cornerstone for his approach to hypnosis and therapy, but there were many other events and observations that led to, reinforced, and added to this insight.

Learning to Walk: Few people have paid more attention to the learning necessary for normal walking than Erickson. As he began to re-learn how to stand and how to walk (an endeavor he undertook in spite of the pronouncement of doctors that he would never again be able to walk) he watched and imitated his baby sister who was busy learning the same thing. In later life he still could describe in minute detail each step in the process, from pulling oneself up, to keeping the feet apart, legs uncrossed, knees straight and hips locked. He was aware of the remarkable range of adjustments necessary to maintain balance as the position of hands, head, or arms is shifted. He could analyze the variety of movements and sensations associated with moving one foot forward and then the other. And having learned to walk again he was able to look around him and say "You all can walk, yet you really don't know the movements or the processes." (Zeig, 1980)

Once again he was confronted by the incredible amount that people know but don't know that they know, by the incredible range of learning that everyone has in their background but seldom recognizes. His infirmities led him to look carefully at what the rest of us tend to take for granted (and thus ignore) and he was mightily impressed by what he saw. In a sense he seemed to be staggered by how little attention people give or need to give to their own behaviors, to their accumulated body of learnings, to their own potentials. People walk, dress, eat, talk, write, sing, and conduct the routine business of their lives without giving it a thought. And yet, as Erickson struggled to understand and re-learn all of these activities he became awed by them and by the richness of learning and the remarkable range of potentials they represented.

Observations Regarding the Meaning of Words

Whether in spite of or because of his failure to begin talking until the age of four, language held a particular fascination for Erickson as a child. He had literally read the unabridged dictionary from front to back by the end of the third grade, a feat that earned him the nickname, "Dictionary." For some reason, however, it never occurred to him that the dictionary was arranged in alphabetical order to facilitate the process of finding words in it. Whenever he wanted to find a word he began at the beginning and looked through every page until he found the word he was looking for. This time-consuming process did not bother him because he enjoyed reading the dictionary and finding out about words. Not until his sophomore year of high school did the purpose of the alphabetical structure occur to him, an insight accompanied by a blinding flash of light and followed by a somewhat sheepish reluctance to admit to his belated recognition of so obvious a fact.

Nonetheless, his ignorance of the structure of the dictionary enhanced his awareness of the meanings, implications, and nature of words. He loved word games, puns, metaphors, and the inherent flexibility of language. At times he would entertain himself by talking to a group of his classmates in terms that he knew would lead one to believe that he was talking about kites, another to believe he was discussing baseball, etc. The multiple implications of words literally fascinated him. For example, he was impressed that the word "run" can have at least 142 different meanings depending upon how it is used and that the word "no" uttered alone can mean at least 16 different things depending upon the voice quality, body language, and inflection employed.

This knowledge of the different meanings and effects of words enabled him not only to say different things to different people at one time, but also to say many things to a single person at one time. He employed his awareness of the multiple implications of words to communicate things that the listener was unaware of on a conscious level. More importantly, he also used it to understand what others were saying unconsciously. It may very well be that his familiarity with the multiple meanings of words allowed him to understand what others were saying in ways that neither they nor other listeners could hear or comprehend. Words were, to him, so flexible in meaning that he tended not to impose his own meaning upon them but rather listened for the specific, perhaps idiosyncratic, unconscious meanings that they had for the speaker.

Observations Regarding Nonverbal Communication

Erickson's awareness of the unconscious levels of communication going on constantly between people was further refined and enhanced by the effects of polio. While still almost totally paralyzed, his interactions with those around him naturally were highly restricted. As a consequence, he was pushed into a role of passive observer of the interactions of others. Once again what he saw and heard became a source of amazement for him because he noticed that the verbal and nonverbal communications between any two people frequently blatantly contradicted one another. Verbal agreement, for example, might be accompanied by a whole range of facial expressions, hand movements, body movements, eye movements, and even voice inflections that implied disagreement. Furthermore, he noticed that such messages of disagreement did not go entirely unnoticed, but often led to an "intuitive" sense that the speaker had not meant what the literal message had conveyed. The reality of this bi-level pattern of communication, perception, and response was overwhelming as he observed his family and friends interacting. This, in turn, added to his awareness that people constantly emit and respond to signals or cues of which they are totally ignorant or unaware.

Observations Regarding Physiological and Behavioral Patterns

Erickson's ability to "read" people, to know things that they did not know about themselves or to see through their attempts to hide information are legendary. When he joined the staff at Worcester State Hospital, the Clinical Director took him aside and advised him to "walk around with a blank face, your eyes open, your ears open." He could not have given this advice to a more receptive, responsive, or astute subject. Erickson immediately began refining his ability to decipher the meaning or implications of minor changes in physiological and behavioral patterns of functioning by writing down his observations about specific people. Later he compared his observations about a person and tried to find out what had occurred in the meantime that might account for any differences. Eventually, he had perfected his observational skills to such an extent that he could tell by a woman's walk or the way she sat in a chair whether she was having an affair; he could listen to his secretary typing and determine whether she had begun menstruating that day; he could determine that a woman was pregnant before she had any idea that she might be and on one occasion (Zeig, 1980) he described in remarkable detail the pattern of minute physiological changes associated with the onset of an active sex life.

In many respects Erickson was a master detective first and a master therapist and hypnotist only as a consequence. He noticed everything about almost everyone he met and he became proficient at organizing clues into meaningful patterns and deciphering their implications. No theory, no catalog of human behavior could possibly convey to an aspiring hypnotherapist the complexity and enormity of information available to Erickson as a result of his lifetime of careful observation. Each movement, each word, each inflection, each physiological characteristic of a person was observed, noted, and interpreted on the basis of his experientially acquired understandings. This book will attempt to convey his general understandings, but it will remain the reader's responsibility to use those understandings to acquire the kind of details Erickson himself found it difficult to convey.

Observations Regarding Cultural Differences

Erickson was thoroughly familiar with the cultural modes and mores of many diverse groups and recommended that all psychotherapists study cultural anthropology both as a way of gaining insights into the behavior of patients from specific cultural backgrounds and as a means of broadening their appreciation for the potential variety of human thought and behavior. Although he acquired a great deal of his familiarity with the idiosyncrasies of diverse groups and nationalities by reading books, he first noticed the impact of various cultural beliefs and attitudes at an early age.

By the age of ten, for example, he had recognized how rigid and unmodifiable were his grandfather's traditional attitudes about planting potatoes. Even after young Erickson had planted a successful potato patch during the "wrong" phase of the moon and with the "eyes" pointed every which way, his grandfather remained unwavering in his original belief that there was a specific phase of the moon during which potatoes should be planted and that they should always be planted with the eyes pointing upwards. He found a similar rigidity in a neighbor who developed headaches whenever Erickson tried to explain the importance of crop rotation to him.

During his sophomore year in college he had the opportunity to observe closely the unusual beliefs and behaviors of an ethnic farming community where the males were expected to (and did) develop headaches the day after sexual intercourse, where married men vomited their breakfasts, and where many aspects of life were governed by similarly atypical patterns of thought and expectation. Erickson was selling books in this rural community and, as such, he ate and slept with a different family each day. He took advantage of this opportunity to observe the intimate details of their lives and did not hesitate to ask questions in an attempt to understand the patterns of thought that led to the unusual events he observed.

In later years Erickson continued to expand his comprehension of the impact of imposed cultural values by studying the do's and don'ts of many different nationalities, ethnic groups, and even regions of the United States. His friendships with Margaret Mead and Gregory Bateson may have contributed to this interest, and his extensive travels on his teaching seminars necessarily exposed him to many diverse groups.

Erickson's interest in cultural differences provided him with more than just an awareness of the conceptual rigidities and learned patterns of response people inherit from their cultural traditions. It also enabled him to perceive psychopathological behavior in a unique light and to derive a unique understanding from those perceptions. For example, while on the Research Service of Worcester State Hospital he interviewed a catatonic schizophrenic who manifested a variety of bizarre behaviors and beliefs which struck Erickson as familiar. Eventually he was able to relate them to those of several primitive tribes, a discovery which puzzled him greatly because the patient obviously was quite unfamiliar with the beliefs and rituals of any of these tribes. These and other observations of the spontaneous development of identical patterns of thought and behavior among separate individuals throughout the world and throughout history led him to conclude that basic human thinking and emotion are very much the same from person to person in spite of individual and regional idiosyncracies. In other words, he observed that the human mind has an incredibly wide but finite range of potential patterns available to it and that everyone has the capacity to function within any one of those patterns. *The particular patterns that any given individual adopts or manifests, he realized, are a result of limitations imposed upon this original pool of potentials by culture and by the individual's unique experiential history.* He determined that given the right circumstances, any individual can and will produce the patterns typical of any disordered state and perhaps of any other individual or culture as well. He also realized that every individual has the capacity to adopt the perspective of others and the ability to adopt new, more useful perspectives under the right circumstances.

Relevant Quotations

The following quotations from various articles and lectures by Milton Erickson are presented to convey his emphasis upon the importance of observation in the development of scientific understanding and in the formation of clinical skills. Examples of his observational capabilities are also included.

It should be noted that many of the quotations used in this and the following chapters were taken from *The Collected Papers of Milton H. Erickson on Hypnosis* (4 volumes), edited by Ernest L. Rossi, published by Irvington Publishers in 1980. Where this is the case, the original date of authorship or publication has been placed in brackets at the end of the quotation in order to provide an orientation regarding the actual dates and sources of the various comments. A complete listing of the original references for this material can be found in the References section.

For the most part our knowledge of psychological processes has been achieved through clinical observations. [1937]

(In Erickson, 1980, Vol. III, chap. 16, p. 145)

Any discussion of hypnotic psychotherapy or hypnotherapy requires an explication of certain general considerations derived directly from clinical observation. [1948]

(In Erickson, 1980, Vol. IV, chap. 4, p. 36)

It is satisfying personally to offer theories and hypotheses, but it would be so much better to investigate actual phenomena. Research should be centered around phenomena, not around achieving fame by placing in the literature a well-argued theory intended to "explain" some unexamined manifestation. [1962]

(In Erickson, 1980, Vol. II, chap. 33, pp. 344–345)

In brief, we need to look upon research in hypnosis not in terms of what we can think and devise and hypothesize, but in terms of what we can, by actual observation and notation, discover about the unique, varying, and fascinating kind of behavior that we can recognize as a state of awareness that can be directed and utilized in accord with inherent but unknown laws. [1962]

(In Erickson, 1980, Vol. II, chap. 33, p. 350)

When I wanted to know something, I wanted it undistorted by somebody else's imperfect knowledge. [1977]

(In Erickson, 1980, Vol. I, chap. 4, p. 114)

Every time I demonstrate something before a professional audience, I tell them, "Now you didn't see, you didn't hear, you didn't think. These are the steps." It is so much easier to think there is something special about me than to learn to really observe and think. "Erickson is mystical," they say.

(Erickson & Rossi, 1981, p. 249)

You haven't been very attentive because I've been going in and out of a trance while I have been talking to you. I've learned how to go into a trance and I can discuss something with you and watch that rug rise up to this level. (Erickson gestures.)... I can go in and out of a trance without any of you knowing it.

(Zeig, 1980, p. 191)

You see, you didn't listen.

(Zeig, 1980, p. 70)

"And so, walk around with a blank face, your mouth shut, your eyes open and your ears open, and you wait to form your judgement until you have some actual evidence to support your inferences and your judgements."

(Zeig, 1980, p. 234)

One's appreciation of, and understanding of the normal or the usual is requisite for any understanding of the abnormal or the unusual. [1977]

(In Erickson, 1980, Vol. II, chap. 18, p. 179)

Anybody doing therapy ought to get to know the range of human behavior.

(Erickson & Rossi, 1981, p. 86)

You must observe ordinary behavior and be perfectly willing to use it.

(Erickson & Rossi, 1981, p. 17)

I knew that you would because everybody else does it!

(Erickson & Rossi, 1981, p. 231)

And you work with patients and you work with your understanding and your understandings come from your knowledge of how you behave. In your observations of the behavior of others you need to have a vivid observation of your own past behavior.

(Erickson, Rossi & Rossi, 1976, p. 289)

Kay Thompson (1975) has reported to me that Milton summed up the essence of good therapy in another single word which I consider equally valid, and that is the command: "Observe!"

(Beahrs, 1977, p. 60)

And therefore you have to have an open mind; not a critical mind, not a judgemental mind, but a curious, a scientific mind wondering what the real situation is. And so you try to appraise it.

(ASCH, 1980, Taped Lecture, 7/16/65)

The wider your understandings of human nature, the biological processes, the history of individual living, the wider your knowledge of your own reactions, of your own potentials, the better you will practice and the better you will live.

(ASCH, 1980, Taped Lecture, 7/16/65)

I think it is tremendously important that you observe everything that's possible and then if you want to use hypnosis you know how to verbalize your suggestions to influence your patient, to elicit their responses.

(ASCH, 1980, Taped Lecture, 7/16/65)

And if you observe a large number of people carefully, you will learn to recognize that.

(Zeig, 1980, p. 161)

When you look at things, look at them.

(Zeig, 1980, p. 169)

And if you learn to observe, you can learn to recognize those changes almost immediately.

(Zeig, 1980, p. 233)

That's why it's so necessary to observe subjects over and over and over again.

(Zeig, 1980, p. 351)

Now the next thing I want to stress is this. For heaven's sakes look at your patient. *Really see* your patient.

(ASCH, 1980, Taped Lecture, 7/16/65)

You meet, you observe your patient — get acquainted with them. To recognize the little things, the little bit of behavior that they're manifesting.

(ASCH, 1980 Taped Lecture, 7/16/65)

My task was that of observing the patient and working with him. [1966]

(In Erickson, 1980, Vol. II, chap. 34, p. 352)

I looked very carefully for everything.

(Zeig, 1980, p. 285)

I'm training him (Dr. Rossi) in observation.

(Erickson & Rossi, 1981, p.107)

Whenever I made an observation, I wrote it down, sealed it in an envelope and put it in a drawer. Sometime later, when I made another observation, I'd write it down, and then compare it with the first observation I made.

(Zeig, 1980, p. 159)

To begin, my first procedure was to make a visual and auditory survey of the interview situation. I wanted to know what my patient could see and hear and how a shift of his gaze or a change of his position would change the object content of his visual field. I also was interested in the various sounds, probable, possible, and inclusive of street noises, that could intrude upon the situation. [1964]

(In Erickson, 1980, Vol. II, chap. 34, p. 352)

I noticed that licking of her lips, the directing of her glance, her general body movements. [1959]

(In Erickson, 1980, Vol. I, chap. 9, p. 222)

I had always been interested in anthropology, and I think anthropology should be something all psychotherapists should read and know about, because different ethnic groups have different ways of thinking about things.

(Zeig, 1980, p. 119)

If you observe children you learn they do this sort of thing all the time. [1976]

(In Erickson, 1980, Vol. I, chap. 21, p. 441)

With my eight children, I've watched each one of them discover their own physical identity. They all follow the same general pattern.

(Zeig, 1980, p. 236)

Don't look at your peers or your family. That's an unwarranted intrusion into the privacy of others.

(Zeig, 1980, p. 161)

When you look at your peers or your family, your own innate sense of courtesy and privacy will stop you from learning.

(Zeig, 1980, p. 162)

I will read faces and if any of you dislike me, I'll know it.

(Zeig, 1980, p. 162)

When a woman begins her sex life, it's a biological function of her body, and all of her body becomes involved. As soon as she begins having sex regularly, her hairline is likely to change slightly, her eyebrow ridges become a millimeter longer, her chin gets a little bit heavier, her lips a little bit thicker, the angle of the jaw changes, the calcium content of the spine changes, the center of gravity changes, breasts and fat pads of the hips become either larger or denser.

(Zeig, 1980, p. 161)

Years ago I'd write out about 40 pages of suggestions that I would condense down to 20 pages and then down to 10. Then I'd carefully reformulate and make good use of every word and phrase so I'd finally condense it down to about five pages. Everyone who is serious about learning suggestion needs to go through that process to become truly aware of just what they are really saying. [1976–1978]

(In Erickson, 1980, Vol. I, chap. 23, p. 489)

I want you to notice how connected everything is even though its all impromptu. *It is a language I've learned, a careful study. I know all the articles of speech and I know the meanings of all the words. Because I learned it carefully, I can speak it easily.*

(Erickson & Rossi, 1979, p. 295)

Nobody seemed to understand my questions about breathing. Soon I began to keep my inquiries to myself, since everybody dismissed them as foolish.

This only enhanced my curiosity. [1960's]

(In Erickson, 1980, Vol. I, chap. 16, p. 363)

Summary

By observing himself and others carefully and objectively throughout his lifetime, Erickson was able to notice things that most of us overlook. He noticed how much people learn and know but forget that they have learned and do not realize that they know. He noticed that people continuously give off and respond to stimuli or communications that occur outside their conscious awareness. He noticed how vast, creative, and orderly are the potential patterns of human thought and behavior and how effectively they are limited and restricted in particular ways by cultural values and by individual experiences. He noticed how unobservant most people are and how many assumptions they impose upon the reality around them. These and other observations formed the foundation for his understanding of people and became the "facts" that guided his hypnotic and psychotherapeutic interventions. Everything he did hypnotically and psychotherapeutically was derived from what he perceived about the particular patient with whom he was working and from what he already knew about people in general from his previous observations.

Thus, everything contained in the remainder of this book, including Erickson's general descriptions of human functioning, his definitions, and his hypnotherapeutic guidelines, rests firmly upon the bedrock of his intelligent critical observation. This point cannot be repeated too often because it is essential to an appreciation of what he had to offer. Only when we stop trying to construct theoretical models or to impose our previously learned constructs upon his words and instead accept what he is saying as a direct description of what *is*, can we effectively comprehend or utilize his wisdom. There is nothing in his words to figure out, though the temptation to do so is overwhelming. There is only a fascinating and humbling description of what people do and of how they can learn to do those things more effectively.

Erickson's general descriptions of human behavior and his guidelines for using what people are and can do will facilitate the process of becoming a more effective hypnotist, therapist, or individual. If we are to follow in Erickson's footsteps we must do more than simply feed upon those of his observations that we can locate and understand; we must obey his injunction to *observe* and examine everything about ourselves and others over and over again in increasingly fine detail. Erickson provided us with a map of the human territory, but eventually we must explore it ourselves in order to develop an accurate picture of it, a feeling for it, and an ability to function effectively within it.

CHAPTER TWO

THE CONSCIOUS MIND

Erickson's observations regarding the basic nature of people eventually led him to a set of general conclusions regarding the conscious and the unconscious minds. This dichotomy apparently served as a shorthand summary for him, a means by which he was able to capture a vast amount of accumulated information within two relatively simple concepts. Even a brief review of his publications suggests that an understanding of the information contained within this dichotomy is necessary for a useful comprehension of his subsequent comments regarding the techniques of psychotherapy and hypnosis. This chapter, therefore, will review the developmental basis and nature of the conscious mind, Chapter 3 will present a description of the unconscious mind, and Chapter 4 will analyze the potential pathological consequences of their functioning and interactions. This observationally based information will then be used as a background for a presentation of his descriptions of the purpose and process of hypnosis and psychotherapy.

Every Person is Unique

One of the most fundamental conclusions drawn by Erickson after his years of observation was that every individual is unique. People differ physiologically and even perceptually. They react differently to the same stimuli and they develop unique personalities as a result.

Erickson's admiration and respect for the qualities specific to each individual prevented him from trying to impose any particular attitudes or behaviors upon his patients and convinced him that no single theory could ever describe all people accurately. He was willing to acknowledge that careful observation of individuals could reveal a pattern or trend of human beings in general and it is this general trend that will be described in the following pages. But he was unwilling to accept the possibility that anyone could ever actually understand, explain, or describe the unique expression of that pattern in any specific person. The best we can hope to do, he maintained, is to develop an appreciation for the general qualities of people and to use that general appreciation as a guidepost in our observations of each individual's particular expression of those general qualities. People behave in accord with their own patterns and they must be responded to with a recognition of their unique individuality. To do otherwise is to impose artificial and arbitrary constraints upon them as individuals, something that Erickson believed patients would justifiably resist.

I think we all should know that every individual is unique... There are no duplicates. In the three and one-half million years that man has lived on earth, I think I am quite safe in saying there are no duplicate fingerprints, no duplicate individuals. Fraternal twins are very,

very different in their fingerprints, their resistance to disease, their psychological structure and personality.

(Zeig, 1980, p. 104)

And so far as I've found in 50 years, every person is a different individual. I always meet every person as an individual, emphasizing his or her own individual qualities.

(Zeig, 1980, p. 220)

Every patient who comes in to you represents a different personality, a different attitude, a different background of experience.

(Haley, 1967, p. 534)

I think any theoretically based psychotherapy is mistaken because each person is different.

(Zeig, 1980, p. 131)

No person can really understand the individual patterns of learning and response of another. [1952]

(In Erickson, 1980, Vol. I, chap. 6, p. 154)

Although each individual is unique in all of his experiential life, single instances often illustrate clearly and vividly aspects and facts of general configurations, trends and patterns. Rather than proof of specific ideas, an illustration or portrayal of possibilities is often the proper goal of experimental work.

(Erickson, 1953, p. 2)

The need to appreciate the subject as a person possessing individuality which must be respected cannot be over-emphasized. Such appreciation and respect constitute a foundation for recognizing and differentiating conscious and unconscious behavior. [1952]

(In Erickson, 1980, Vol. I, chap. 6, p. 146)

The Primary Joy of Life is Freedom

Erickson believed that freedom or self-determination, being able to do what you want to do, is one of the primary pleasures of life. Being inept, confused, or unnecessarily constrained creates a lack of freedom and a lack of freedom is something everyone necessarily resists, tries to avoid, or reacts to with discomfort.

> **It might be well to keep in mind the small child's frequent demonstration of the right to self-determination.**
>
> *(Erickson, 1954a, p. 173)*

> **A small child always asks, "Can I do it when I want to?" The feeling of comfort and freedom is very important.**
>
> *(Erickson & Rossi, 1979, p. 215)*

> **If you tell anyone they *have* to do something, they invariably come back with they *don't*.**
>
> *(Erickson & Rossi, 1979, p. 253)*

> **When you are duty bound, you don't like it.**
>
> *(Zeig, 1980, p. 317)*

> **And I was really doing it! And what greater joy is there than doing what you want to do? [1977]**
>
> *(In Erickson, 1980, Vol. I, chap. 4, p. 130)*

> **I always find when I can do something, it's pleasurable. [1977]**
>
> *(In Erickson, 1980, Vol. I, chap. 4, p. 130)*

> **If you are uncertain about yourself, you can't be certain about anything else.**
>
> *(Erickson, Rossi & Rossi, 196., p. 106)*

Anything is better than that state of doubt.
(Erickson, Rossi & Rossi, 1976, p. 106)

If the surrounding reality becomes unclear, they want it cleared up by being told something.
(Erickson, Rossi & Rossi, 1976, p. 107)

Since it is awfully uncomfortable to lose reality, you have to replace that reality with another.
(Erickson, Rossi & Rossi, 1976, p. 87)

If you are uncertain about something, you tend to avoid it.
(Erickson, Rossi & Rossi, 1976, p. 106)

You know, ordinarily, what is what about yourself and the other person. When confused you suddenly become concerned about who you are and the other person seems to be fading.
(Erickson, Rossi & Rossi, 1976, p. 106)

In real life, as one grows up through puberty, one naturally goes through periods of great uncertainty; believing and unbelieving.
(Erickson, Rossi & Rossi, 1976, p. 185)

But everybody likes to put together things that belong together. [1977]
(In Erickson, 1980, Vol. I, chap. 21, p. 435)

Experience is the Source of Learning

The initial obstacle confronted by the child in its pursuit of freedom through mastery is its lack of experience. Mastery and understanding, even the simple act of perceiving, all require a history of experiences in that arena. The child lacks experience, its only source of learning and knowing; hence it lacks knowledge and freedom. But it has a tremendous capacity to accumulate experiences, to decipher them, and to utilize them. The human infant is endowed with a brain composed of billions of interactive nerve cells that continually receive information from many diverse sources. These complex quantities of stimuli must be organized and deciphered if mastery is to begin. Thus the child's first order of business probably is to learn how to focus its attention upon, to become aware of, or to respond selectively to *one* kind of input at a time. In other words, it probably must begin with a mastery of its attentional processes.

Actually, as Erickson noted, no one really knows what a child learns first. But it seems evident that every child must, of necessity, first orient itself largely toward the realities of its senses and its body. The child must learn to focus its attention upon sights, sounds, and tastes. It must learn where its hands and arms are and how to move them. It must learn to walk, to talk, and to think.

> **And you need to realize in each first experience, not knowing prevents us from noticing even though we do record.**
>
> *(Erickson & Rossi, 1979, p. 308)*

> **This uncertain bobbing up and down, trial and error, is typical of all learnings. You try to do something new, but there are many partial and abortive efforts.**
>
> *(Erickson & Rossi, 1981, p. 78)*

> **Early learning is a long, hard task, and all kids go through that.**
>
> *(Erickson & Rossi, 1981, p. 187)*

You don't learn all at once. You learn in segmented fashion.
(Erickson & Rossi, 1981, p. 93)

Experience can be very informative.
(Erickson & Rossi, 1981, p. 92)

Experience is the only teacher. [1952]
(In Erickson, 1980, Vol. I, Chapter 6, p. 148)

We really don't know what any one person learns first.
(Erickson & Rossi, 1981, p. 198)

There was a time when you didn't even know you were a people.
(Erickson & Rossi, 1979, p. 231)

One of the important things you learn when you are first born... is that you don't know you've got a body.
(Zeig, 1980, p. 41)

Now, one thing about a child is that he is unacquainted with his body. He doesn't know that his hands are his. He doesn't know that he is moving them. He doesn't recognize his knees or his feet. They are just objects. So he has to feel them over and over again. And learning to recognize your body is really a very difficult thing.
(Zeig, 1980, p. 236)

One time you didn't know those were your hands, so you tried to pick up your right hand with your right hand.
(Erickson & Rossi, 1979, p. 231)

And little Johnny has to locate and identify every part of his body.
(Zeig, 1980, p. 238)

I have personally experienced polio, and I know something about the things that can happen to a person who has had polio. You can forget your body, you can lose your awareness of the various parts of your body. [1960]

(In Erickson 1980, Vol. II, chap. 31, p. 323)

It took a long, long time for me to learn where my feet were, and to recognize the individual parts of my body.

(Zeig, 1980, p. 236)

So the relative distance to various parts of the body differs almost from day to day — at least from week to week.

(Zeig, 1980, p. 238)

He has to know it from the front, from below, from above and from in back. Then he is secure in his knowledge.

(Zeig, 1980, p. 237)

The Importance of Expectation and Reward

Learning is a difficult and complex process at best, one that always involves some pain, failure, and risk, and people can be lazy beings who tend to avoid pain or difficulties whenever possible. Accordingly, people must hope or expect to succeed eventually or they may refuse to try or may give up too soon. Similarly, their successes must be recognized or acknowledged for the same reason. Children are no different from adults in this respect, and many children seem to fail to learn things simply because their parents do not expect them to do so, do not recognize their strides in that direction or do not motivate them effectively.

Most children are expected to be able to learn how to walk and most do a reasonably good job of mastering their muscles. The motivation to do so seems to be quite intrinsic and intense. They usually do such a good job, in fact, that eventually they can pay less and less attention to these overlearned activities and can turn their conscious attention instead to the environment, with which their mobility has brought them increased contact.

All I did was give a look of confident expectation. Now that's the important thing. An infant learning to walk, you know he can learn to walk, but the infant doesn't know. You give the infant the confident support of your expectation.

(Erickson, Rossi & Rossi, 1976, p. 282)

Similarly, respect must be given to the child's ideational comprehension with no effort to derogate or minimize the child's capacity to understand. It is better to expect too great a comprehension than to offend by implying a deficiency. [1958]

(In Erickson, 1980, Vol. IV, chap. 15, p. 176)

Full regard must be given to the human need to succeed and to the desire for recognition by the self and others of that success. [1952]

(In Erickson, 1980, Vol. I, chap. 6, p. 151)

Deeds are the offspring of hope and expectancy.

(Erickson, 1954c, p. 261)

People always have that tendency to put off working on a problem to tomorrow.

(Erickson, Rossi & Rossi, 1976, p. 196)

People can be lazy. If I started teaching by precision, I'd bore them.

(Zeig, 1980, p. 354)

And one usually starts with rather simple things. Because human beings are essentially, fundamentally, rather simple creatures.

(Erickson & Rossi, 1981, p. 12)

Now another thing that you ought to bear in mind is this matter of escape reactions. What do you do when something painful comes along? You want to escape from it.

(ASCH, 1980, Taped Lecture, 7/18/65)

Yes. People like to escape from things. You'd better bear that in mind. And their escape is a very generalized reaction. And so the question is "How much escape do they really want?" And bear in mind that normally, naturally we have a wealth of ways of escaping that are normal and that hypnotically you can use the same mechanisms.

(ASCH, 1980, Taped Lecture, 7/16/65)

Integrating With Reality

Mastery of the basic physiological equipment occurs fairly rapidly even though it is a complex and difficult process. Mastery of and effective functioning within the external physical and social environment, however, is a much more challenging process requiring constant vigilance and continual learning throughout one's life.

People, as a consequence, ordinarily have their conscious awareness rather diffusely focused upon external realities. They must scan one thing after another if they are to monitor the complex variety of events around them. Unless they are aware of the significant events and processes occurring around them, they will be unable to respond in those self-protective or self-enhancing ways that promote freedom and survival. Hence their awareness flits from this to that in a continual scanning of internal and external circumstances.

However, awareness of events by itself is insufficient. The *meaning* of those events must be determined on the basis of the ever-increasing accumulation of experientially based learnings acquired by the child. Events must be understood, not just noticed, if the child is to determine to what to respond and how to respond to it. Furthermore, the simpler and more painless this understanding is, the more likely the child is to acquire it. Parsimony is not just a scientific preference.

> **You tend to orient to reality and to give your attention in a diffuse way. [1959]**
>
> *(In Erickson, 1980, Vol. III, chap. 4, p. 28)*

> **Now the conscious mind is your state of immediate awareness. Consciously, you are aware of the wheelchair, the rug on the floor, the other people present, the lights, the bookcases, the night-blooming cacti flowers, the pictures on the wall, Count Dracula on the wall right behind you. ("Count Dracula" is a dried skate that hangs on one wall.) In other words, you are dividing your attention between what I say and everything around you.**
>
> *(Zeig, 1980, p. 33)*

> **In the ordinary state of conscious awareness, however, we are constantlly orienting ourselves to the concrete reality around us. We do this as a matter of biological preservation... You remain well aware of these facts, and from moment to moment you reinforce this orientation to reality. [1960]**
>
> *(In Erickson, 1980, Vol. II, chap. 31, p. 321)*

People in the nontrance state do not lose complete general awareness of the immediate reality surroundings nor of the general context of thinking and speaking; and should they do so in partial fashion, they "come to" with a start, explaining (usually without a request to do so), "For a moment or two there I absentmindedly forgot everything except what I was thinking," reorienting themselves as they speak to their general environment. But it is to the actual reality that they orient themselves. [1967]

(In Erickson, 1980, Vol. I, chap. 2, p. 40)

In the ordinary waking state, however, it appears that the responsive functioning occurs in relationship to the stimulus as emerging from, and constituting only a part of, a much greater and seemingly more significant reality background. [1958]

(In Erickson, 1980, Vol. II, chap. 19, p. 194)

Waking responsiveness tends to be goal-directed towards an integration with objective reality in some form. [1958]

(In Erickson, 1980, Vol. II, chap. 19, p. 192)

Learning the Constraints of Reality

Obviously, absolute freedom is an impossibility because reality imposes restrictions, limitations, and consequences that cannot or should not be ignored. The process of growth and development, therefore, is the process of learning what those limitations, restrictions, and possibilities are.

Thus, the newborn infant is confronted with a monumental task. In order to navigate freely within its environment, and yet to be so well integrated into the environment that it will survive, it must learn how to attend to, to decipher and to utilize the tremendously complex influx of sensations from its senses in a way that enhances its purposes and goal attainments. It must accumulate organized memories of previous experiences and develop an understanding of the rules of reality from them. It must learn how to control its muscles and it must learn what its own abilities and weaknesses are. In short, it must develop an organized view of its internal and external environments and it must learn how to respond appropriately and freely within the constraints and rules of those environments.

In the process of living, the price of survival is eternal vigilance and the willingness to learn. The sooner one becomes aware of realities and the sooner one adjusts to them, the quicker is the process of adjustment and the happier the experience of living. When one knows the boundaries, restrictions and limitations that govern, then he is free to utilize satisfactorily whatever is available. [1962]

(In Erickson, 1980, Vol. IV, chap. 57, p. 514)

Reality, security, and the definition of boundaries and limitations constitute important considerations in the growth of understanding in childhood. To an eight year old child, the question of what constitutes power and strength and reality and security can be a serious matter. When one is small, weak, and intelligent, living in an undefined world of intellectual and emotional fluctuations, one seeks to learn what is really strong, secure, and safe. [1962]

(In Erickson, 1980, Vol. IV, chap. 57, p. 507)

Reality, security, definition of boundaries and limitations all constitute important considerations in the childhood growth of understandings. There is a desperate

need to reach out and to define one's self and others. [1975]

(In Erickson, 1980, Vol. I, chap. 20, p. 419)

There governs children, as growing, developing organisms, an ever-present motivation to seek for more and better understandings of all that is about them. [1958]

(In Erickson, 1980, Vol. IV, chap. 15, p. 174)

Children have a driving need to learn and to discover, and every stimulus constitutes, for them, a possible opportunity to respond in some new way. [1958]

(In Erickson, 1980, Vol. IV, chap. 15, p. 174)

Building a Frame of Reference

As the child interacts with its environment and gains experience, it gradually builds an overall view of its reality context. At first, this context is objectively based (though naive) and fairly fluid. The child lacks experience but is open to new information that will improve its understanding.

Reality, however, is enormously complex and difficult to observe or to analyze effectively. Because people tend to avoid difficult or painful circumstances or to transform them into simpler and more pleasing ones, most children will accept shorter, easier, more straightforward descriptions of reality if they are offered. Adults provide these shorthand versions of reality in the form of arbitrary classification systems, attitudes, beliefs, theories, culturally based rules of conduct, and even a predefined categorization and naming system called language.

Because each child is physiologically unique and has unique experiences, the shorthand rules or images of reality eventually adopted by each individual will be relatively unique as well. Once the child has picked up the general rules and principles that the members of its culture have agreed to use, it will begin applying these general rules in its own unique manner and will develop a unique model of reality.

Over time the child constructs an increasingly well-organized shorthand view or model of reality through which the world is viewed and analyzed. This model of reality enables the child to understand the meaning of events quickly and easily and also allows it to determine quickly what appears to be an appropriate response. The objective direct view of reality is gradually replaced by the simpler, more straightforward (though less accurate) conscious model. The complex, demanding, and time-consuming qualities of objective observation and analysis make this development of a shorthand model appealing and adaptive. Even adults opt for simple theories and universally applicable techniques although careful observation of complex circumstances might eventually provide a more accurate awareness and a more effective response.

The accumulated shorthand model or context of understandings that acts as a filter between the person's conscious awareness and objective reality and that subsequently dictates the meaning of events and provides the organizations for responses *is what Erickson referred to as the conscious mind.* Almost everything an individual thinks, perceives and does at a conscious level of awareness is a reflection of or is influenced by this conscious frame of reference.

> **Children are small, young people. As such, they define the world and its events in a different way than does the adult, and their experiential learnings are limited and quite different from those of the adult. [1958]**
> *(In Erickson, 1980, Vol. IV, chap. 15, p. 174)*

Children have their own ideas and need to have them respected, but they are readily open to any modification of those ideas intelligently presented to them. [1958]
(In Erickson, 1980, Vol. IV, chap. 15, p. 176)

And philosophers of old have said, "As a man thinketh, he is."
(Erickson & Rossi, 1979, p. 262)

And all philosophers say, reality is all in the head.
(Zeig, 1980, p. 90)

A central consideration in the proposed experimental project was suggested by the well known Biblical saying, "As a man thinketh in his heart, so is he." [1964]
(In Erickson, 1980, Vol. I, chap. 1, p. 4)

Waking subjects are restricted to their general conscious concepts of how to function intellectually. [1962]
(In Erickson, 1980, Vol. III, chap. 13, p. 117)

Because consciously you behave in accord with the conscious universe, the conscious patterns of behavior.
(ASCH, 1980, Taped Lecture, 2/2/66)

The subjects accept those ideas in terms of their own frames of reference and a lifetime of experiential learning. These experiential learnings may be unusual and quite unexpected. [1960]
(In Erickson, 1980, Vol. II, chap. 31, p. 313)

Language Development

At first a child's conscious understandings or framework can be expressed only behaviorally through the organization of its responses to its environment. Eventually, however, these experientially acquired understandings of the conscious mind begin to be influenced by and expressed within a language system. Learning to understand language and to speak is a slow, trial-and-error process just as most learning seems to be. It is also an individual-specific process in the sense that every person develops unique experientially based definitions or meanings for each word. Thus, for example, the word "mother" conjures up a slightly different set of associations and responses for each person — usually associations derived from the unique patterns of interaction with the person's own mother. Every word has a unique implication or meaning for each individual that stems from and defines their unique frame of reference.

A newly born baby is extremely ignorant. It has a sucking reflex and it can cry. But it is a meaningless cry. It is, I expect, the discomfort with the new environment.

(Zeig, 1980, p. 234)

After a while, mother begins to notice that the meaningless cries acquire a meaning.

(Zeig, 1980, p. 235)

Each cry is altered as the child begins to comprehend various things.

(Zeig, 1980, p. 235)

There's another thing to be taken into consideration: how all of us learn to talk. There's a long, long experience of making errors... There's a wealth of learning you get from making mistakes.

(Zeig, 1980, p. 336)

The problem in learning to speak well is in your willingness to learn slowly.

(Erickson & Rossi, 1981, p. 82)

We always translate the other person's language into our own language.

(Zeig, 1980, p. 64)

Because when you talk to people, they hear you in their language.

(Zeig, 1980, p. 70)

I had to wait until I understood *her* words.

(Zeig, 1980, p. 158)

You o ight to be acquainted with the linguistic patterns of your patients. And we all have our own personal understandings.

(Zeig, 1980, p. 78)

All of you will apply what I say in accordance with your own specific understandings.

(Zeig, 1980, p. 64)

Now, every word in any language has usually a lot of different meanings.

(Zeig, 1980, p. 78)

Rigidity and Non-objectivity of Conscious Frames of Reference

At first the ordinary person's mind or brain is relatively unstructured, objective, flexible, and open to new learnings. Over time, however, it naturally becomes increasingly rigid, biased, idiosyncratic, and unable to accept perceptions, learn-ings, or responses that cannot be accommodated by its previously adopted structure. Increases in "understanding" or the acceptance and utilization of specific culturally imposed conscious frames of reference necessarily leads to less flexibili-ty and more tightly organized perceptions and responses. Eventually the entire conscious awareness of the individual may become restrictively governed or dictated by the very structure that originally developed to allow an increased freedom of response. Obviously, the degree of rigidity and bias of conscious frames of reference will vary from person to person and from culture to culture but the general trend is in the direction of increased organization and rigidity of struc-ture.

> **Now, Dr. Rossi here is somebody who is trained in psychology. He has been oriented to place individual meanings or interpretation on everything according to his past teachers.** *He does not know very much about* **look-ing at or** *experiencing reality.* **He must experience reality in terms of what he has been taught and read.**
>
> *(Erickson & Rossi, 1981, p. 193)*

> **The author has encountered such rigidity of frames of reference. [1967]**
>
> *(Erickson, 1980, Vol. I, chap. 2, p. 38)*

> **These are all conscious biases. You can broaden your activity, however, if you recognize the bias. Experimen-talists in hypnosis ought to know about the unlimited number of biases that everybody builds up.**
>
> *(Erickson, Rossi & Rossi, 1976, p. 179)*

> **Biases are a part of our conscious living.**
>
> *(Erickson, Rossi & Rossi, 1976, p. 180)*

They are not just biases, they are part of the way we experience the world.
(Erickson, Rossi & Rossi, 1976, p. 180)

When you use the word "bias" it is so easily misunderstood. It is actually a *common set*.
(Erickson, Rossi & Rossi, 1976, p. 180)

I want to make her aware that she has many many rigid sets. Everybody has.
(Erickson, Rossi & Rossi, 1976, p. 213)

People say, "But I always eat cereal for breakfast! But we always have chicken on Sunday." These are all conscious biases.
(Erickson, Rossi & Rossi, 1976, pp. 178–179)

A young man says, "It's a nice day today." His frame of reference is a picnic with his sweetheart. A farmer says, "It's a nice day today." His frame of reference is that it is a good day to mow hay... Totally different meanings, yet you could understand them when you knew their frame of reference.
(Erickson & Rossi, 1981, p. 255)

Complexity of Conscious Frames of Mind

As the child grows older it moves into new settings and situations which often place the child in totally new contexts of demands and expectations. In essence, the child is confronted by new realities. Such circumstances often dictate the development of somewhat new and different conscious frames of reference. Consequently, over time the conscious mind may develop a number of separate frameworks or perspectives, each of which may be utilized in special circumstances in response to special contextual demands. Usually these various frameworks are coherently organized or interrelated and aspects of one may blend into or even become the foundation for another. In some sense they each usually represent variations on a basic underlying theme rather than a totally separate or unique perspective. Subjectively the individual experiences a smooth and almost automatic transition from one perspective to another as the external circumstances change and conscious awareness shifts from one perspective or filter to another. However, when one of these conscious frameworks of perception, thought, or response contains something completely unacceptable to the others it may become completely severed or isolated from the rest of the conscious mind, a phenomenon seen at various times in true multiple personalities.

As the complex structure of the whole conscious mind becomes more tightly or completely organized, it becomes an increasingly distinct and exclusive set of patterns of perception, thought, and response. The brain remains capable of numerous other patterns and may engage in them at times, but if events or thoughts do not "fit" into the acceptable patterns of the structure of the adopted conscious mind, then they usually are excluded from consideration and do not become available to the person who is aware only of those things allowed through the filter of the conscious mind. The conscious mind, therefore, eventually becomes a dissociated, unique, and complex entity that provides rather specific, exclusive views and ways of thinking about the world.

The human personality is characterized by infinite varieties and complexities of development and organization, and it is not a simple limited unitary organization. It is, rather, to be regarded as having as complicated a

structure, organization, and development as has the individual's experiential background. [circa 1940's]

(In Erickson, 1980, Vol. III, chap. 24, p.262)

There can be separate states of awareness that develop spontaneously in ordinary life. [circa 1940's]

(In Erickson, 1980, Vol. III, chap. 8, p. 61)

From this realization of the complexity of the structure of the personality there has developed the understanding of the possibility — and the actual probability — of separate and specific integrations within the total organization as a common characteristic...In this regard Oberndorf has spoken of "that galaxy of personalities which constitute the individual." [circa 1940's]

(In Erickson, 1980, Vol. III, Chap. 24, p. 263)

Nor is there as yet sufficient evidence at hand to establish how many degrees of such multiple formations may exist. [1939]

(In Erickson, 1980, Vol. III, chap. 23, p. 256)

In fact one must ask whether one is justified in dismissing the possibility that all acts of repression involve the creation of a larval form of a secondary personality. [1939]

(In Erickson, 1980, Vol. III, chap. 23, pp. 256 — 257)

So little has been said about the varying role of the patient who may present to the analyst not one personality but many. [1939]

(In Erickson, 1980, Vol. III, chap. 23, p. 256)

Summary

All unique individuals attempt to maintain their freedom to respond by extending their awareness and understanding of the nature of the rules of their reality. Their slowly accumulated, experientially, and culturally based conscious frame of reference eventually provides the understanding of what can or should be done and these understandings guide their responses. As long as their awareness is directed toward the world through that frame of reference, perspective, set or state of mind, all thoughts, perceptions, and responses are influenced, limited, or directed by it.

CHAPTER THREE

THE UNCONSCIOUS MIND

It is unfortunate, perhaps, that so much of what Erickson observed and knew about human functioning was reduced to a shorthand reference to the unconscious and the conscious. In spite of his frequent declarations that this bifurcation of people into conscious and unconscious levels of functioning was a "conceptual convenience," it is potentially a very confusing and misleading oversimplification. Not only does the term "unconscious" carry a host of undesirable and inaccurate connotations from numerous theoretical systems, the conscious-unconscious duality itself fails to convey adequately Erickson's complex understanding of human personality.

The term "unconscious," for example, conjures up Freudian and Jungian implications for most of us almost automatically, none of which have any relevance to Erickson's observations at all. Even when these traditional theoretical connotations are overcome, there remains the problem of eliminating the implied mystical notions of an all-knowing, infallible unconscious and other everyday interpretations related to the process of being "knocked unconscious" by a blow to the head or by drugs. As a careful review of the material presented in this chapter should suggest, none of these uses of the term are relevant to what Erickson meant by the "unconscious."

Erickson was not unaware of these potential sources of conceptual confusion. Early in his career he sometimes substituted the term subconscious and often put the term unconscious in quotes in an apparent attempt to suggest an idiosyncratic definition. On later occasions he referred instead to "a different level of awareness," to "one's own actual potentialities," and to "useful unrealized self-knowledge." Generally, however, he simply used the term "unconscious" without specific qualification, although it must be reemphasized that what he meant by the term "unconscious" was something vastly different from what most authors have meant by it. A genuine appreciation for what he had to offer requires the adoption of his understandings and the avoidance of imposed assumptions.

The unwarranted and misleading implications of the term "unconscious" are not the only roadblocks to a comprehension of the fundamental concepts underlying Erickson's approach. As indicated earlier, the conscious-unconscious dichotomy itself also is a potential source of confusion. Aside from the unavoidable fact that it almost necessarily leads some people into a questionable application of the right-left hemisphere paradigm that is now being used to account for almost all dichotomous human behavior, it also fails to capture the complexity of human functioning that Dr. Erickson actually observed. Multiple levels of awareness, information processing and responding from within a multitude of conceptual conscious and unconscious frameworks or perspectives were apparent to him. Care must be taken, therefore, to avoid confusing this "conceptual convenience" with a completely accurate description of reality. Although accurate as far as it goes, Erickson saw many more dimensions to people than this dichotomy implies.

Having prefaced this presentation with what may seem to be an inordinate number of qualifications or cautions, an attempt now will be made to summarize or to review the term "unconscious" from Erickson's perspective.

The Reality of the Unconscious

It is important at the outset to recognize that when Erickson referred to the unconscious mind he was referring to a very real, observable, demonstrable, phenomenon. He was not merely using the term as a metaphor or as a construct. He meant that people actually *have* an unconscious mind or unconsicous levels of awareness in the same sense that they have an arm or a leg. The unconscious, in Erickson's view, is a necessary, observable, and very real component of every human personality.

> Now what I'd like to have you understand is this: that you have a conscious mind, and you know that and I know that, and you have an unconscious mind or subconscious mind, and you know that I mean by that, do you not?
>
> *(Erickson & Rossi, 1981, p. 157)*

> [Hypnosis] is characterized by various physiological concomitants, and by a functioning of the personality at a level of awareness other than the ordinary or usual state of awareness. For convenience in conceptualization, this special state, or level of awareness, has been termed "unconscious" or "subconscious". [1948]
>
> *(In Erickson, 1980, Vol. IV, chap. 4, p. 37)*

> **The activity involved in this (i.e. in automatic writing and crystal-gazing) is perhaps one of the best "proofs" of the existence of the "subconscious" mind. [1943]**
>
> *(In Erickson, 1980, Vol. III, chap. 1, p. 10)*

> **Furthermore, the unconscious as such, not as transformed into the conscious, constitutes an essential part of psychological functioning.**
>
> *(Erickson, 1953, p.2)*

The Separate Abilities of the Unconscious

Not only is the unconscious real, it also is distinct and separate from the conscious mind. It coexists with the conscious mind as totally separate, mutually exclusive processes of awareness, learning, and response. Its activities continue in parallel with the activities of the conscious mind, although there are influence processes from one system to the other.

The unconscious can listen to or perceive things that the conscious mind ignores. It can think about one thing while the person is consciously thinking about something else. The unconscious has its own separate interests, memories, and understandings. The unconscious can control physical activities without the conscious mind being aware of it and, as a result, it can communicate with others and express ideas that are outside the range of conscious perception or awareness.

Usually, but not always, the processes and activities of the unconscious mind support or extend the activities and desires of the conscious mind. Under the right circumstances, however, the unconscious mind may act in a more or less autonomous manner, expressing its own desires or understandings only and initiating activities that are unrelated to the processes of the conscious frame of reference.

As indicated previously, one of the principal outcomes of

Erickson's careful observations of himself and others was his cumulative appreciation for the fact that people know much more than they are consciously aware that they know, do much more than they are consciously aware that they do, perceive much more than they are consciously aware of perceiving and have a whole variety of intellectual, behavioral, and physiological capacities about which they also are oblivious. His lifetime of observations consistently led him to the conclusions that humans have and continually use a vast reservoir of experientially acquired learnings of which they are largely unaware, have unused or overlooked capacities, potentials and experientially acquired knowledge, and engage in interactions or communication exchanges with no awareness that they are or have done so. Because all of these events and potentials exist outside the range of ordinary conscious awareness, he naturally referred to them as "unconscious" and to the separate system within which they occurred or existed as the "unconscious mind." By definition therefore, the unconscious is all of those elements of our functioning to which we do not pay attention for one reason or another or about which we are consciously unaware.

Thus, the separateness of the unconscious from the conscious and the actuality or reality of the unconscious are almost definitional necessities as well as objectively observable or demonstrable qualities. Like light and dark, the unconscious and the conscious are defined in terms of each other, although in Erickson's perspective this light-dark dichotomy should probably be applied in the reverse of its typical application with the light representing the unconscious instead of the dark. But no matter how this comparison is made, it is clear that the existence in conscious awareness of only selected features of the overall input and activity of the brain as interpreted from within a particular frame of reference or perspective leaves a lot left over to be accounted for. This accounting is the unconscious, a phenomenon which logic dictates and that careful observation demonstrates.

> **Your unconscious knows all about it — probably more than your conscious mind does — and your unconscious mind can keep from you, from your conscious mind, anything it doesn't want you to know consciously.**
>
> *(Erickson & Lustig, 1975, Vol. 1, p. 9)*

> **Because you are dealing with a person who has both a conscious mind and an unconscious mind.**
>
> *(Erickson & Rossi, 1981, p. 6)*

> **R: [Rossi] So the conscious and unconscious really are separate systems.**
> **E: [Erickson] Yes, they are separate systems.**
>
> *(Erickson, Rossi & Rossi, 1976, p. 258)*

> **Yes, I seem to bifurcate the individual into the conscious and unconscious. When I say something, I may say it to the conscious or I may say it to the unconscious.**
>
> *(Erickson & Rossi, 1981, p. 103)*

> **The first idea I want to impress upon you is one way of thinking about your patients clinically. It is desirable to use this framework because of the ease of concept formation for the patient. I like to regard my patients as having a conscious mind and an unconscious mind. I expect the two of them to be together in the same person, and I expect both of them to be in the office with me. *When I am talking to a person at the conscious level, I expect him to be listening to me at an unconscious level, as well as consciously.***
>
> *(Erickson & Rossi, 1981, p. 3)*

Also, it became apparent that there were multiple levels of perception and response, not all of which were necessarily at the usual or conscious level of awareness, but were at levels of understanding not recognized by the self, often popularly described as "instinctive" or "intuitive."

(Bandler & Grinder, 1975, Preface, p. viii)

Now you don't really need to listen to me because your unconscious mind will hear me. You can let your conscious mind wander in any direction it wants to.

(Erickson & Rossi, 1981, p. 189)

I know his unconscious is listening. It has to. He's only a few feet away from me, my voice is loud enough. It will!

(Erickson & Rossi, 1981, p. 200)

Your unconscious mind can listen to me without your knowledge and also deal with something else at the same time.

(Erickson, Rossi & Rossi, 1976, p. 38)

The patient's unconscious mind is listening and understanding much better than is possible for his conscious mind. [1966]

(In Erickson, 1980, Vol. IV, chap. 28, p. 277)

I don't know if you have any conscious idea, but always the unconscious mind has its own thoughts. Its own desires.

(Erickson, Rossi & Rossi, 1976, p. 285)

I'm making it apparent here that there are two sets of interests, and the unconscious is going to have its interests.

(Erickson, Rossi & Rossi, 1976, p. 207)

You demonstrate that the conscious can think one way and the unconscious another. You're going to have a chance to see and prove within yourself that they think differently.

(Erickson, Rossi & Rossi, 1976, p. 171)

Your unconscious learned a lot yesterday. It also learned that we could learn a lot without intruding upon the personality.

(Erickson, Rossi & Rossi, 1976, p. 207)

You let them know that they do know a lot more than they realize. They have that knowledge in their unconscious.

(Erickson, 1980, Vol. IV, p. 98)

It is not necessary for you to remember consciously, because your unconscious mind will remember what I say and what it means, and that is what is necessary. [1953]

(In Erickson, 1980, Vol. IV, Chapter 42, p. 376)

Also, it is explained that thinking can be done separately and independently by both the conscious and unconscious mind, but that such thinking need not necessarily be in agreement. [1961]

(In Erickson, 1980, Vol. I, chap. 5, p. 138)

I tell them that no matter how silent they are, their unconscious mind is beginning to think, beginning to understand, that they themselves do not need to know consciously what is going on in their unconscious mind.

(Erickson & Rossi, 1981, p. 18)

Your unconscious can know the answer, but you don't have to know the answer.

(Erickson & Rossi, 1979, p. 203)

It's important for you to realize that your unconscious mind can start a train of thought, and develop it without your conscious knowledge — and reach conclusions, and let your conscious mind become aware of those conclusions.

(Erickson & Lustig, 1975, Vol. 2, p.4)

I wanted your unconscious mind to have the liberty of doing something while your conscious mind was filled with other things.

(Erickson, Rossi & Rossi, 1976, p. 206)

Your unconscious can try anything it wishes. But your conscious mind isn't going to do anything of importance.

(Erickson, Rossi & Rossi, 1976, p. 9)

And it really doesn't matter what your conscious mind does because your unconscious automatically will do just what it needs to.

(Erickson, Rossi & Rossi, 1976, p. 67)

Consciously chosen words, thoughts, and acts can mean more than one thing at a time: their conscious or manifest content on the one hand, and a latent, unconscious content on the other. [1939]

(In Erickson, 1980, Vol. III, chap. 16, p. 156)

They have had a lifetime of experience in which talking is done at a conscious level, and have no realization that talking is possible at a purely unconscious level of awareness. [1952]

(In Erickson, 1980, Vol. I, chap. 6, p. 145)

His unconscious mind can communicate directly and adequately and is free to make whatever communication it wishes, **whether by sign language, verbally or in both manners. [1964]**

(In Erickson, 1980, Vol. I, chap. 13, p. 309)

It is impressive to see how ready the unconscious seemed to be to communicate with the examiner by means of this accessory sign language of drawing, while at the same time the consciously organized part of the personality was busy recounting other matters. [1938]

(In Erickson, 1980, Vol. III, chap. 17, p. 174)

She was able to execute consciously an act which in itself was fully expressive and complete, but which simultaneously possessed an additional unrecognized significance at another level of mentation. [1937]

(In Erickson, 1980, Vol. III, chap. 16, p. 150)

With another hypnotic subject, it was possible to carry on a written conversation having a conscious import but which was developed entirely in accord with an import known only to the unconscious mind of the subject and to the investigator without the subject becoming aware consciously of the actual nature of the conversation. [1939]

(In Erickson, 1980, Vol. IV, chap. 1, p. 12)

It would seem, therefore, that humorlessly and quite without conscious comic intent the unconscious can use irony, punning, and the technique of the puzzle. In short, the techniques of conscious humor are an earnest and serious matter in unconscious psychic processes. This is particularly disconcerting when weighty and significant problems are treated by means of unconsciously chosen representatives and devices which to our conscious judgements seem ridiculous and trivial. [1937]

(In Erickson, 1980, Vol. III, chap. 16, p. 157)

As in dreams, puns, elisions, plays on words and similar tricks that we ordinarily think of as frivolous, all play a surprising and somewhat disconcerting role in the communication of important and serious feelings... It is ever a source of fresh amazement when the unconscious processes express weighty and troublesome problems in a shorthand which has in it an element of levity. [1940]

(In Erickson, 1980, Vol. III, chap. 18, p. 186)

[This] served to convince me further that people communicate with each other at "breathing" levels of awareness unknown to them. [circa 1960's]

(In Erickson, 1980, Vol. I chap. 16, p. 364)

Communication can be verbal, but it is also quite obvious that there is a great deal of nonverbal communication. Communication can be an angry look, a lovely look — all kinds of looks and all kinds of gestures. [1960]

(In Erickson, 1980, Vol. II, chap. 31, p. 328)

When do you kiss a pretty girl?... When she is ready, not when you are ready. You wait for that undefinable behavior that she manifests. You don't ask a girl for a kiss, but in her presence you just gaze thoughtfully at the mistletoe. You are just being thoughtful. She gets the idea, and she starts thinking about the kiss.

(Erickson & Rossi, 1981, p. 230)

One student can brush back her hair with a deliberateness that says "I hope that son-of-a-bitch reaches the end of the lecture soon." Then there's that unconscious brushing back of the hair that indicates they are attending to you.

(Erickson & Rossi, 1981, p. 70)

Certain patients, while explaining their problems, will unwittingly nod or shake their heads contradictorily to their actual verbalizations. [1961]

(In Erickson, 1980, Vol. I, chap. 5, p. 138)

There stands a baby, dirty face, tousled of hair, runny nose, wet, smelly, dirty, and its face lights up and it toddles to you so happily because it *knows* its a nice baby and *that you will be glad to like it and that you will want to pick it up.* You know what you will do! So does the baby! *You can't help yourself.* ...Beautiful little child, hair combed, clean, neat, in a state of perfection, but its face says, "Who just who on earth would *ever* want to pick me up?" Certainly you don't, you agree with the child, and you want to find the parents and slap them around for mistreating that child, because you don't want to be greeted again, ever again, by that child in that manner.

(Erickson & Rossi, 1979, p. 437)

You are saying that their unconscious mind can now work, and work secretly, without the awareness of the conscious mind.

(Erickson & Rossi, 1981, p. 18)

The unconscious works without your knowledge and that is the way it prefers.

(Erickson & Rossi, 19⁻5, p. 163)

The Unconscious is a Storehouse

Because Erickson's primary goal in hypnosis and therapy was to help others learn how to use their unconscious capacities to resolve their problems and to respond more freely in new ways, it is not surprising that he emphasized the fact that the unconscious represents a reservoir of unrecognized experientially acquired learnings or knowledge. This feature of the unconscious was of primary interest to him therapeutically and he almost invariably described the unconscious in this way.

Erickson was genuinely impressed by how much people know but do not know that they know. Some of this knowledge consists of psychological, emotional, physical, or intellectual information that originally was consciously and intentionally acquired but later dropped out of conscious awareness. The complex learning underlying walking is an example. The learning that was required to begin to walk is unavailable to most adults, even though they continue to utilize and to rely upon it. Other learning can occur without conscious awareness or purpose. People can learn without consciously knowing that they have learned and can use that learning later without recognizing that they are doing so. This significant type of learning can occur because the unconscious is a separate, parallel system of awareness and information processing.

Finally, unconscious learning can be unused. Even though a large proportion of human behavior is unconscious or automatic and most of what we do intentionally or consciously is dependent upon the use of unconsciously held learnings, a tremendous amount of what we have learned and know is never applied or utilized effectively by us because of our conscious repressions and rigidities.

The unconscious mind or level of awareness, therefore, is a vast storehouse of unrecognized, unused or misused memories and learnings, a storehouse that can provide the basic information and learning necessary for psychotherapeutic or hypnotic responses to occur. The unconscious probably already knows what the person's problem is, the source of the problem, and how to alleviate the problem. As such, it obviously is a potentially beneficial ally in many respects.

Now, the unconscious mind is a vast storehouse of memories, your learnings. It has to be a storehouse because you cannot keep consciously in mind all the things you know. Your unconscious mind acts as a storehouse. Considering all the learning you have acquired in a lifetime, you use the vast majority of them automatically in order to function.

(Zeig, 1980, p. 173)

In hypnosis we utilize the unconscious mind. What do I mean by the unconscious mind? I mean the back of the mind, the reservoir of learning. The unconscious mind constitutes a storehouse. [1959]

(In Erickson, 1980, Vol. III, chap. 4, p. 27)

The body learns a wealth of unconscious psychological, emotional, neurological, and physiological associations and conditionings. These unconscious learnings, repeatedly reinforced by additional life experiences, constitute the source of the potentials that can be employed through hypnosis. [1967]

(In Erickson, 1980, Vol. IV, chap. 24, p. 238)

Common experience has demonstrated repeatedly that unconscious attitudes toward the body can constitute potent factors in many relationships. Learning processes, physical and physiological functioning, and recovery

from illness are, among others, examples of areas in
which unrecognized body attitudes may be of vital
significance to the individual. [1960]

(In Erickson, 1980, Vol. II, chap. 21, p. 203)

Yet as a result of experiential events of his past life,
there has been built up within his body — although all
unrecognized — certain psychological, physiological, and
neurological learnings, associations, and conditionings
that render it possible for pain to be controlled and even
abolished. [1967]

(In Erickson, 1980, Vol. IV, chap. 24, p. 237)

Your unconscious does know much more about you
than you do. It's got a whole background of years of
learning, feeling, thinking, and doing. And all our days
we are learning things — learning how.

(Erickson & Lustig, 1975, Vol. 2, p. 3)

Human beings, once they have learned anything,
transfer this learning to the forces that govern their
bodies. [1959]

(In Erickson, 1980, Vol. III, chap. 4, p. 27)

The next thing I wish to call to your attention is the
matter of the experiential learning that we all absorb during a lifetime of experiences. Little children practice
walking and getting up and sitting down, lying down,
rolling over, using every muscle and action of their ex-
tremities and torso. They get acquainted with the various
parts of their bodies and learn the full extent of their
capabilities. They learn these things so thoroughly that
years later, when they are full-grown adults and have
forgotten the process through which they learned their
actions they will respond promptly when a mosquito
lands on any part of their body. [1959]

(In Erickson, 1980, Vol. III, chap. 4, p. 27)

You do a lot of things automatically.

(Zeig, 1980, p. 222)

You see movements without complete conscious awareness in kids all the time.

(Erickson & Rossi, 1981, p. 77)

There is a lot of your behavior you don't know about.

(Zeig, 1980, p. 42)

When you listen to a radio program of music, for instance, if you want to single out the instruments, you don't look at a bright light or thumb through a book. You close your eyes, you unconsciously turn your dominant ear toward the music, and you carefully shut out visible stimuli. If you are holding a cold glass in your hand, you put it down so that the coldness does not divert your attention away from the music. You are not necessarily aware of performing these actions because your unconscious mind has directed their performance. It knows how you can best hear the music.

(Erickson & Rossi, 1981, p. 24)

In the course of living, from infancy on, you acquired knowledge, but you could not keep all that knowledge in the foreground of your mind. In the development of the human being learning in the unconscious became available in any time of need. When you need to feel comfort, you can feel comfort.

(Erickson, Rossi & Rossi, 1976, p. 155)

And that is something you need to teach your patients, when the appropriate time comes to respond with a certain kind of behavior you can do so. You do not have to know consciously that you already know that behavior.

(ASCH, 1980, Taped Lecture, 7/16/65)

Because the important understanding that you need is this, that any knowledge acquired by your unconscious mind is knowledge that you can use at any appropriate time. But you need not necessarily be aware that you have that knowledge until the moment comes to use it. And then you just quite naturally respond with the appropriate behavior.

(ASCH, 1980, Taped Lecture, 7/16/65)

Your body is a lot wiser than you are.

(Zeig, 1980, p. 63)

A child's body tells him how many swallows for a good drink before he has a chance to absorb much of that water.... So you don't need to be more aware of your learning than a child is of the number of swallows of water.

(Erickson & Rossi, 1981, p. 99)

We are usually unaware of all the automatic responses we make on the basis of the locus of sound and the inflections of voice. [1976–1978]

(In Erickson, 1980, Vol. I, chap. 23, p. 481)

You all can walk, yet you really don't know the movements or the processes.

(Zeig, 1980, p. 37)

Joint sensation and kinesthetic memories are as valid as any other kinds of memories. You can substitute them and modify them. I think there is need for a great deal of research on the characteristics of these different types of learnings and memories, the conditions for change, and the way in which they undergo spontaneous alterations during life. [1960]

(In Erickson, 1980, Vol. II, chap. 31, p. 324)

> **I had long forgotten that, but my unconscious had remembered it.**
>
> *(Erickson, Rossi & Rossi, 1976, p. 288)*

> **You see, you are never given a course in accent learning, yet you pick up those accents. You don't know you are picking them up, but you are learning them and you learn how to recognize them.**
>
> *(Zeig, 1980, p. 314)*

The Unconscious is Unknown Potentials

Every normal individual enters this world with a neurological and biophysical system capable of perceiving, thinking, and responding in an incredible variety of ways. As discussed in the previous chapter, during growth and development only a fraction of these potential patterns of perception, understanding, and response become actualized within the conscious mind. The remainder remain hidden from view, unused and generally unavailable. A host of mental frames of reference, beliefs, attitudes, understandings, perceptions, somatic and physical response capabilities and emotions are effectively cut off from ordinary conscious awareness and are relegated to the province of the unconscious.

All of the various phenomena or responses that can be manifested during a hypnotic trance are based upon abilities normally excluded from conscious awareness. A good hypnotic subject is merely a person who has learned how to accept and to use these unconscious capacities. Hypnosis does not create something that was not there previously, it just enables people to use their unconscious capacities. Most of these hidden, unconscious capacities are utilized in one form or another in the normal course of events, but examples of their use are usually overlooked. For example, experiences of amnesia, anesthesia, automatic movement, and even hallucinations occur very frequently, but in a manner that the conscious mind ignores or accepts as ordinary without recognizing the reservoir of abilities that must underlie such occurrences. Hypnosis merely brings these underlying abilities to the surface of awareness and uses them directly.

The unconscious outstrips the conscious in all of its perceptual, conceptual, emotional, and response capabilities. It is or contains everything that the conscious mind overlooks, ignores or rejects *plus* everything that the conscious mind contains as well. The unconscious has access to and can use almost everything that occurs or exists within the conscious mind but the conscious mind generally is excluded from or protected from the contents and potentials of the unconscious.

> **Most people do not know of their total capacities for response to stimuli. They place mystical meanings on much of the information they get by subtle cues.**
> *(Erickson, Rossi & Rossi, 1976, pp. 247–248)*

> **All of us have a tremendous number of generally unrecognized psychological and somatic learnings and conditionings. [circa 1950's]**
> *(In Erickson, 1980, Vol. IV, chap. 21, p. 224)*

> **The average person is unaware of the extent of his capacities of accomplishment which have been learned through the experiential conditionings of this body behavior through his life experiences. [1967]**
> *(In Erickson, 1980, Vol IV, chap. 24, p. 237)*

> **Every person has abilities not known to the self, abilities that can be expressed in trance.**
> **Memories, thoughts, feelings, sensations completely or partially forgotten by the conscious mind. Yet they are**

available to the unconscious and can be experienced within trance now or later whenever the unconscious is ready. [1976]

(In Erickson, 1980, Vol. I, chap. 22, p. 468)

The unconscious mind is made up of all your learnings over a lifetime, many of which you have completely forgotten, but which serve you in your automatic functioning. Now, a great deal of your behavior is the automatic functioning of these forgotten memories.

(Zeig, 1980, p. 33)

It's very charming, the capacity that we have if we'll only learn to use other areas of our brain.

(ASCH, 1980, Taped Lecture, 7/16/65)

When you stop and think about it, nobody does know his capacities.

(Erickson, Rossi & Rossi, 1976, p. 36)

Little is really known of the actual potentials of human functioning. [1970]

(In Erickson, 1980, Vol. IV, chap. 6, p. 53)

Every person has abilities not known to the self. [1976–78]

(In Erickson, 1980, Vol. I, chap. 22, p. 468)

Consciousness does not have available all the knowledge that is in the unconscious, which actually governs our perceptions and behavior.

(Erickson & Rossi, 1979, p. 367)

That patient may actually be governed by unconscious forces and emotions neither overtly shown nor even known. [1965]

(In Erickson, 1980, Vol. IV, chap. 20, p. 212)

The problem yet remaining is to ensure that the members of the medical profession fully realize that the thinking, the emotions, and the past experiential learnings of each person can play a significant role in his psychological and physiological functionings. [1970]
(In Erickson, 1980, Vol. IV, chap. 6, p. 58)

The Unconscious is Brilliant

Given the above attributes of the unconscious in comparison to the conscious mind, it is not surprising that Erickson observed the unconscious to be "...much smarter, wiser and quicker" than the conscious mind. It has access to more information than does the conscious mind and can analyze and review that information without the biasing influences of pride, prejudice, or expectation. In a sense, it represents the innate intellectual potential of each individual were that individual to function at peak capacity.

It must be mentioned that in spite of its comparative brilliance, the unconscious is not infallible. On occasion it can and does arrive at erroneous or illogical conclusions. Also, it is not surperhuman and is subject to normal physiological and perceptual limitations. It cannot and does not know what it has no reason to know on the basis of experience. Although it may seem miraculous at times, it is not. It only seems so in comparison to what we generally believe to be the normal capacities and abilities of people.

Now what people don't *know*...it's infinite...things that they actually do know but believe that they don't know.
(Zeig, 1980, p. 179)

We all have so much knowledge of which we are unaware.

(Erickson, Rossi & Rossi, 1976, p.247)

The unconscious mind is very brilliant.

(Erickson & Rossi, 1979, p.312)

The unconscious is much smarter, wiser, and quicker. It understands better.

(Erickson & Rossi, 1979, p. 302)

The Unconscious is Aware

One of the most significant and paradoxical aspects of the unconscious mind is that it is not unconscious at all. It is, on the contrary, extremely aware of and responsive to everything that occurs. It is unconscious only in the sense that the conscious mind is oblivious to its presence, to its ongoing operations, to its attempts to communicate, and to its influences upon ordinary thought, perception and behavior. Our awareness or unconsciousness of it gives it its name, not any lack of awareness on its part.

Erickson often noted that people are unconsciously aware of much more than they are consciously. Of particular significance is the ability of an individual to be much more aware unconsciously of the unconscious activities and responses of another person that either of them can be consciously. In an interaction between two people, the unconscious mind of each is busy being aware of the unconscious activities of the other while, in all probability, neither person is consciously aware of those activities. What this amounts to is an ongoing, surreptitious level of communication that may end up having as much influence on the interaction as the conscious level of communication. Obviously, anyone interested in being a therapist would do well to learn how to become aware of and to use this unconscious ability to decipher the unconscious communications of another. They should know what their own unconscious is communicating to the patient's unconscious as well. Such exchanges could have a significant impact on the progress of therapy and should be monitored carefully.

There also should be a ready and full respect for the patient's unconscious mind to perceive fully the intentionally obscured meaningful therapeutic instructions offered them. [1966]

(In Erickson, 1980, Vol. IV, chap. 28, p. 277)

One should also give recognition to the readiness with which one's unconscious mind picks up clues and information. [1966]

(In Erickson, 1980, Vol. IV, chap. 28, p. 277)

Because a person's unconscious mind tends to listen and tends to single out those things. Any six-months-old baby can look at mother's face as mother spoons some pablum toward the baby and read in great big headlines on mother's face "Who on Earth could stand the taste of that stuff?" And the baby agrees and spits it out.

(ASCH, 1980, Taped Lecture, 2/2/66)

Your unconscious mind understands very well and can work hard. [1964]

(In Erickson, 1980, Vol. I, chap. 13, p. 323)

Respectful awareness of the capacity of the patient's unconscious mind to perceive meaningfulness of the therapist's own unconscious behavior is a governing principle in psychotherapy. [1966]

(In Erickson, 1980, Vol. IV, chap. 28, p. 277)

The Unconscious Perceives and Responds Literally

Conceptual frameworks, perceptual categorizations, biases, judgements, and expectations are the province of the conscious mind. The unconscious level of awareness or mentation usually is characterized by the absence of these influences. As a consequence, the unconscious typically involves a more objective and less distorted awareness of reality than the conscious.

Erickson described the unconscious perception and knowledge of reality as direct, unbiased, and literal. The unconscious absorbs and knows about reality on the basis of simple, concrete experiences rather than on the basis of complex interpretations or explanations. It does not filter or distort material to suit its perspective or framework because it does not have one. It is not constrained by a specific context and can respond to events without the limitations imposed by contextually derived meanings. It simply perceives, processes, and reacts to whatever *is* in a direct or literal manner. Its perceptions, understandings, and responses are, therefore, more akin to those of a child who has yet to learn the rigid rules, judgements, biases, and filters of an adult. It does not "read meaning into" a statement or an event, but responds in a literal or multi-contextual manner. Normally, it does not impose contexts, although it may allow the event to determine the context or it may impose a context suggested to it by a hypnotist. All contexts or perspectives are available to it, although, generally, unconscious awareness is simple, direct, and literal, as are unconscious responses.

Paradoxically, the literal awareness that occurs at an unconscious level is probably responsible for the ability of the unconscious to understand and utilize complex metaphors, puns, analogies, and symbolism of all kinds in ways that may seem to be astoundingly creative to our restricted conscious intellects. It seems illogical that literalism would provide a creative outcome, but the relationship may be clarified by reiterating the point that to be literal means not to be constrained by or responsive to contextually implied meanings.

For example, when we hear the word "run," we normally determine what is meant by the context within which it occurs. The unconscious response to the word "run," however, is not contextually bound because it does not abide by or impose any particular perspective or cognitive contexts upon the word. The significance of this fact becomes more apparent when the following sentence is considered: "The watch runs." Everyone recognizes and tends to respond to the implied meaning of "run" in this statement but notice what happens if we allow ourselves to respond to it literally, i.e. without contextual restraints. We may, as a result, imagine a watch with legs running, a watch running like water out of a faucet, a watch running like the dye in cloth, etc. Any of these images is a possible literal interpretation; from a literal standpoint each is a legitimate visual representation of what was said. Even more creative expressions of this statement can occur is we free ourselves from the contextually implied meaning of "watch."

Erickson's recognition of the literalism of the unconscious evidently enabled him to communicate a literal message unconsciously via metaphors and puns while the patient responded consciously to the surface meaning of his statements. It also apparently enabled him to understand the so-called "symbolism" of dreams by reacting to their literal meanings, rather than to their contextual or implied meanings.

Finally, the literalism available at the unconscious level of awareness provides a source of objective, detached perception. Events or memories that might be impossible to consider because of their personal significance or their conflict with conscious beliefs, values, and attitudes becomes interesting and informative when viewed from within the objective perspective of the unconscious.

> **The unconscious is literal and tends to accept only what is said.**
>
> *(Erickson & Rossi, 1979, p. 431)*

> *R:* **The unconscious knows reality from concrete experiences.**
> *E:* **Yes.**
>
> *(Erickson, Rossi, & Rossi, 1976, p. 218)*

> **The secondary-level suggestion depends upon the literalism of the unconscious.**
>
> *(Erickson & Rossi, 1979, p. 162)*

> **He answered questions simply and briefly, giving literally and precisely no more and no less than the literal significance of the questions implied. [1965]**
>
> *(In Erickson, 1980, Vol. 1, chap. 3, p. 94)*

The Unconscious is Childlike

It is not surprising that children are more in touch with or more able to utilize their unconscious minds than are adults. Their conscious minds have yet to dissociate completely as rigidly structured and separate systems of functioning so children necessarily continue to participate in and to utilize their unconscious levels of literal awareness and learning. As a result, the behavior and styles of children represent the basic character of an adult's unconscious. The unconscious is childlike.

Erickson remarked on several occasions that children are much more responsive to unconscious processes and are much more observant than adults. He also noted that they are more responsive to hypnosis, an observation that has been supported consistently by empirical research.

How many of us really appreciate the childishness of the unconscious mind? Because the unconscious mind is decidedly simple, unaffected, straightforward and honest. It hasn't got all of this facade, this veneer of what we call adult culture. It's rather simple, rather childish.

(ASCH, 1980, Taped Lecture, 2/2/66)

A parallel can be drawn between those infants who have not yet learned the realities of life and the putting aside of learned realities that can be observed as an entirely spontaneous manifestation in the hypnotic trance, most clearly so in the somnambulistic state. [1967]

(In Erickson, 1980, Vol. I, chap. 2, p. 76)

When you have a patient in a trance, the patient thinks like a child and reaches for an understanding.

(Erickson, Rossi & Rossi, 1976, p. 255)

The unconscious is much more childlike in that it is direct and it is free.

(Erickson, Rossi & Rossi, 1976, p. 255)

The Unconscious is the Source of Emotions

Emotions often burst forth into awareness unbidden, unwanted, and usually not understood. In general, emotions come from the unconscious. As psychophysiological expressions they typically are reflections of unconscious feelings about or reactions to the situation, usually as that situation relates to the conscious personality. Emotions are not logical, rational, or conscious, but they are a natural and potentially useful form of unconscious communication. They tell us how we feel about something even when we are unaware of how we feel.

> *R:* **Feelings come from our unconscious.**
> *E:* **Yes.**
> *(Erickson, Rossi & Rossi, 1976, p. 182)*

> **Emotional reactions are not necessarily rational, especially so at an unconscious level of reaction. [1952]**
> *(In Erickson, 1980, Vol. 1, chap. 6, p. 151)*

> **Explosiveness is a sudden welling up of the unconscious and everyone has had that experience.**
> *(Erickson & Rossi, 1979, p. 227)*

The Unconscious is Universal

Erickson reached the conclusion that the unconscious is a fairly uniform, similar set of processes from one individual to another on the basis of his observations of multiple personalities, hypnotized subjects and the similarities of rituals and beliefs across cultural and historical contexts. He was, for example, much impressed by the similarities of the drawings of psychotics from different cultures and different centuries.

Even though tentative and not easily observable, the universality of the unconscious, its similarity from one person to another, formed an important aspect of his general understanding of people. The unconscious, it would appear, knows no national, cultural, or historical boundaries; it speaks in a literal manner and uses a form of thought that understands the unconscious of another much more effectively than could the conscious mind of either person. Obviously, the more similar the life experiences of any two people are, the more true this is, but any two people growing up in this world would have enough similar experiences to make it more true than not.

The unconscious seems to reflect the fact that all people are, originally, just plain human beings with essentially identical neurophysiological capacities and an innate tendency to learn, to respond, and to perceive in particular ways. In many respects, most of Erickson's comments regarding the unconscious might be considered to be descriptions of the basic nature of, the innate capacities of, and the response tendencies of human beings in general. His description of the unconscious seems to be a description of a fundamental aspect of people; a description that is neither psychoanalytic, nor humanistic, nor behavioral but is simply an objective description of what all people are, do, and are capable of doing originally and continuously beneath the level of their divergent conscious frames of reference.

There must be individual differences in the contents of the unconscious because every unconscious contains only the information or impressions provided by the unique experiential learning history of the particular unique individual. But the fundamental form, structure, or pattern of response of every human unconscious may be very similar indeed. It would appear that people are both fundamentally different and fundamentally similar.

> **Your unconscious behaves in accord with its own code of behavior.**
>
> *(ASCH, 1980, Taped Lecture, 2/2/66)*

Human thinking and human emotion the world over through all of our records is very much the same, that we can all get the same ideas in various disordered states.

(ASCH, 1980, Taped Lecture, 8/14/66)

Underneath the diversified nature of the consciously organized aspects of the personality, the unconscious talks in a language which has a remarkable uniformity; further, that that language has laws so constant that the unconscious of one individual is better equipped to understand the unconscious of another than the conscious aspects of the personality of either. [1938]

(In Erickson, 1980, Vol. III, chap. 19, p. 186)

The similarities [between various pictures and dreams] were amazing, until one realizes that the dreams and the pictures come from essentially similar minds even though from different mental states and cultures. [1964]

(In Erickson, 1980, Vol. I, chap. 14, p. 338)

Thus, the common dream symbolism of the mentally ill patients of India and the United States; the common symbolism in the art work of the mentally ill German patients of an earlier era and those of newly admitted mentally ill patients in the United States; the translation of cryptic automatic writing of one hypnotic subject by another subject; along with this report on the Pantomime Technique in hypnosis, all suggest the following: That a parallelism of thought and comprehension processes exists which is not based upon verbalizations evocative of specified responses, but which derives from behavioral manifestations not ordinarily recognized or appreciated at the conscious level of mentation. [1964]

(In Erickson, 1980, Vol. I, chap. 14, p.338)

In other words, this boy was simply a human being, with a human mind competent and capable of working along the patterns that the human mind is capable of working. And it was utterly amazing the way this boy's productions could be paralleled.

(ASCH, 1980, Taped Lecture, 8/14/66)

Summary

Erickson's observations led him to the conclusion that people actually have an unconscious mind that is separate from conscious awareness. This unconscious mind perceives, thinks and responds to the world in a literal or objective fashion unimpaired by the rigidities and biases of the conscious mind. It sees things the conscious mind ignores, it knows things the conscious mind overlooks, and it remembers things the conscious mind has forgotten. It takes responsibility for many complex activities such as walking, driving a car, reading, etc. It often influences the thoughts, perceptions, and behavior of the conscious mind by providing "intuitive" hunches, educated guesses, dream experiences, and emotional responses. Although childlike in many respects, it actually is wiser and more perceptive than the conscious mind. It contains a vast range of unrecognized capabilities and potentials, some of which are used in an unnoticed fashion on a daily basis. Many of these capabilities, however, lie dormant and unused because of the restraints and concerns of the conscious mind.

Finally, the unconscious is a universal attribute. No matter how different people are in their conscious realms of existence, they remain linked by the qualities and capacities of their unconscious minds. Diverse cultural backgrounds do not seem to prevent clear communication and understanding at the unconscious level of awareness.

CHAPTER FOUR

NORMALCY AND PATHOLOGY

It should be apparent from the descriptions presented in the previous chapters that Erickson did not view people as inherently or typically perfect. On the contrary, the normal development of the conscious mind and the general inability to use many of the processes and capabilities of the unconscious mind would seem destined to produce a population of rather imperfect, illogical, prejudiced, and even downright strange individuals. Indeed, this appears to be exactly what Erickson saw as he looked about him. Rather than becoming depressed or upset about the universal imperfection of people, however, he accepted and embraced it as a desirable quality. He even warned therapists not to strive for or demand perfection in their patients, but to accept and utilize the unique and often bizarre qualities that they presented.

If imperfection is an acceptable and normal trait, then we may well wonder exactly what therapists should strive to cure.

What aspects of human behavior are undesirable or abnormal and in need of improvement or change? The material in this chapter provides Erickson's answer to that question. The quotations reviewed below define the nature and source of psychopathological phenomena, thereby setting the stage for an understanding of his goals and strategies of psychotherapy. This material derives directly from his basic orientation toward life, that people should observe and use what *is* in order to meet their needs, attain their goals or accomplish their purposes, and relies upon his observations regarding conscious and unconscious functioning. As a result, what is presented here is not really new but, like much of the material in the remainder of this book, is merely a natural extension of his more fundamental observations. It is, nevertheless, of paramount importance to the development of an overall comprehension of an Ericksonian approach to hypnosis and psychotherapy.

What is Abnormal?

Abnormality was a relative term for Erickson. He maintained that the same behavior could be viewed as abnormal in one situation but as normal in another. The temper tantrum of one child could be an intelligent and adaptive response, while the purposeless temper tantrum of another might be a sign of abnormality. Similarly, the various phenomena of hypnosis are desirable abilities when manifested under the direction of a hypnotist but are potentially unproductive pathological occurrences under uncontrolled circumstances.

The differentiating features of abnormal and normal behavior were specified clearly by Erickson. *Any behavior that does not serve a useful and meaningful goal for the person, that is at variance with that individual's personality, or that actually interferes with that person's ability to attain reasonable personal goals is abnormal or undesirable.* This emphasis upon the nonutilitarian features of abnormal behavior appears to be a natural extension of his basic orientation toward life and it gives a special flavor to his hypnotherapeutic approach. Interestingly enough, however, it is a view that he rarely expressed in a direct manner and, consequently, all but one of the following quotes were taken from the same source.

And so, when recognition is given to the fact that everyone is queer in some respects, the question arises, "By what means, criterion or yardstick may judgement of abnormality be passed effectively and correctly?"

(Erickson, 1941a, p. 100)

Abnormal behavior, on the other hand, is not purposeful in a clearly understandable, recognizable, and effective fashion, and it is primarily directed to goals that are not in keeping or harmony with what one properly expects of that individual.

(Erickson, 1941a, p. 101)

However, this does not necessarily mean that the purpose and goal of human behavior must necessarily be legitimate and desirable, since human nature is not perfect. Normal human behavior can be subject to prejudices, misunderstandings, ignorance, and to all the weaknesses of mankind, and yet have purposes and goals readily understood and appreciated as being harmonious to an individual possessed of normal desires and strivings, regardless of any errors of judgement and the lack of common sense in his behavior.

(Erickson, 1941a, p. 101)

Thus, behavior that does not serve a readily understandable and useful goal for the individual, that is not in
keeping with what may reasonably be expected of that
person, that is persisted in to such an extent that it interferes with the person's other and understandably
useful behavior, is definitely abnormal.

(Erickson, 1941a, p. 101)

In other words, to be abnormal, behavior must
necessarily be lacking in purposeful useful qualities so far
as the reasonably average goals of the specific individual
person are concerned.

(Erickson, 1941a, p. 101)

The general practitioner needs primarily to judge his
patient's behavior in terms of what may reasonably be
expected of that particular individual, in terms of what is
purposeful and useful to the individual and in terms of
what behavior is in keeping and harmony with the general established patterns of behavior of the specific person.

(Erickson, 1941 a, p. 108)

As one views the schizophrenic patient and looks over
his life history, one is impressed repeatedly by the lack of
understandable purposefulness in his behavior, the use-
lessness of many things that he does and the general tendency toward infantile and childish behavior, which
would be suggestive in a small child of a behavior
disorder.

(Erickson, 1941a, p. 107)

On the basis of my knowledge of psychiatry, psychotic
behavior is disturbed, uncontrolled, and misdirected
behavior which the individual has limited ability to
change, modify, or understand. ...In psychosis there is

the wrong behavior, in the wrong place, usually at the wrong time. [1960]

(In Erickson, 1980, Vol. II, chap. 31, p. 326)

The neurotic's complaints, however unreal physically, do dominate, limit and restrict normal functioning as much as does actual physical disease.

(Erickson, 1941a, p. 106)

These symptoms are real to the patient, and when they interfere seriously with that person's social, economic and personal adjustments, when they cause his behavior to become purposeless and useless, adequate recognition and attention should be given to these complaints.

(Erickson, 1941a, p. 106)

Conscious Sources of Abnormality

Although Erickson rarely provided direct statements of his definition of abnormality, he did allude to it whenever he discussed the pathological consequences of conscious attitudes or mental sets. Conscious sets or biases were viewed as the typical source of difficulties or abnormalities in learning and performance by Erickson. The behavior of the conscious mind often leads to bias, confusion, and even interference with unconscious capacities and can result in a disruption of performance, an inability to profit from experience and an inability to attain one's goals. Abnormality, therefore, often stems directly from the interfering, inept and non-objective activities of the conscious mind which too often strives for understandings, even erroneous or limiting understandings, at the expense of a general awareness of experiences and an unconscious "feeling" for how best to conduct oneself.

As an aside, it may be worth noting that the comments contained in the following section probably could be used to explain the lack of specificity of Erickson's various presentations. They suggest that Erickson was concerned that others develop a "feeling" for or "sense" of his perspective rather than a conceptual explanation or understanding of it or of his techniques.

In the ordinary state of conscious awareness performance is too often limited by considerations which may actually be unrelated to the task. [1970]
(In Erickson, 1980, Vol. IV, chap. 6, p. 55)

Ideas, understandings, beliefs, wishes, hopes, and fears can all impinge easily upon a performance in the state of ordinary awareness — disrupting and distorting even those goals which may have been singly desired. [1970]
(In Erickson, 1980, Vol. IV, chap. 6, p. 55)

Their failure in the waking state resulted not from incapacity, since capacity had been demonstrated, but from a mental set, contingent upon wakefulness, precluding the initiation of the remote preliminary mental processes leading to the actual performance. [1938]
(In Erickson, 1980, Vol. II, chap. 10 p. 99)

The blinding effects of emotional bias. [1948]
(In Erickson, 1980, IV, chap. 4, p. 44)

Don't let conscious frames of reference occlude your vision.
(Erickson, Rossi & Rossi, 1976, p. 209)

People assume so much.
(Zeig, 1980, p. 354)

You are letting your intellect interfere with your learning.

(Zeig, 1980, p. 42)

The conscious mind understands the logic of it, and the unconscious understands the reality.

(Erickson, Rossi & Rossi, 1967, p. 218)

Confusion results from trying to impose some form of regimentation upon natural processes.

(Erickson, Rossi & Rossi, 1976, p. 243)

R: That rational approach is good for certain intellectual things, but for total human functioning it is not good.
E: It's *not* good!

(Erickson, Rossi & Rossi, 1976, p. 251)

It would spoil the magician's art if you knew how he did that trick. If you want to enjoy swimming, do not analyze it. If you want to make love, don't try to analyze it.

(Erickson, Rossi & Rossi, 1976, p. 255)

The feeling is the essential thing. Knowing about it is not the essential thing.

(Erickson & Rossi, 1976, p. 164)

The best way of learning, to use folk language, is by getting the feel of it. You get the feel of a poem, the feeling of a picture, the feeling of a statue. Feeling is a very meaningful word. We do not just feel with the fingers, but with the heart, the mind. You feel with the learnings of the past. You feel with the hopes for the future. You feel the present.

(Erickson, Rossi & Rossi, 1976, p. 253)

Too often the conscious behavior keeps you too busy so you deprive the unconscious of an opportunity to express itself. It's another scientific truism.

(Erickson, Rossi & Rossi, 1976, p. 38)

This illustrates the biasing influence of a conscious set on true knowledge.

(Erickson, Rossi & Rossi, 1976, p. 209)

Rigidity of Abnormality

Given that much of the abnormality confronting a psychotherapist is the manifestation or consequence of certain conscious biases or sets, the obvious solution would be to alter or eliminate those biases and sets. This sounds easy but every experienced therapist knows that it is not. The conscious mind evolves into a very rigid structure, one that resists experiencing things that cause it to change. The earlier a pathology-inducing attitude was absorbed into that structure the more resistant it seems to be to change and the more likely the individual is to persist in the abnormal behavior. Any attempt to argue somebody out of a deeply ingrained conscious mental set that probably was initiated and supported by the family or the culture usually will prove to be a futile endeavor. If anything, such attempts will initiate frantic efforts to further defend the pathology-inducing ideation.

When we were very young, we were willing to learn. And the older we grow, the more restrictions we put on ourselves.

(Zeig, 1980, p. 75)

And for human behavior — we start from childhood to become rigid, very rigid in our behavior, only we don't know that. We think that we are being free, but we are not. And we ought to recognize it.

(Zeig, 1980, p. 117)

Those early maladjustments serve to establish and to fix within the individual unhealthy and abnormal ways of behaving so that the individual becomes progressively more handicapped in his general life situation.

(Erickson, 1941a, p. 102)

Those deviations from the normal in children do lead to a greater susceptibility to mental illness.

(Erickson, 1941a, p. 104)

Their complaints constitute essentially the childhood behavior disorders grown older and larger.

(Erickson, 1941a, p. 106)

The reader should bear in mind that the hold of social conventions upon the patients also played a significant role in both their illness and their therapy.

(Erickson, 1980, Vol. IV, p. xxii)

And people are so very, very rigid. And each ethnic group has its do's and don'ts.

(Zeig, 1980, p. 120)

We have billions of brain cells that have the capacity to respond to billions of different stimuli, and the brain cells are very specialized. When you come from people who generation after generation only use certain brain cells, every signal that you get as an infant centers you around that.. ...You see, while we're born with similar brain cells, there's a pattern of response that's inherent in our behavior.. ...Ingrained so that you indirectly warn the child away from their natural response.

(Zeig, 1980, p. 340)

The tendency for one pattern of thinking to persist, and the difficulty in shifting to another type, are generally recognized. [1937]

(In Erickson, 1980, Vol. III, chap. 16, p. 149)

I discussed in general the fixity of the subject's beliefs and the general imperviousness to any reasoning approach to her delusional ideas. A parallel was drawn between this behavior and the general attitude taken by the psychotic patient when a reasoning approach is made to any form of abnormal ideation. [1939]

(In Erickson, 1980, Vol. III, chap. 20, p. 205)

When you understand how man really defends his intellectual ideas and how emotional he gets about it, you should realize that the first thing in psychotherapy is not to try to compel him to change his ideation; rather you go along with it and change it in a gradual fashion and create situations wherein he himself willingly changes his thinking. [1977]

(In Erickson, 1980, Vol. IV, chap. 36, p. 335)

The Protection of Abnormality

Part of the problem with direct frontal assaults upon the pathology-inducing ideation of the conscious mind is that the ideation and structure of the conscious mind are thoroughly protected. Even before patients enter the therapist's office, they will probably have constructed a rather massive system of conscious and unconscious protections for the particular pattern of thought that supports or initiates their pathological symptoms. In fact, many of the symptoms presented by patients actually are devices constructed or used by them to protect the structure of their conscious minds from potentially profitable but threatening experiences and understandings.

The unconscious automatically protects the conscious mind when conscious vulnerabilities make it necessary to do so, even to the point of preventing the conscious from becoming unpleasantly aware of the ideas or behaviors underlying emotional problems. Patients, therefore, are people who have been unwilling or unable to view themselves, others or their situation objectively and who even may have unconsciously constructed a more or less elaborate set of protective responses that will enable them to continue in their distorted and ineffectual awareness of reality.

Those personality traits disliked by the self are easily repressed from conscious awareness and are rapidly recognized in others or projected upon others. [1948]
(In Erickson, 1980, vol. IV, chap. 4, p. 43)

The conscious mind already has its own set ideas about the neurosis. It has its fixed, rigid perceptions that constitute a neurotic set. It's very difficult to get people at the conscious level to accept an alteration of their general thinking about themselves. [1973]
(In Erickson, 1980 Vol. III, chap. 11, p. 100)

The neurotic is self-protective of the neurosis. [1973]
(In Erickson, 1980, Vol. III, chap. 11, p. 100)

Man is characterized not only by mobility but by cognition and by emotion, and man defends his intellect emotionally. [1977]
(In Erickson, 1980, Vol. IV, chap. 36, p. 335)

No two people necessarily have the same ideas, but all people will defend their ideas whether they are psychotically based or culturally based, or nationally based or personally based. [1977]

(In Erickson, 1980, Vol. III, chap. 36, p. 335)

The development of neurotic symptoms constitutes behavior of a defensive protective character. Because it is an unconscious process, excluded from conscious understandings, it is blind and groping in nature, does not serve personality purposes usefully, and tends to be handicapping and disabling in its effects.

(Erickson, 1954d, p. 109)

Unconscious conflict and indecision within the psyche gives rise to anxiety against which defenses are erected. [1944]

(In Erickson, 1980, Vol. III, chap. 21, p. 216)

The unconscious always protects the conscious.

(Erickson, Rossi & Rossi, 1976, p. 13)

R: Does the unconscious *always* protect the person?
E: Yes, but often in ways that the conscious mind does not understand.

(Erickson & Rossi, 1979, p. 296)

Unconsciously you don't have to do what you consciously say you will. In everyday life, you may accept an invitation for dinner, and later your unconscious lets you forget it.

(Erickson & Rossi, 1979, p. 315)

Good unconscious understandings allowed to become conscious before a conscious readiness exists will result in conscious resistance, rejection, repression and even the loss, through repression, of unconscious gains. [1948]
(In Erickson,, 1980, Vol. IV, chap. 4, p. 41)

The unconscious is going to be protective of consciousness. It is going to try to reassure the conscious mind with "You don't have to be depressed if you didn't do things." The unconscious won't say "You did something even though you didn't know it." It doesn't function that way. It just says "You don't have to worry because you failed."
(Erickson, Rossi & Rossi, 1976, p. 208)

Utilizing the patient's own neurotic irrationality to affirm and confirm a simple extension of his neurotic fixation relieved him of all unrecognized unconscious needs to defend his neuroticism against all assaults. [1965]
(In Erickson 1980, Vol. IV, chap. 20, p. 218)

A remarkable illustration of the intensity and effectiveness with which the body can provide defenses for psychological reasons. [1954]
(In Erickson, 1980, Vol. IV, chap. 14, p. 170)

By this utterance the patient demonstrated the protectiveness of the unconscious for the conscious. [1948]
(In Erickson, 1980, Vol. IV, chap. 4, p. 40)

Your unconscious mind knows what is right and what is good. When you need protection, it will protect you.
(Erickson & Rossi, 1979, p. 296)

You have all the protection of your own unconscious, which has been protecting you in your dreams, permitting you to dream what you wish, when you wish, and keeping that dream as long as your unconscious thought necessary, or as long as your conscious mind thought would be desirable.

(Erickson, Rossi & Rossi, 1976, p. 35)

And your unconscious mind can keep from you, from your conscious mind, anything it doesn't want you to know consciously.

(Erickson & Lustig, 1975, Vol. 1, p. 9)

You don't know just how much your unconscious wants you to know.

(Erickson & Rossi, 1977, p. 50)

These defenses prevent both unconscious resolution of the conflict and its emergence into consciousness, and may result in inhibition of thinking, confusion, interference with activity. [1944]

(In Erickson, 1980, Vol. III, chap. 21, p. 216)

The conscious mind downgrades unconscious accomplishments, and you can't allow that downgrading to continue because conscious emotions filter down to the unconscious.

(Erickson, Rossi & Rossi, 1976, p. 208)

Yes, it [conscious] can limit itself. The things I say are consciously heard but are understood on an unconscious level only. But the unconscious can keep those sexual connotations to itself. You don't allow the self to become aware of it.

(Erickson & Rossi, 1979, p. 154)

We all realize that personality reactions and emotional attitudes may manifest themselves directly or indirectly, consciously or at a level at which people are unaware of their conduct, or if they become aware of their conduct, may be unaware of their motivations. [1939]
(In Erickson, 1980, Vol. IV, chap. 1, p. 12)

"A patient himself is a person who is afraid to be direct."
(In Beahrs, 1977, p. 57)

Forms of Abnormality

Pathological symptoms and complaints are either expressions of a faulty underlying conscious set or the results of mechanisms used to defend the person against the recognition of something unpleasant. Erickson often employed the Freudian classifications of such defense mechanisms and seemed to be especially intrigued by the processes of repression and dissociation. He postulated that all acts of repression may generate new and separate personalities, a postulate that may further explain the development of the conscious and unconscious minds. In many respects, the conscious/unconscious dichotomy seems to be a dissociation created by repression. Consequently, it is not unreasonable to conclude that Erickson's observations indicated that everyone is a dual personality. The typical separation between the conscious and the unconscious minds seems to be comparable in source and effect to the division that occurs in multiple personalities.

The dissociative process also was of interest to Erickson because he found that it could be a valuable circumstance in the hypnotherapeutic process. He actually used the hypnotic trance to enhance the conscious/unconscious dissociation of a patient so that he could communicate directly with the unconscious mind while the conscious awareness was focused elsewhere.

Be that as it may, the following comments are offered as an expression of his perception of various psychopathological conditions and symptoms, including multiple personalities.

I don't know what the mechanism of displacement is, but I do know that human beings make use of that mechanism. [1960]

(In Erickson, 1980, Vol. II, chap. 31, p. 317)

However, the history of psychopathology is replete with evidence to show that the human mind, however lacking it may be in fundamental endowments, needs little instruction in devising complex escape mechanisms. [1932]

(In Erickson, 1980, Vol. I, chap. 24, p. 497)

Against this, she originally defended herself by a partial dissociation and an attempted identification with her grandfather. [1939]

(In Erickson, 1980, Vol. III, chap. 23, p. 258)

Clearly, in the production of the multiple personality, a process must occur in which certain psychological events are rendered unconscious. [1939]

(In Erickson, 1980, Vol. III, chap. 23, p. 256)

In fact, one must ask whether one is justified in dismissing the possibility that all acts of repression involve the creation of a larval form of a secondary personality. [1939]

(In Erickson, 1980, Vol. III, chap. 23, pp. 256-257)

The "repression" which would result in a multiple personality would be a vertical division of one personality into two more or less complete units like the splitting of a paramecium. [1939]

(In Erickson, 1980, Vol. III, chap. 23, p. 256)

The states of conscious and unconscious mentation existing in cases of multiple personality *coexist* quite as truly as in simpler repressions. [1939]

(In Erickson, 1980, Vol. III, chap. 23, p. 257)

The person with dual or multiple personalities must necessarily have constructed them out of a single experiential background. Hence, any differences in the personalities constructed must reflect differing uses, differing qualities of activeness or passiveness for the same items in this experiential background. [circa 1940's]

(In Erickson, 1980, Vol. III, chap. 24, p. 267)

Hence, I would stress as an adequate measure of discovery for multiple personalities any procedure of systematic clinical observation that would permit the recognition of different sets and patterns of behavior integration and a determination of the interrelationships between various organizations of behavior reactions. [circa 1940's]

(In Erickson, 1980, Vol. III, chap. 24, p. 263)

Inevitably, this raises the question of how frequent such unrecognized dual personalities may be, either as partial or complete formations. [1939]

(In Erickson, 1980, Vol. III, chap. 23, p. 255)

It is possible also that the unsuspected presence of just such dual personalities, closely knit and completely segregated from the rest of the personality, may account for certain analytic defeats. [1939]

(In Erickson, 1980, Vol. III, chap. 23, p. 252)

Not infrequently in neurotic difficulties, there is a surrender of the personality to an overwhelming symptom-complex formation, which may actually be out of proportion to the maladjustment problem.

(Erickson, 1954d, pp.116-117)

Psychopathological manifestations need not necessarily be considered expressive of combined or multiple disturbances of several different modalities of behavior. Rather, they disclose that a disturbance in one single modality may actually be expressed in several other spheres of behavior as apparently unrelated coincidental disturbances. Hence, seemingly different symptoms may be but various aspects of a single manifestation for which the modalities of expression may properly be disregarded. [1943]

(In Erickson, 1980, Vol. II, chap. 14, p. 156)

Recovery from one illness (or conflict) frequently results in the establishment of a new physiological equilibrium (or "resolution of libido") thereby permitting the favorable resolution of a second concurrent and perhaps totally unrelated illness (or conflict).

An intercurrent disease may exercise a favorable effect upon the original illness, for example, malaria in paresis. [1935]

(In Erickson, 1980, Vol. III, chap. 28, p. 320)

The psychotherapeutic approach and the hypnotic approach [to stuttering], in my experience, are most effec-

tive if you recognize one general factor. Stuttering is a
form of aggression against society, and people in general.
(Erickson, 1977b, p. 32)

The extreme obsessional character of their behavior,
thought, and emotions was most marked. They seemed,
as persons, to be sound, yet caught in a situation they
could not handle.
(Erickson & Rossi, 1979, p. 362)

Minimizing Abnormality

It seems appropriate to conclude this brief chapter on abnormality and this introductory section on the general nature
of people with some words about the ideal form of human
functioning from Erickson's point of view. The following collection of quotations offers a straightforward and optimistic
summary of his prescriptions for ideal, albeit imperfect functioning. The essence of his message seems to be that if people
were able to confront and experience the realities of life openly
and objectively and were able to accept and to use these experiences and the full range of their conscious and unconscious capacities, then generally they would be able to
learn how to do the right thing, in the right way at the right
time as defined by their unique goals and circumstances. They
could overcome a majority of life's obstacles and problems
and could live a creative, comfortable, and joyful existence
full of wonderment at the unfolding of their own capacities.

Erickson's comments on the human potential to overcome
adversities and to learn from them provides an effective
backdrop for the subsequent presentation of his goals and
strategies of psychotherapy in the next section of this book
because many of the statements quoted here actually are the

comments and suggestions he offered to his patients during hypnotherapy. They were not uttered as mere speculations on how nice life could be but were presented to open up new ways for his patients to think, act, and feel. They represent his goals for his patients and his prescription for effective living.

Among our patients here we can demonstrate many who were such model children that they never learned the realities of life. In other words, the diet of social development and health must include a reasonable amount of "roughage."

(Erickson, 1941a, p 104)

The Erickson family, in large part, looks upon illness and misfortune as part of the roughage of life.

(Zeig, 1980, p. 185)

Life is much better if sometimes it rains and sometimes it doesn't.

(Erickson & Rossi, 1979, p. 266)

"Erickson, you better face life as it really is.... You better face it, Erickson. All your life, you are going to be confronted with the unfairness of life."

(Zeig, 1980, p. 210)

I had to learn to reconcile myself to the unfairness of life.

(Erickson & Rossi, 1977, p. 42)

There are plenty of alternatives in any situation.... When you attend a session of group therapy, what on earth are you going to see? That is what you go there for.

(Erickson & Rossi, 1981, p. 206)

In other words, reacting to the good and the bad, and dealing with it adequately — that's the real joy in life.

(Erickson & Lustig, 1975, Vol. 2, p. 7)

Too many of us have the attitude, "It can happen to you but it can't happen to me." [Deleted name] took the attitude, "If it can happen to someone else it can happen to me," which is a very nice, intelligent attitude.

(ASCH, 1980, Taped Lecture, 8/8/64)

Because we all start dying when we are born. Some of us are faster than others. Why not live and enjoy, because you can wake up dead. You won't know about it. But somebody else will worry then. Until that time — enjoy life.

(Zeig, 1980, p. 269)

Life isn't something you can give an answer to today. You should enjoy the process of waiting, the process of becoming what you are. There is nothing more delightful than planting flower seeds and not knowing what kind of flowers are going to come up.

(Erickson & Rossi, 1979, p. 389)

Yes, you encourage patients to do all those simple little things that are their own right as growing creatures. You see, we don't know what our goals are. We learn our goals only in the process of getting there. "I don't know what I'm building but I'm going to enjoy building it and when I get through building it I'll know what it is." In doing psychotherapy you impress this upon patients. You don't know what a baby is going to become. Therefore, you take good care of it until it becomes what it will.

(Erickson & Rossi, 1979, p. 389)

What I want you to do is to begin being yourself. Accepting yourself. And knowing that you can control yourself. You want to do something. You control yourself. You focus your efforts. And it is a wonderful thing to explore, to discover the self.

(Erickson & Rossi, 1979, p. 387)

And we should be willing to feel, fully, the pleasures and the happiness that we want, as all our feelings are done by ourselves.

(Erickson & Lustig, 1975, Vol. 2, p. 6)

Everybody is like his fingerprints. They're one of a kind. And never will be another like you. And you need to enjoy, always being you. And you can't change it — just as fingerprints can't be changed.

(Erickson & Lustig, Vol. 1, p. 7)

The important thing always is to do the right thing at the right time. To know that you can rely on yourself. To let your unconscious feed to you the right information that permits you to do the right thing at the right time.

(Erickson, Rossi & Rossi, 1976, p. 260)

People who accomplish a great many things are people who have freed themselves from biases. These are the creative people.

(Erickson, Rossi & Rossi, 1976, p. 179)

The ideal person would be one who had a readiness to accept the interchange between the conscious and unconscious. Children are uncluttered by rigid conscious sets, and therefore children can see things that adults cannot.

(Erickson, Rossi & Rossi, 1976, p. 258)

Juvenility is far superior to senility.

(Erickson, Rossi & Rossi, 1976, p. 256)

There is nothing wrong with having rigid sets. But if you want to alter yourself in some way, you must be unashamedly aware that you do have sets and it's better to have a greater variety of sets.

(Erickson, Rossi & Rossi, 1976, p. 213)

It's a nice thing to learn because it will teach you objectivity which will enable you to do right things at the right time in the right way.

(Erickson, Rossi & Rossi, 1976, p. 158)

Summary

Erickson defined abnormal behavior as any behavior that did not serve a useful purpose for the individual. Furthermore, he concluded that abnormality usually is a consequence of rigid, highly protected, non-objective conscious mental sets which resist experiential learning. Normal behavior is productive and appropriate for the individual involved, although it need not be totally unprejudiced or reasonable because people are not inherently perfect. On the other hand, people do have the capacity to function very creatively, competently, and joyfully if they can overcome the self-limiting and destructive components of their rigid mental sets.

SECTION II
PSYCHOTHERAPY

SECTION II
PSYCHOTHERAPY

It should come as no surprise to learn that the goals, attitudes, and interventions used by Erickson in psychotherapy were derived from his observations on the basic nature of people and from his firm belief that effective living requires awareness, acceptance, and responsivity to the objective realities of life. What may come as a surprise is the depressing realization that one cannot become an Ericksonian psychotherapist simply by learning a specific set of Ericksonian therapy techniques.

In a very real sense, Ericksonian psychotherapy cannot be defined as a specific set of techniques nor can a therapist become an Ericksonian simply by memorizing and applying a particular group of techniques to patients. Erickson's underlying orientation and wisdom formed the well-spring from which his words and behaviors emerged. His techniques were tailored by his past and present observations to fit the peculiar demands of each moment; they were not firmly fixed or stylized routines.

What Erickson did in therapy was derived from his underlying framework and is definable as Ericksonian only because of this fact. Similarly, whatever is done by any therapist who has a similar orientation could be categorized as Ericksonian and, more importantly, any therapist who adopts an Ericksonian perspective probably will tend to engage in Ericksonian therapy automatically. Becoming an Ericksonian psychotherapist does not necessarily mean learning to *do* what Erickson did, but it does mean learning to think like Erickson thought. It means adopting an Ericksonian attitude toward people, toward therapy, and toward oneself as a therapist. It means developing an appreciation for the implications of an Ericksonian perspective and then accumulating the experientially and observationally based resources necessary to act upon those implications.

Obviously, the techniques used by a novice who only recently has developed an Ericksonian perspective will not be particularly unique or effective because that individual will not yet have acquired the requisite background of observations and experiences from which to respond effectively. The Ericksonian orientation provides the goals and attitudes, but not the means to the desired ends. Knowing what to do is not the same as knowing how to do it. For this reason, the observations, verbal and nonverbal skills, and general instructions provided by Dr. Erickson over the years may be useful tools for neophyte Ericksonians until they develop the observational and experiential basis for doing the right thing at the right time in their own way. The essential ingredients in becoming an Ericksonian, however, are the comprehension and incorporation of an Ericksonian orientation. Erickson stressed this point on numerous occasions and, accordingly, the material provided in the following chapters emphasizes the development of an overall, universally applicable sense or flavor of his approach rather than an accumulation of linguistically, culturally, or individually bound techniques. This material does not tell therapists exactly what to do in therapy, but it does tell them how to think so that they will know or be able to learn what to do. Such a teaching approach may demand a greater tolerance for ambiguity than the presentation of specifics and may require a greater dedication to conceptual and behavioral flexibility than the presentation of any answers. However, as the old saying goes, you can give a person a fish and feed him for a day or you can teach him how to fish and feed him for a lifetime. Erickson preferred to do the latter.

CHAPTER FIVE

THE GOAL OF PSYCHOTHERAPY

What happens during a therapy session is dependent to a large extent upon the goals and purposes of the therapist. The questions asked, the responses given, and the strategies used invariably are reflections of the underlying purpose of the psychotherapist. In fact, one of the major sources of differentiation between the various "schools" of therapy is the different goals that they have established for the patient and, by implication, for the therapist. Some strategies are designed to promote insight, others to maximize self-actualization, some to facilitate integration, and others simply to change inappropriate or undesirable responses. Whatever the goal, a great deal of the therapist's behavior is determined by it.

Erickson's goal for the therapeutic process was to facilitate the change to a new, preferably objective, perspective upon the presenting problem which would enable the person to use his or her own experientially acquired learnings in order to emit a more adaptive response to the situation. He often ignored insight and generally avoided perfectionism. Objective perception of an effective response to life's current situations was what he expected of himself and it was what he believed his patients required as well. The material presented below emphasizes these points and provides additional details regarding the general purposes of the Ericksonian psychotherapy process.

Focus on the Possible, Not on Perfection

Erickson did not expect his patients to be more than they were. He realized that nobody is perfect and that human faults are necessary and even desirable. His goal in therapy was not to create a perfect human being, but to help people learn how best to use their existing abilities and potentials, limited or faulty as they might be. By recognizing and accepting his patients' handicaps, he maintained an atmosphere of acceptance, protection, and trust and provided patients with attainable goals.

> **I object very seriously to this attitude of perfection that some physicians and dentists and psychologists have when dealing with human beings. I've never met a perfect human being yet and I never expect to meet one. I think the faults that you recall in human beings give their charm to that individual that enable you to recognize and remember that individual.**
>
> *(ASCH, 1980 Taped Lecture, 7/18/65)*

Long experience in psychotherapy has disclosed the wisdom of avoiding perfectionistic drives and wishes on the part of patients and of motivating them for the comfortable achievement of lesser goals. This then ensures not only the lesser goal but makes more possible the easy output of effort that can lead to a greater goal. Of even more importance is that the greater accomplishment then becomes more satisfyingly the patient's own rather than a matter of obedience to the therapist. [1965]

(In Erickson, 1980, Vol. IV, chap. 17, p. 190)

The writer recognizes that complete awareness of absolute truth is much less available than happy adjustments based upon those partial understandings acceptable to individuals and available and suitable to their own unique limitations. [circa 1950's]

(In Erickson, 1980, Vol. IV, chap. 40, p. 368)

The purpose of psychotherapy is to enable a patient to achieve a legitimate personal goal as advantageously as is possible. [circa 1930's]

(In Erickson, 1980, Vol. IV, chap. 54, p. 482)

It is imperative that recognition be given to the fact that comprehensive therapy is unacceptable to some patients. Their total pattern of adjustment is based upon the continuance of certain maladjustments which derive from actual frailties. Hence, any correction of those maladjustments would be undesirable if not actually impossible. Therefore, a proper therapeutic goal is one that aids the patient to function as adequately and constructively as possible under those internal and external handicaps that constitute a part of his life situation and needs.

(Erickson, 1954d, p. 109)

Indeed, it often seems absurd to attempt to reeducate patients when all that may be needed may be a redirection of their endeavors, rather than a change or a correction of their behavior. [1973]

(In Erickson, 1980, Vol. IV, chap. 38, p. 348)

Nor should therapists have so little regard for their patients that they fail to make allowance for human weaknesses and irrationality. [1965]

(In Erickson, 1980, Vol. IV, chap. 20, p. 212)

One does not try to force upon his patient a new pattern, but rather to reestablish the old unused and forgotten pattern of behavior the patient had previous to the development of his phobia.

(Erickson, 1941b, p. 17)

One takes the attitude that the patient is there to benefit *eventually* — perhaps in a day, a week, a month, six months, but within some reasonable period — *not* in the immediate moment. This tendency to correct the immediate behavior must be avoided because the patient really needs to show you that particular behavior.

(Erickson & Rossi, 1981, p. 18)

Focus on the Future, Not on the Past

Erickson was concerned only with the adequacy of a patient's present and future adjustments to reality. Insight into the mistakes of the past or into the past causes of present problems were of minor interest to him. He pointed out that the past is over and cannot be changed. His only concern with the past was that patients develop the ability to look at it carefully and objectively in order to overcome whatever misperceptions, or irrational beliefs, or limitations from the past were influencing their present behavior. He stated that insight into causal connections with prior events may be useful to the extent that it enables the therapist to guide the patient's attention toward relevant memories, but insight on the part of the patient was not the goal.

> **Insight into the past may be somewhat educational. But insight into the past isn't going to change the past. If you were jealous of your mother, it is always going to be a fact that you *were* jealous of her. If you were unduly fixated on your mother, it is always going to be the fact. You may have insight, but it doesn't change the fact. Your patient has to live in accord with things of today. So you orient your therapy to the patient living today and tomorrow, and hopefully next week and next year.**
>
> *(Zeig, 1980, p. 269)*

> **You have those learnings, in adult life, you can correct them. But there is no real need to correct them. They should be appreciated.**
>
> *(Erickson, Rossi & Rossi, 1976, p. 214)*

> **Well, the deed is done and cannot be undone, so let the dead past bury its dead. [1964]**
>
> *(In Erickson, 1980, Vol. 1, chap. 13, p. 325)*

> **Emphasis should be placed more upon what the patient does in the present and will do in the future than upon a mere understanding of why some long-past event occurred.**
>
> *(Erickson, 1954d, p. 127)*

> *You present new ideas and new understandings and you relate them in some indisputable way to the remote future.* **It is important to present therapeutic ideas and post hypnotic suggestions in a way that makes them con-**

tingent on something that will happen in the future.

(Erickson & Rossi, 1975, p. 148)

The rest of the hour was spent in an "explanation of the importance of reordering the behavior patterns for tomorrow, the next day, the next week, the next year, in brief, of the future, in order to meet the satisfactory goals in life that are desired." [1964]

(In Erickson, 1980, Vol. I, chap. 13, p. 315)

It's so ridiculous to pore over what you did when you were five years old because it belongs to the unchangeable past and any present understandings of that are different than that of the five year old. The adult level of understanding precludes any real understanding of the child's or the adolescent's world.

(Rossi, 1973, p. 15)

The problems were remote in origin, recent only in manifestation. To search for those remote origins would have been impossible until the traumatic course of stressful emotional events rendered the patients more accessible and probably more permanently damaged. Past experience with many similar patients suggests the importance of a ready approach to the immediate problem by dealing with it directly.

(Erickson & Rossi, 1979, p. 358)

Yes, take them from where they are now. That's where they are going to live today. Tomorrow, they live in tomorrow...next week, next month and next year. You might as well forget your past. Just as you forgot how you learned how to stand up, how you learned to walk, how you learned to talk. You have forgotten all that.

(Zeig, 1980, p. 221)

If your patient has something covered up, she's got it covered up for a very good reason, and you'd better respect that fact. You ask the patients to respect the fact that you personally do not think it needs to be covered up but that you are going to abide by their needs, *their actual needs.* Now you've told them you will abide by their needs, but they don't hear you qualify it to their "actual needs."

(Erickson & Rossi, 1979, p. 347)

It is essential that the therapist understand it [the patient's past] as fully as possible but without compelling the patient to achieve the same degree of special erudition. It is out of the therapist's understandings of the patient's past that better and more adequate ways are derived to help the patient to live his future.

(Erickson, 1954d, p. 128)

To assume that the original maladjustment must necessarily come forth again in some disturbing form is to assume that good learnings have neither intrinsic weight nor enduring qualities, and that the only persisting forces in life are the errors.

(Erickson, 1954d, p. 127)

From the point of view of analytic therapy, it is particularly interesting to emphasize that the obsessional phobia was relieved merely by the recovery of these specific conditioning events and without any investigation or discharge of underlying patterns of instinctual oedipus relationships, castration anxiety, or the like. [1939]

(In Erickson, 1980, Vol. III, chap. 23, p. 255)

Familiarity breeds contempt. When you go through a painful situation again and again in a dream, changing it a bit each time, it becomes less painful. [circa 1940's]

(In Erickson, 1980, Vol. IV, chap. 35, p. 334)

Objectivity Cures

Erickson noticed that people automatically respond more effectively when they are able to view the past, the present, and even the future in an objective, detached manner. As noted earlier, he attributed disordered or ineffectual behavior to a lack of exposure to accurate objective data about something, whether the environment, the past, or oneself. In a similar manner, he maintained that the provision of accurate, experientially based information or an objective appraisal would initiate growth-oriented responses from a majority of patients.

There is a natural tendency to overemphasize the importance of immediate understandings and subjective attitudes in preference to a thoughtful, objective consideration of eventual probabilities and possibilities. [circa 1940's]

(In Erickson, 1980, Vol. IV, chap. 46, p. 424)

This comprehensive, objective viewing of stressful matters is thus carried out against suggested backgrounds of various possible understandings. Ideally, objective thinking is possible in the ordinary waking state, but emotional stress is likely to constitute a serious interference, if not an actual barrier. [circa 1940's]

(In Erickson 1980, Vol. IV, chap. 46, p. 424)

The pressing emotional urgency of the actual current situation can be altered by the interjection or interpolation of a sense of perspective in time, thereby creating an opportunity conducive to more comprehensive and objective thinking. [circa 1940's]

(In Erickson, 1980, vol. IV, chap. 46, p. 424)

Thus he was enabled to see himself in an objective, detached fashion and, from unrecognized inner knowledge, to appreciate exactly what was occurring. [1937–38]

(In Erickson, 1980, Vol. IV, chap. 55, p. 493)

I gave Louise one nice look at her childish behavior. That was enough. I had her see her childish behavior in the behavior of other people who should know better. That was all the therapy that was needed.

(Zeig, 1980, p. 226)

Inducing and compelling an open-mindedness or mental receptiveness to new, inexplicable, curiosity-evoking ideas in settings causing the patient to look forward with hopeful anticipation and not to expend her energies in despondent despair over the past. [1963]

(In Erickson, 1980, Vol. IV, chap. 30, p. 311)

The overlay of neuroticism, however extensive, does not distort the central core of the personality, though it may disguise and cripple the manifestations of it. [1952]

(In Erickson, 1980, Vol. I, chap. 6, p. 146)

Objectivity Requires Reorganization

In order for patients to develop the more accurate and objective view of themselves and of reality that will enable them to cope more effectively, they obviously must change their present orientations toward that reality. This change in orientation was described by Erickson as a reordering, a resynthesis or a restructuring of the rigid and inhibiting conscious mental sets that patients have. *The initiation or facilitation of this restructuring process was his primary therapeutic goal.*

In some ways, Erickson was not concerned about where this restructuring began because he had discovered that once a patient experiences anything in a new way or from a new perspective, this new orientation will spread throughout the system. The destruction of any segment of a rigid and limiting mental set will initiate reverberating alterations and reassociations throughout the person's experiential life. Getting patients to experience something that would violate or disrupt their habitual conscious patterns of perception, thought, and response was what he wanted to accomplish. Once that had been accomplished, patients were allowed to grow and to develop in their own unique ways.

It is the experience of reassociating and reorganizing his own experiential life that eventuates in a cure, not the manifestation of responsive behavior which can, at best, satisfy only the observer. [1948]
(In Erickson, 1980, Vol. IV, chap. 4, p. 38)

Therapy results from an inner resynthesis of the patient's behavior achieved by the patient himself. [1948]
(In Erickson, 1980, Vol. IV, chap. 4, p. 38)

Not until he goes through the inner process of reassociating and reorganizing his experiential life can effective results occur. [1948]
(In Erickson, 1980, Vol. IV, chap. 4, p. 39)

The induction and maintenance of a trance serve only to provide a special psychological state in which the patient can reassociate and reorganize his inner psychological complexities and utilize his own capacities in a manner in accord with his own experiential life.... therapy

results from an *inner resynthesis* of the patient's behavior achieved by the patient himself. ...It is this experience of reassociating and reorganizing his own experiential life that eventuates in a cure. [1948]

(In Rossi, 1973, p. 19)

Hence, no more than was necessary was said to initiate those inner processes of her own behavior, responses and functionings which would be of service to her. [1964]

(In Erickson, 1980, Vol. I, chap. 13, p. 330)

It altered the place they could go for pleasure. It was a breakdown of a narrow, limited, restricted life existence. You can't be rigid in one area alone, it always spreads.

(Rossi, 1973, p. 15)

Providing the patient with alternatives sets the stage for inner search and creative problem-solving.

(Erickson, 1980, Vol. IV, p. 148)

To break her inhibitions, really break them! Notice how I engineered that: first the left shoe, then the right, the left stocking, then the right. I carefully built up a momentum of an affirmative character so she finally took off all her clothes and followed all my suggestions designed to shatter her lifelong inhibitions.

(Rossi, 1973, p. 13)

There results then a new psychological orientation of compelling force, effecting a new organization of thinking and planning. The writing of the letter constituted an initiation of action, and an action once initiated tends to continue.

(Erickson, 1954c, p. 283)

Thus he was placed in a situation permitting the development of a new frame of reference at variance with the repressed material of his life experience, but which would permit a reassociation, an elaboration, a reorganization, and an integration of his experiential life. [1948]
(In Erickson, 1980, Vol. IV, chap. 4, p. 43)

You always have patients experience as much of themselves and their limiting sets as possible within therapy. *The most important thing in therapy is to break up the patient's rigid and limiting mental sets.*
(Erickson & Rossi, 1979, p. 343)

I facilitate a certain flexibility in mental functioning when I remind her how easily her pleasure and fear can be "removed and reassumed."
(Erickson & Rossi, 1979, p. 347)

We are giving the patient new possibilities and we are taking away the undesirable qualities.
(Erickson & Rossi, 1979, p. 330)

And when I shattered that rigid idea it shattered the hell out of them. It even led them to try other positions. I hadn't told them there were other positions, they started investigating other positions on their own.
(Rossi, 1973, p. 15)

R: So you can actually enhance physical abilities by breaking through conscious bias about limitations.
E: Yes, unrecognized conscious bias.
(Erickson, Rossi & Rossi, 1976, p. 178)

Yes, it disrupted the rigidity that governed her entire life. Just as the first break in the shell pecked by a newly emerging chick immediately shatters the whole shell so

her whole life opened up. I just gave her simple statements. You do this, do that. No questions, just do it
silently.

(Rossi, 1973, p. 12)

He's placed a bad interpretation on a loss of erection.
Why should he keep that forever and ever?

(Erickson & Rossi, 1979, p. 266)

I am getting her away from her own habitual conscious
patterns.

(Erickson & Rossi, 1981, p. 80)

I'm asking her to adopt a frame of reference that is
totally new and different.

(Erickson & Rossi, 1979, p. 344)

R: That's the therapeutic response...
E: Yes, getting a new frame of reference.

(Erickson & Rossi, 1981, p. 255)

R: You are structuring a learning set for therapeutic
change.
E: Yes, new and different learnings for psychotherapeutic change. Without saying "Now I'm going to cram
down your throat some new understanding."

(Erickson, Rossi & Rossi, 1976, p. 33)

I want you to read the last chapter first and then you
sit down and try to think, wonder and speculate on what
was in the preceding chapter. Think in all directions, and
read that second to last chapter and see in how many
ways you were wrong; and you will be wrong in a lot of
ways. Then you read that second to the last chapter and
by the time you read a good book from the last chapter
to the first chapter, wondering and speculating, imagi-

ning, and figuring out, you'll learn to think freely in all directions.

(Zeig, 1980, p. 128)

The patient comes to you with a certain mental set and they expect you to get into that set. If you surprise them, they let loose of their mental set and you can frame another mental set for them.

(Erickson, Rossi & Rossi, 1976, p. 128)

When patients find something new, never again can they function in the old incomplete way. Their world is permanently changed.

(Erickson & Rossi, 1979, p. 392)

Therapy is often a matter of tipping the first domino. All that was needed was the correction of one behavior and if that one behavior was corrected....

(Rossi, 1973, p. 14)

Because once you break that restrictive, phobic pattern, the person will venture into other things.

(Zeig, 1980, p. 255)

When you get that wrongly directed energy turned in another direction, the patient heals.

(Zeig, 1980, p. 110)

When you get the patient to do the main work, all the rest of it falls in place.

(Zeig, 1980, p. 159)

You depend upon the patient's natural associative process to put things together.

(Erickson & Rossi, 197 , p. 386)

You start patients in a train of association, but they drift along on their own currents of thought and frequently leave the therapist stranded far behind.

(Erickson, Rossi & Rossi, 1976, p. 93)

This also gets the person into their own individuality. In psychotherapy we are looking for individualities. A patient, all too often, does not have much.

(Erickson & Rossi, 1979, p. 390)

R: The cure is to let that individuality come out and flower in all its particular genius.

E: That's right. That's what you need to do, and that is why they are seeing you.

(Erickson, Rossi & Rossi, 1976, p. 39)

You let the subject grow!

(Erickson, Rossi & Rossi, 1976, p. 265)

And remember always that you're unique. And all that you have to do is let people see that you are you.

(Erickson & Lustig, 1975, Vol. 2, p. 6)

Only Experiences Can Initiate Reorganization

As mentioned previously, people learn from experience. Only experientially acquired learning can be used to guide behavior and only internal or external events that are experienced directly can disrupt old patterns and initiate new ones. Reorganization or resynthesis, therefore, is the production of a new perspective as the result of new internal or external experiences. Generating such experiences and helping the patient become able to learn from them is the task of the therapist.

Erickson's verbal interactions with his patients were designed to initiate experiences which would facilitate the resynthesis process. He often worded reorganizational statements vaguely or even incorrectly so that patients would restate his basic points to themselves in a clearer, more correct, or more personally meaningful manner. By this device he was able to elicit an internal experience that would have more impact than something heard but not experienced in a personal way. Words, phrases, or statements that trigger internal responses or that touch upon and move attention toward one's own experiential background evidently have a more significant effect than those that are understood on an intellectual but not an experiential level.

Similarly, Erickson's frequent use of metaphors, analogies, and personal anecdotes apparently was *partially* motivated by the desire to force the patient to personalize the meaning of his words. The import of his statements could become an experiential event which then would be translated automatically by patients into terms related to their own thoughts and previous experiences. He believed that these strategies were more likely to convey a meaning that could be experienced and internalized by the listener than simple or direct statements of his basic points.

Patients can only respond out of their own life experiences.

(Erickson & Rossi, 1979, p. 258)

Therefore, his response could derive only from his own experiential associations and learned activities. [1938]

(In Erickson, 1980, Vol. II, chap. 1, p. 9)

You give many examples so that patients are more likely to find one that's personally convincing and actually helps alter their behavior. The only things I say to you that cling are those that touch upon your experience in some way. You always study your patients for evidence that they are accepting what you say.

(Erickson & Rossi, 1979, p. 346)

Now when you want to prove something to a subject, and really prove it to them, try to let the proof come from within them. And let it come from within them in a most unexpected way. [1959]

(In Erickson, 1980, Vol. I, chap. 9, p. 239)

It is this internalization of the suggestion that makes it an effective agent in behavior change.

(Erickson & Rossi, 1975, p. 146)

You are avoiding saying to the subject but get the subject to say themselves.

(Erickson, Rossi & Rossi, 1976, p. 86)

There is a need to give the patient an earnest, compelling desire to protect and to respect that which is accepted. Therefore, let patients reword the presented ideas to please themselves. Then they become the patients' own ideas!

(Erickson & Rossi, 1979, p. 436)

To grasp such an analogy requires a creative effort on his part. Because it is his own creative effort, he is less likely to reject it than if it was simply thrust upon him as a direct statement.

(Erickson & Rossi, 1979, p. 259)

Behavior Generates Experiences

Although Erickson relied heavily upon the effects of verbal interaction in his therapy and teaching to initiate internal experiences, his ultimate goal was to get his patients and students to do something, *anything*, that would generate an experientially based challenge to their rigid, maladaptive, conscious patterns of response. Behavior provides experiences that cannot be easily overlooked.

It is at this point that his psychotherapeutic strategies often become difficult to understand or to imitate effectively. He used a variety of behavioral prescriptions for his clients, including climbing mountains, racing a bike, squirting water between the front teeth, eating a ham sandwich, and removing every stitch of clothing while standing in his office. Each of these behaviors had immediate and beneficial effects upon the patients involved and these benefits rapidly spread to all areas of their lives. Obviously, however, the behaviors themselves are not universally applicable as therapeutic interventions. They were selected and prescribed for individual patients because of the particular needs, personalities, and areas of conceptual rigidity of these patients. Climbing mountains or stripping off all of one's clothes are not magical techniques that would be effective with everyone. Erickson clearly stated that what he had patients do was only a relatively straightforward response to the needs and personalities of his patients.

Whether he used behavioral prescriptions or complex metaphors, he was simply attempting to get his patients to experience something that would force them to confront the reality of themselves and their situations either directly or symbolically. If the symbolism was appropriate and blatant enough or if the patient could be induced to undergo the experience directly, then the destruction of repressive barriers, rigidities, or biases would become a *fait accompli* and the process of reorganization would continue apace.

It clearly illustrates the need and the value of actual behavior in enabling a patient to make therapeutic progress. [1935]

(In Erickson, 1980, Vol. IV, chap. 58, p. 521)

I believe that patients and students should do things. They learn better, remember better.

(Zeig, 1980, p. 72)

The important thing is not so much bookwork, following the rules you read in books. The important thing is to get the patient to do the things that are very, very good for him.

(Zeig, 1980, p. 195)

In psychotherapy for you, I want action and response not words, ideas, theories, concepts. I want responses, desirable, good, informative responses of action and change, not contemplation of change, but change and action of a constructive sort. [circa 1930's]

(In Erickson, 1980, Vol. IV, chap. 54, p. 484)

The thing to do is to get your patient, any way you wish, any way you can, to do something.

(Zeig, 1980, p. 143)

Then, as a result of some concrete or tangible performance, the patient develops a profound feeling that the repressive barriers have been broken, that the resistances have been overcome, that the communication is actually understandable and that its meaning can no longer be kept at a symbolic level.

(Erickson, 1954, p. 128)

And I had them do something. And he got a new perspective upon life and she got a new perspective upon the
boresomeness of something she didn't like.

(Zeig, 1980, p.148)

When you have a patient with some senseless phobia,
sympathize with it, and somehow or other, get them to
violate that phobia.

(Zeig, 1980, p. 253)

Leading the patient to, "See what I [the patient] can
do," is much more effective than letting the patient see
what things the therapist can do with or to the patient.
[1963]

(In Erickson, 1980, Vol. IV, chap. 30, p. 291)

The rest of the hour was spent in an "explanation of
the importance of reordering the behavior patterns for
tomorrow, of the future, in order to meet the satisfactory
goals in life that are desired." This was all in vague gen-
eralities, seemingly explanations, but actually cautious
post-hypnotic suggestions, intended to be interpreted by
him to fit his needs. [1964]

(In Erickson, 1980, Vol. I, chap. 13, p. 315)

After exploration of the underlying causes of her problem, the next step in therapy was to outline in great
detail, with her help, the exact course of activity that she
would have to follow to free herself from past rigidly established habitual patterns of behavior. [1952]

(In Erickson, 1980, Vol. I, chap. 6, p. 164)

Patients Can and Must Do the Therapy

Erickson's position with regard to the desired role of the patient was simple and direct. He maintained that the patient has

the ability to do something that will be beneficial and that it is the patient's responsibility to do it. The therapist can create conditions conducive to change, can attempt to motivate the patient to change and can even provide a change-inducing experience, but change must occur within the patient. Change cannot be forced upon patients and patients cannot be expected to change in ways that are inappropriate for their needs or foreign to their experiential backgrounds. Unfortunately, this also implies that some patients cannot or will not experience change under any conditions the therapist can create. Therapists who keep the burden of responsibility for change on the shoulders of their patients will have less difficulty recognizing and accepting their impotence in such circumstances.

> **People come to you for help when they could furnish their own help.**
>
> *(Zeig, 1980, p. 195)*

> **Well, you've got a lot of things to help you. And keep them handy — handy in every possible way. And know that your own brain cell responses can meet your needs.**
>
> *(Erickson & Lustig, 1975, Vol. 2, p. 5)*

> **If you can utilize the great variety of brain cells that exist in the human being and depend upon them to function in their own way of thinking you can rely upon your patient to be able to furnish you with the ways and means and methods of dealing with intricate problems of everyday living.**
>
> *(ASCH, 1980, Taped Lecture, 8/14/66)*

> **Now the important thing for all of you is to recognize that when a patient comes in to you tremendously handicapped, how handicapped is he really? What brain cells does he have unused?**
>
> *(ASCH, 1980, Taped Lecture, 7/16/65)*

People do any number of things against themselves, and they do it in a very intelligent way to defeat themselves, to destroy themselves and that's what you need to know. Because if anybody can destroy the self intelligently then they can also use their brains to build things up intelligently.

(ASCH, 1980, Taped Lectures, 8/14/66)

Therapy for both was predicated upon the assumption that there is a strong normal tendency for the personality to adjust if given an opportunity. [1955]

(In Erickson, 1980, Vol. IV, chap. 56, p. 505)

The potentials within a person can restore well-being. [1970]

(In Erickson, 1980, Vol. IV, chap. 6, p. 58)

You reach an understanding that every happiness is earned and, if given to you, it's merited. Because there is no such thing as a free gift; you have to earn it or you have to merit it. And merit requires labor and effort on your part.

(Erickson & Lustig, 1975, Vol. 2, p. 4)

The burden of responsibility was hers, the means was hers. [1964]

(In Erickson, 1980, Vol. 1, chap. 13, p. 325)

Whatever he does has to be on his own responsibility.

(Erickson & Rossi, 1981, p. 195)

The patient himself must put the recommended regime into action. [1957]

(In Erickson, 1980, Vol. IV, chap. 5, p. 49)

R: You are continually putting the responsibility for change back on the patient.

E: On to them always!

(Erickson, Rossi & Rossi, 1976, p. 37)

You never give the patient the impression that you must be constantly alert. You give them the impression that they are always sharing in the responsibility for the success of the work.

(Erickson, Rossi & Rossi, 1976, p. 264)

No matter what the author said, she was dependent upon her own resources only. **[1964]**

(In Erickson, 1980, Vol. I, chap. 13, p. 330)

"You're here to get whatever benefit you can get. And I think you're reasonably intelligent and if you exercise your intelligence you really ought to find some way of getting some kind of benefit. And I really don't care what kind of benefit you receive so long as you take the benefit that is available to *you*." Now I was able to give the burden upon her. *She* had to take the benefit that *she* could get, the benefit that she could derive from the situation. I challenged her intelligence.

(ASCH, 1980, Taped Lectures, 2/2/66)

She came to me with a problem, and I tell her she is going to have to do some thinking. And then I demonstrate to her exactly the kind of thinking.

(Erickson & Rossi, 1979, p. 210)

All therapy occurs within the patient, not between the therapist and patient.

(Erickson & Rossi, 1979, p. 160)

Bear in mind that it is the patient who is the important element.

(Haley, 1967, p. 535)

What your patient does and what he learns must be learned from within himself. There is not anything you can force into the patient.

(Haley, 1967, p. 535)

Reliance was placed upon the patient's own thinking and intelligence to make the proper psychological interpretation of her symptom when she became ready for that realization. [1944]

(In Erickson, 1980, Vol. IV, chap. 2, p. 25)

In a learning situation you have to do your own learning. I want you to learn a lot faster than I did, It took me about 30 years to learn, and there is no sense in that.

(Erickson, Rossi & Rossi, 1976, p. 264)

When I see patients, I really want them to do a great deal of thinking, because I don't know what's right for them. They have to reach that through an understanding of what they know, have experienced.

(Erickson & Lustig, 1975, Vol. 2, p. 5)

Yes, I think Joe's a very competent young man. I think he was competent in his psychotherapy. I think my competence lay in the fact that I knew enough to induce the trance and sit back and encourage Joe to follow out his own inclinations and understandings.

(ASCH, 1980, Taped Lecture, 8/14/66)

I gave that boy an understanding of his own capacity to be his own therapist. I told him "Never overextend yourself, just be cautious."

(ASCH, 1980, Taped Lecture, 8/14/66)

The experienced therapist makes clear to patients that responses must be in accord with their own potentialities, even though those potentialities may as yet be unrealized, misused, or misunderstood. [1973]

(In Erickson, 1980, Vol. IV, chap. 38, p. 348)

And some people love their illness and keep their illness, so you force them to do something to be frank.

(Zeig, 1980, p. 324)

There are some people you can't help. You can try.

(Zeig, 1980, p. 284)

Any young man who will impose upon his wife in the first seven years in that fashion is not going to change.

(Zeig, 1980, p. 201)

He is a born loser. Born to lose. Born to be a failure.

(Zeig, 1980, p. 210)

There is no hope for those people — they are professional patients. That is their sole goal in life.

(Zeig, 1980, p. 209)

There are other patients whose goal is no more than the continuous seeking of therapy but not the accepting of it. With this type of patient hypnotherapy fails as completely as do other forms of therapy. [1964]

(In Erickson, 1980, Vol. IV, chap. 19, p. 211)

Summary

Erickson emphasized the natural healing power of objectivity and avoided the seeking of insight. He accepted human imperfection but attacked and undermined conscious biases whenever they interfered with accurate objective awareness. His goal of psychotherapy was simple — a breakdown of biases to allow objectivity and freedom of action — but attainment of the goal often called for a complex restructuring of conscious understandings and responses. The initiation of these restructuring processes was accomplished by the creation of experiences, experiences that symbolically or indirectly moved patients toward more objective awareness of these abilities, thoughts, and situations. He generated internal experiences with his words and he generated external experiences with behavioral prescriptions. In all instances, however, he remained aware that the purpose of therapy is to allow patients to use their own potentials in whatever unique way is most productive and possible for them. Change, however, remains the patient's reponsibility. Some people cannot or will not be helped. Such is the reality of the therapy situation.

CHAPTER SIX

CREATING A PSYCHOTHERAPEUTIC CLIMATE

Although Erickson has been memorialized as a powerful and effective clinician who could cure even the most resistant or hopeless patients, he was exceedingly modest about the importance of the therapist within the therapy process. He challenged the "primacy of the therapist" attitude that pervades most other approaches and argued vehemently that it is the *patient's* needs, beliefs, abilities, and welfare which should define the character of therapy. He questioned the value and validity of pre-packaged, technique-oriented approaches to therapy that specify how a therapist should conduct a therapy session or what should be accomplished in therapy without reference to the individual patient. He rejected the use of a general theory to prescribe specific goals or techniques and he attacked the prejudices and professional inhibitions that often prevent therapists from recognizing or doing those things that are most responsive to a patient's needs.

In short, Erickson insisted that it must be the patient who provides the goals, defines the process, and actually does the therapy. Because he realized that it is up to the patient to undergo the desired changes, he recognized that the therapist can do little more than provide a setting conducive to those changes. The attitudes and behaviors necessary to create such a setting were the subject of many of his comments and form the bulk of the material contained in this chapter.

Therapists Provide Therapeutic Climates

According to Erickson, the therapist is a relatively unimportant component of the therapy process, merely the creator of a catalytic situation. Thus, the first and most important thing that a therapist can do is create a setting that will permit and motivate patients to undergo the restructuring events necessary to enable them to apply their experientially acquired learnings effectively within a more objective view of themselves and of the world. Therapists do not even have to know the nature of the presenting problem or understand what needs to be done to resolve it. All therapists really need to know is how to create a situation or relationship that will motivate patients to use their own experiences and capacities to accomplish their own therapy.

> **I don't think the therapist is *the* important person; I think the patient is *the* important person in the situation.**
>
> *(Erickson, 1977b, p. 22)*

> **The therapist is really unimportant. It is his ability to get his patients to do their own thinking, their own understanding.**
>
> *(Zeig, 1980, p. 157)*

What the therapist knows, understands, or believes about a patient is frequently limited in character and often mistaken. What he is willing to let patients discover about themselves and to use effectively is of exceedingly great therapeutic importance. [1973]

(In Erickson, 1980, Vol. IV, chap. 38, p. 349)

It is the patient who does the therapy. The therapist only furnishes the climate, the weather. That's all. The patient has to do all the work.

(Zeig, 1980, p. 148)

I didn't know what her problem was. She didn't know what her problem was. I didn't know what kind of psychotherapy I was doing. All I was was a source of a weather or a garden in which her thoughts could grow and mature and do so without her knowledge.

(Zeig, 1980, p. 157)

I don't think the therapist does anything except provide the opportunity to think about your problem in a favorable climate.

(Zeig, 1980, p. 219)

I don't need to know what your problem is for you to correct it.

(Erickson & Rossi, 1979, p. 172)

The therapist merely stimulates the patient into activity, often not knowing what that activity may be, and then guides the patient and exercises clinical judgement in determining the amount of work to be done to achieve the desired results. [1948]

(In Erickson, 1980, Vol. IV, chap. 4, p. 39)

How to guide and to judge constitute the therapist's problem, while the patient's task is that of learning through his own efforts to understand his experiential life in a new way. [1948]

(In Erickson, 1980, Vol. IV, chap. 4, p. 39)

In psychotherapy you teach a patient to use a great many of the things that they learned, and learned a long time ago, and don't remember.

(Zeig, 1980, p. 38)

What they [therapists] say or do serves only as a means to stimulate and arouse in the subjects past learnings, understandings and experiential acquisitions, some consciously, some unconsciously acquired. [1964]

(In Erickson, 1980, Vol. I, chap. 13, p. 326)

What is needed is the development of a therapeutic situation permitting the patient to use his own thinking, his own understandings, his own emotions in the way that best fits him in his scheme of life. [1965]

(In Erickson, 1980, Vol. IV, chap. 20, p. 223)

I think that in hypnotherapy and in experimental work with subjects you have no right to express a preference; that it is a cooperative venture of some sort, and that the personality of the subject or the patient is the thing of primary importance. What the hypnotist or the therapist thinks, or does, or feels is not the important thing; but what he can do to enable the subject or the patient to accomplish certain things is important. It's the personality involved and the willingness of the therapist or the hypnotist to let the subject's personality play a significant role.

(Erickson, 1977a, p. 14)

> **Thus, a favorable setting is evolved for the elicitation of needful and helpful behavioral potentialities not previously used, not fully used, or perhaps misused by the patient. [1966]**
>
> *(In Erickson, 1980, Vol. IV, chap. 28, p. 263)*

Therapists Provide Motivation

Therapists do whatever is necessary to motivate patients. They serve as sources of comfort, hope, confidence, or inspiration and they serve as sources of frustration, discomfort, anger, and fear. They provide whatever it takes to initiate therapeutic movement. They do not instruct patients in the "proper" modes of thought or response; they merely create a therapeutic setting within which patients will be motivated, confident, and comfortable enough to do things that will help them discover, though their own experiences, whatever modes of thought or behavior are appropriate for their unique circumstances.

Erickson did not give pep talks to his patients to motivate them; he simply noticed the things that already motivated or interested them and used those. Once he had created a therapeutic atmosphere of trust, confidence, and an expectation of success, he could stimulate his patients into action using their natural sources of motivation as the trigger or impetus. More will be said about this crucial triggering component of the therapy process in the next chapter.

> **The psychological aspect of medicine constitutes the art of medicine and transforms the physician from a skillful mechanic or technician into a needed human source of faith, hope, assistance, and, most importantly, of motivation toward physical and mental health and well-being. [1959]**
>
> *(In Erickson, 1980, vol. IV, chap. 27, p. 255)*

He didn't need a direction about what to do. But he did need motivation. And that is one of the things in psychotherapy and the use of hypnosis — the motivation of a patient to do things. Not the things that you necessarily think they ought to do, but the things that they as personalities have the feeling that they really ought to do.

(Erickson & Rossi, 1981, p. 12)

When you talk toughly to the patient you give them an inspiration. They think they *can* do things. And you state it so simply and so earnestly you'd better believe what you are saying. How else are you going to get a patient who is despairing to do things? When you convey an understanding and an earnest and sincere belief.

(ASCH, 1980, Taped Lecture, 7/16/65)

My attitude towards patients is: You are going to accomplish your purpose, your goal. And I am very confident. I look confident. I act confident. I speak in a confident way, and my patient tends to believe me.

(Zeig, 1980, p. 61)

I was utterly confident. A good therapist should be utterly confident.

(Zeig, 1980, p. 61)

That is what my family says: "Why do your patients do the crazy things you tell them to do?" I say, "I tell it to them very seriously. They know I mean it. I am totally sincere. I am absolutely confident that they will do it. I never think, 'Will my patients do that ridiculous thing?' No, I know that they will."

(Zeig, 1980, p. 196)

Therapists Solicit Trust and Cooperation

In order to function as sources of inspiration, support, and motivation, therapists first must secure the trust and then the cooperation of patients. The atmosphere confronting a patient within the therapy setting must be conducive to the development of a sense of trust and cooperation. The essential ingredient of such an atmosphere is the therapist's genuine awareness of, respect for, and willingness to be responsive to the needs, fears, beliefs, and general personality of the patient. Patients do not enter therapy to be ridiculed, rejected, ignored, or dominated; they enter therapy to be protected, understood, and aided in their attempts to cope with the realities of their internal or external situations.

In dealing with patients, your entire purpose is to secure their cooperation and to make certain that they respond as well as they can.
(Erickson & Rossi, 1981, p. 43)

All techniques of procedure should be oriented about the subjects and their needs in order to secure their full cooperation. [1952]
(In Erickson, 1980, Vol. I, chap. 6, p. 148)

Merely to make a correct diagnosis of the illness and to know the correct method of treatment is not enough. Fully as important is that the patient be receptive of the therapy and cooperative in regard to it. Without the patient's full cooperativeness, therapeutic results are delayed, distorted, limited, or even prevented. [1965]
(In Erickson, 1980, Vol. IV, chap. 20, p. 212)

Actually, the real purpose was to develop in her a receptiveness, a responsiveness, a feeling of complete acceptance and a willingness to execute adequately any suggestion offered to her. [1965]
(In Erickson, 1980, Vol. IV, chap. 20, p. 220)

And, it is important to give them (*patients*) the opportunity of discovering that they can trust you.
(Erickson & Rossi, 1981, p. 5)

It is this that the patient comes in for, not to have the therapist take charge, but to give the therapist an opportunity of doing something, and doing something in accord with the needs of the patient, not in accord with the needs of the therapist.
(Erickson, 1977b, p. 22)

The primary problem is how to treat the patient so that his human needs may be met as much as possible. [1959]
(In Erickson, 1980, Vol. IV, chap. 27, p. 256)

In dealing with any type of patient clinically there is a most important consideration that should be kept constantly in mind. this is that the patient's needs as a human personality should be an ever-present question for the therapist to insure recognition at each manifestation. [1965]
(In Erickson, 1980, Vol. IV, chap. 20, p. 212)

That sense of goodness and adequacy is not to be based upon a sense of superiority of one's own attributes, but upon a respect for the self as an individual dealing rightfully with another individual, with each contributing a full share to a joint activity of significance to both. [1958]
(In Erickson, 1980, Vol. IV, chap. 15, p. 175)

> **Hence the therapist aids the patients to express quickly and freely their unpleasant feelings and attitudes, encouraging the patients by open receptiveness and attentiveness, and by the therapist's willingness to comment appropriately in a manner to elicit their feelings fully in the initial session. [1964]**
>
> *(In Erickson, 1980, Vol. I, chap. 13, pp. 299–300)*

Therapists Recognize and Accept Each Patient's Limitations

No therapist can create a therapeutic atmosphere if the realities of the patient's current condition are ignored, overlooked, or distorted. Therapists must learn to perceive and to respond to the reality confronting them, just as patients must.

Appearances and presentations aside, therefore, therapists must begin therapy with a full realization that the people they meet in therapy are not completely rational, sensible, or capable of responding in an adult manner to the obvious purposes of the situation. They may sound like reasonable and rational adults and they may present their problems in a manner that sounds mature, but the fact of the matter is that they are probably functioning in a very childish manner in many respects. This childish aspect of their functioning must be recognized and responded to if a therapeutic atmosphere is to be created. Unreasonable or childish beliefs and emotions should not be challenged as irrational, but must be respected and perhaps used. Patients should be treated with a certain amount of care and with a due consideration for and acceptance of all of the childish fears and foibles that they bring into therapy with them.

Too often the therapist regards patients as necessarily logical, understanding, in full possession of their faculties — in brief, as reasonable and informed human beings. [1965]

(In Erickson, 1980, Vol. IV, chap. 20, p. 212)

Nor should seemingly intelligent, rational, and cooperative behavior ever be allowed to mislead the therapist into an oversight of the fact that the patient is still human and hence easily the victim of fears and foibles, of all those unknown experiential learnings that have been relegated to his unconscious mind and that he may never become aware of or ever show just what the self may be like under the outward placid surface...Too often it is not the strengths of the person that are vital to the therapeutic situation. Rather, the dominant forces that control the entire situation may derive from weaknesses, illogical behavior, unreasonableness, and obviously false and misleading attitudes of various sorts. [1965]

(In Erickson, 1980, Vol. IV, chap. 20, p. 212)

But all of your patients have their own rigidities.

(Zeig, 1980, p. 121)

And our patients tend to restrict themselves and really cheat themselves out of a lot of things.

(Zeig, 1980, p. 255)

Patients often can't think for themselves. You start them thinking in some good reality way.

(Zeig, 1980, p. 288)

Patients can be silly, forgetful, absurd, unreasonable, illogical, incapable of acting with common sense, and very often governed and directed in their behavior by

emotions and by unknown, unrecognizable and perhaps undiscoverable unconscious needs and forces which are far from reasonable, logical, or sensible. [1965]
(In Erickson, 1980, Vol. IV, chap. 20, p. 212)

Adults are only little children grown a little older, and a lot taller. And they still behave like infants in the medical or dental or psychological office.
(ASCH, 1980, Taped Lecture, 7/16/65)

And another thing all patients should keep in mind, adults are only children grown tall.
(Erickson, Rossi & Rossi, 1976, p. 254)

So far as the patient is concerned you do not remind yourself of adult understandings. Nor do you look at behavior with adult understandings.
(Erickson, Rossi & Rossi, 1976, p. 215)

There was no other way for the patient to understand except in terms of intense childish beliefs and emotions with all their attitudes of acceptance.
(Erickson & Rossi, 1979, p. 435)

Such presentation [of ideas] needs to be in accord with the dignity of the patient's experiential background and life experience — there should be no talking down to, or over the head of, the patient. [1958]
(In Erickson, 1980, Vol. IV, chap. 15, p. 175)

Patients Are Ambivalent About Therapy

Patients enter the therapy setting with mixed emotions and conflicting desires. On the one hand they desire help and guidance, but on the other they are afraid to do what they know they must do. They may want nothing more than to have the therapist understand their situation perfectly, and yet they may do everything they can in order to hide their real problems or thoughts from the therapist.

Patients are people who have an injury; a painful, sore, uncomfortable, or embarrassing area of life. For one reason or another they have not been able to face these injuries and handicaps directly, which is why they have developed into problems. Accordingly, it is unreasonbable to expect patients to be willing or able to discuss their problems openly and objectively at first blush and it may be equally unreasonable and naive for therapists to believe what patients tell them initially. Therapists should not confuse the accepting attitude necessary for the creation of a therapeutic climate with absolute belief in what the patient says.

Every patient that walks into your office is a patient that has some kind of a problem. I think you'd better recognize that problem, that problems of all patients — whether they are pain, anxiety, phobias, insomnia — every one of those problems is a painful thing subjectively to that patient, only you spell the pain sometimes as p-a-i-n, sometimes you spell it p-h-o-b-i-a. Now, they're equally hurtful. And therefore, you ought to recognize the common identity of all of your patients. And your problem is, first of all, to take this human being and give him some form of comfort. And one of the first things you really ought to to is to let the patient discover where he really does have that pain...So that he can actually identify the pain and put it where it really belongs and not have it radiate to his total personality.

(ASCH, 1980, Taped Lecture, 7/18/65)

You should recognize that your patient is a totality whose toothache hurts clear down to the soles of his feet. And hurts clear back to the earliest learning that he acquired about how to grow up to be a big strong man. And that encompasses an awful lot of territory. And the same way with every other kind of distress.

(ASCH, 1980, Taped Lecture, 7/18/65)

Patients do come to you with tremendous anxiety. And it's all important that you recognize that anxiety, that you ought not to be led astray.

(ASCH, 1980, Taped Lecture, 2/2/66)

When a patient does a peculiar thing, when a patient gives a peculiar history, I think you ought to be very, very curious about it. Anxiety will show itself. You ought to be able to recognize it.

(ASCH, 1980, Taped Lecture, 2/2/66)

He [the patient] is both willing and unwilling to secure help from you.

(Erickson & Rossi, 1981, p. 4)

There always exists, whether recognized or not, a general questioning uncertainty about what will happen or what may or may not be said or done. [1952]

(In Erickson, 1980, Vol. I, chap. 6, p. 149)

They will hide that anxiety very carefully.

(ASCH, 1980, Taped Lecture, 2/2/66)

When you deal with patients they always want to hang onto something.

(Zeig, 1980, p. 93)

Any statesman can tell us that most of the world's troubles derive from a lack of communication. So it is with matters of human illness and health. [1970]

(In Erickson, 1980, Vol. IV, chap. 6, p. 75)

Mental disease is the breaking down of communication between people. [1970]

(In Erickson, 1980, Vol. IV, chap. 6, p. 75)

I think too often physicians overlook the meaningfulness of communication. They are listening to words, to stories, to general accounts and not listening to the actual communications that the patient is offering. And the actual communications concern the things that the patient is too afraid to face, too unwilling to face. That's why they are seeking professional help.

(ASCH, 1980, Taped Lecture, 2/2/66)

Why do patients have psychiatric problems? It's because they do not want to face them. Why do they have anxiety problems? Because they do not want to face the problems they have. And it's necessary for you to be willing to point out something. They want you to understand things that they do not know consciously that they are depending upon you to understand.

(ASCH, 1980, Taped Lecture, 2/2/66)

Now your patients come to you and tell you their problems. But do they tell you their problems or do they tell you what they *think* are problems? And are they problems only because they *think* that the things are problems?

(Zeig, 1980, p. 79)

How many patients come into your office convinced that this is the way it is and will be forever, when you in

your own knowledge know, "Yes, for a time you're going to be depressed. But it's not forever."

(ASCH, 1980, Taped Lecture, 7/16/65)

Most neurotic ills come from people feeling inadequate, incompetent. And have they really measured their competence?

(Zeig, 1980, p. 222)

Your patients in the psychiatric field are often exceedingly difficult. They are fearful to begin with, they are distressed — they do not know how to handle themselves or they would not be your patient.

(Erickson & Rossi, 1981, p. 8)

Patients Are Unreliable Sources

Even after the inhibiting anxieties of the first encounter have diminished, what patients say during therapy should not be accepted at face value. To do so is to ignore the obvious fact that patients do not necessarily even know the most important details about their situation and the added fact that patients will try to protect themselves at all costs. Patients will often lie, distort, conceal, rationalize, and resist all efforts to help them. Such behavior may be childish and irrational, but it is typical and, from the patient's perspective, necessary. Therapists who recognize the patient's need to engage in such tactics will not be led astray by them and therapists who respect or accept the validity of this need will not be infuriated or frustrated by such avoidant actions. Recognition, acceptance, and even utilization of whatever the patient presents will accomplish far more than a narrow-minded or biased rejection or challenge of it. Even the most sophisticated forms of resistance and distortion can be used to create a therapeutic atmosphere of trust and cooperation if the therapist recognizes them and comprehends their necessity at the moment.

Even subjects who have unburdened themselves freely and without inhibition to the author as a psychiatrist have manifested this need to protect the self and to put their best foot forward no matter how freely the wrong foot has been exposed. [1952]

(In Erickson, 1980, Vol. I, chap. 6, p. 149)

Again the senior author reached the conclusion that the psychiatric portrayal she offered of herself was no more than a symptomatic screen to conceal her actual problem.

(Erickson & Rossi, 1979, p. 444)

And yet I do know that patients will conceal things.

(ASCH, 1980, Taped Lecture, 2/2/66)

Now, when a patient comes in you ought to be aware of the fact that the patient cannot face certain things at all and they are going to distract you. This matter of anxiety, they may distract you because they are resistant.

(ASCH, 1980, Taped Lecture, 2/2/66)

Patients come to you for help. They may resist help, but they hope desperately you'll win.

(Zeig, 1980, p. 333)

Now then, patients can resist and they will resist.

(Zeig, 1980, p. 93)

This adverse attitude [resistance] is part and parcel of their reason for seeking therapy; it is the manifestation of their neurotic attitude against the acceptance of therapy and their uncertainty about their loss of their defenses

and hence it is a part of their symptomatology. Therefore this attitude should be respected rather than regarded as an active and deliberate or even unconscious intention to oppose the therapist. Such resistance should be openly accepted, in fact graciously accepted since it is a vitally important communication of a part of their problems and often can be used as an opening into their defenses. This is something that the patients do not realize; rather they may be distressed emotionally since they often interpret their behavior as uncontrollable, unpleasant, uncooperative rather than as an informative exposition of certain of their important needs. [1964]

(In Erickson, 1980, Vol. I, chap. 13, p. 299)

Often patients come to you not knowing why they are unhappy or distressed or disturbed in any way. All they know is that they are unhappy, and they give you a wealth of rationalizations to explain it.

(Erickson & Rossi, 1981, p. 7)

Consciously they will tell you any story that seems to be reasonable, that seems to be well founded. And they'll tell it to you with great intensity. They will make you believe it. But they are using that particular thing.

(ASCH, 1980, Taped Lecture, 2/2/66)

A person seeking therapy comes in and tells you one story that is believed fully at the conscious level and in nonverbal language can give you a story that is entirely different.

(Erickson, Rossi & Rossi, 1976, p. 68)

The patient is going to come in and withhold some vital information, tremendously vital information. And you see them laboriously sit down and assume a certain position that you have come to recognize as meaning

"I'm going to tell you everything except..." You'd better know that they're telling you everything except...and
you'd better respect that and you'd better tell them right
away "Now, while I expect you to tell me your entire history, certainly I don't want you to do it *today*. I want
you to be willing to withhold a certain thing *until* you are
really ready to tell me *more*.

(ASCH, 1980, Taped Lecture, 7/16/65)

Now I cite these two cases as actual instances of the
need to listen to patients, always, and to form your own
conclusions, and to form your conclusions from what
you notice, from what *you* see, from what you understand and *never* to take your patient's word for anything.

(ASCH, 1980, Taped Lecture, 2/2/66)

Therapists Must Decipher What Patients Say

No matter what patients say, even if they are being as open
and honest as possible and even if what they say makes perfect
sense to the therapist, the wise therapist realizes the necessary
gap between the real meaning of the patient's verbalizations
and the perceived meaning. In order to avoid misunderstandings and misinterpretations, therapists should reserve judgement or belief until they are certain that they understand the
personal meanings of the patient's vocabulary. As indicated
previously, every person has a different perspective or orientation to the world and each underlying perspective gives words
a slightly different meaning. Understanding can occur only
after the therapist has managed to adopt the perspective of the
patient and has listened to the patient's words and observed
the patient's behavior from that perspective.

This is not an easy task. Adopting someone else's orientation to the world and seeing events from that perspective

requires considerable effort, close attention, and continual practice. The conceptual flexibility required does not come automatically but must be developed by the therapist through continual practice.

To complicate matters further, the actual meaning of a communication or a behavior may reside within the patient's unconscious. Patients may say one thing at a conscious level and be oblivious to the unconscious communications inherent in their phrasings or intonations. The therapist's task, therefore, is not only to determine and adopt the patient's conscious perspectives and to decipher the meanings of communications from that orientation, but also to assume the orientation or framework of the patient's unconscious and to respond to the meanings of communications from that level of functioning as well.

The patterns or orientations of the unconscious are almost universal, which means that a therapist's unconscious probably can comprehend and respond to the meaning of the communications from the patient's unconscious reasonably well with little or no training. The difficulty, of course, lies in nurturing the therapist's ability to do so at a conscious level. Erickson's ability to do this may be attributable, in part, to his physiological anomalies which prevented him from being distracted by irrelevancies and, in part, to the years he spent carefully observing patients in order to learn the meanings of these unconscious verbal and nonverbal signals. Perhaps the only potential shortcut to the process of gaining increased access to the perceptions and understandings of the patient's unconscious is hypnosis. As will be discussed later, hypnosis can facilitate the therapist's understandings of and responses to the messages sent by the patient's unconscious.

Even if therapists do not fully comprehend the exact meaning of the patient's words or behaviors, the simple expedient of adopting the dominant or significant verbal and non-verbal mannerisms of the patient can provide the patient with a sense of comfort and understanding. The patient's concepts and vocabulary, not those of the therapist, should dominate the situation. As the therapist utilizes the patient's style of communication to convey meaning, the patient begins to feel understood, secure, and relieved of the burden of deciphering what the therapist says. A therapeutic atmosphere results and cooperation increases.

I never believe anything that I hear from that chair over there until I've confirmed and reaffirmed it. 'Cause it is interesting to listen to but you should not believe it until you really know. And that sort of an attitude toward your patients is utterly important.

(ASCH, 1980, Taped Lecture, 2/2/66)

Now I have the right to be as stupid as possible. It isn't requisite for me to understand all. There can be progressive understanding on your part.

(Erickson, Rossi & Rossi, 1976, p. 132)

I don't have to believe anything that anybody tells me. I don't believe it until I understand her words.

(Zeig, 1980, p. 158)

Whenever you see patients, you really ought to consider, "What type of orientation do they have?"

(Zeig, 1980, p. 232)

Every patient poses problems that need understanding from more than one point of view. [1957]

(In Erickson 1980, Vol. IV, chap. 5, p. 51)

You have to look at your patient as if you were sitting on a seat higher than his. You also have to look at him from a much lower seat. You need to look at him from the other side of the room. Because you always get a totally different picture from different points of view. Only by such a total look at the patient can you gain some objectivity.

(Erickson, Rossi & Rossi, 1976, p. 212)

Your approach to him must be in terms of him as a person with a particular frame of reference for that day and the immediate situation.

(Haley, 1967, p. 535)

And when you listen to the patient, listen to what you hear, then get over in that chair and listen again, because there is another side to the story.

(Zeig, 1980, p. 169)

When you listen to patients, listen carefully and try to think what is the other side of the story. Because if you just hear the patient's story, you really don't know all the story.

(Zeig, 1980, p. 169)

And so, your patients tell you many things and your tendency is to put your meaning upon the patient's words.

(Zeig, 1980, p. 174)

So, I warn all of you, don't ever, when you are listening to a patient, think you understand the patient, because you're listening with your ears and thinking with your own vocabulary. The patient's vocabulary is something entirely different.

(Zeig, 1980, p. 58)

And in psychotherapy you listen to your patient knowing that you don't understand the personal meaning of his vocabulary.

(Zeig, 1980, p. 158)

Now in psychotherapy — if you want to do psychotherapy — you have to learn, first of all, that each of us has a different meaning to the words used in common.

(Zeig, 1980, p. 173)

When you are doing psychotherapy, you listen to what the patients say, you use their words, and you can understand those words. You can place your own meaning on those words, but the real question is what is the meaning that a patient places on those words. You cannot know because you do not know the patient's frame of reference.

(Erickson & Rossi, 1981, p. 255)

So you listen to your patient knowing he has personal meaning for his words and you don't know his personal meaning. And he doesn't know your personal meanings for words. You try to understand the patient's words as *he* understands them.

(Zeig, 1980, p. 158)

I emphasized the importance of understanding the patient's words and really understanding them. You don't interpret your patient's words in *your* language.

(Zieg, 1980, p. 78)

I usually do not take a complete history. I want to listen to that first presentation that the patient offers.

(ASCH, 1980, Taped Lecture, 2/2/66)

You let the patients use their own words to describe the process.

(Erickson & Rossi, 1979, p. 381)

You search out for those things that are peculiar to the person.

(Erickson & Rossi, 1981, p. 100

Never forget folk language. You should always recognize how the folk language is related to symptom formation.

(Erickson & Rossi, 1979, p. 277)

The method by which a story is told may be even more important than its content. [1944]

(In Erickson, 1980, Vol. III, chap. 29, p. 355)

I hope I've taught you something about psychotherapy. The importance of seeing and hearing and understanding, and getting your patient to do something.

(Zeig, 1980, p. 158)

How many times does a patient need to state his complaint? Only that number of times requisite for the therapist to understand. [1966]

(In Erickson, 1980, Vol. IV, chap. 28, p. 277)

Yet experience has taught me the importance of my assumption of the role of a purely passive inquirer, one who asks questions solely to receive an answer regardless of its content. An intonation of interest in the meaning of the answer is likely to induce subjects to respond as if they had been given instructions concerning what answer to give. [1965]

(In Erickson, 1980, Vol. I, chap. 3, p. 94)

Therapists Must Acknowledge the Patient's Reality

There is a natural tendency, perhaps, to downplay the seriousness of a patient's condition or to employ euphemisms when referring to the more unpleasant and painful aspects of the situation. However, an important part of all patients' desires to be understood and accepted is the desire to find someone who will be honest with them, someone who will acknowledge with brutal frankness the validity of their accurate perceptions. This does not mean that their irrational fears and irrational beliefs must be given credence, but it does mean that the therapists should not argue with them and obviously should agree fully when there is some truth to what they say. The therapy situation must be an island of truth, a setting wherein two people can be honest with each other. Patients trust therapists who tell them the truth, though it must be remembered that it is largely the patient who determines what is true and what is not. Almost everything Erickson ever said to his patients was either an axiomatic, necessary truism, an objectively verifiable fact, or something that the patient already believed to be true. The development of trust depends upon honesty and acceptance. Once patients have learned that the therapist can be trusted, then the therapist can begin to direct them toward topics and experiences that they otherwise would have avoided.

> **She wanted understanding and recognition; not a falsification, however well-intended, of a reality comprehensible to her. [1958]**
>
> ***(In Erickson, 1980, Vol. IV, chap. 15, p. 176)***

At no time was he given a false statement, nor was he forcibly reassured in a manner contradictory to his understandings. [1958]

(In Erickson, 1980, Vol. IV, chap. 15, p. 179)

He was told seriously and impressively, "You are entirely right, absolutely right..." [1965]

(In Erickson, 1980, Vol. IV, Chapter 20, p. 217)

Such a brutal beginning, with such negative statements only partially balanced by a final qualified favorable statement, could have no other effect than to convince her of my utter sincerity of purpose.

(Erickson & Rossi, 1979, p. 432)

That is a fact and you pause to let them reflect on the factual nature of that statement. They have a chance to recognize that you are really speaking the truth.

(Erickson, Rossi & Rossi, 1976, p. 39)

Calling a spade a spade, especially in the patient's own language, however unrecognized at the time, often expedites therapy by convincing the patient that the therapist is unafraid of his task and recognizes it clearly.

(Erickson & Rossi, 1979, p. 433)

If you're afraid ever to say a word or to name a condition to a patient, you're going to alert the patient to the fact that you are afraid.

(ASCH, 1980, Taped Lecture, 2/2/66)

But this matter of using metaphors, analogies, allegorical statements and so on to direct your patient's attention from one mood to another — and you never avoid what the patient says.

(ASCH, 1980, Taped Lecture, 7/16/65)

There is no more important problem than so speaking to the patient that he can agree with you and respect your intelligent grasp of the situation as judged by him in terms of his own understandings. [1958]

(In Erickson, 1980, Vol. IV, chap. 15, p. 177)

Every care was taken to ensure the desired understanding of it by the patient.

(Erickson, 1954d, p. 110)

You see, all I want to do is *to find out if we can understand each other.* [1964]

(In Erickson, 1980, Vol. I, chap. 13, p. 319)

Therefore he could listen respectfully to me, because I had demonstrated that I understood the situation fully. [1958]

(In Erickson, 1980, Vol. IV, chap. 15, p. 177)

A community of understandings was first established with him, and then, one by one, items of vital interest to him in his situation were thoughtfully considered and decided, either to his satisfaction or sufficiently agreeably to merit his acceptance. His role in the entire situation was that of an interested participant, and adequate response was made to each idea suggested. [1958]

(In Erickson, 1980, Vol. IV, chap. 15, p. 179)

I am taking over control of the total situation. I haven't offered anything with which he can take issue.

(Erickson & Rossi, 1981, p. 183)

Therapists Protect Patients

By accepting, understanding, and utilizing the productions of the patient, the therapist expresses a genuine concern and respect for the personality and needs of another individual.

Therapists must protect patients in every way possible rather than challenging or threatening them. Patients will relax and place their trust in a therapist who respects them and protects them by not expecting more from them than they can produce. Therapy will occur only if the therapist allows it and allows it to occur in a protective atmosphere as slowly or quickly as is necessary for the patient.

All this is an introduction to one important thing, and I think it is paramount in any approach to hypnotic therapy. That is that one must always protect the subject or the patient. The patient does not come to you just because you are a therapist. The patient comes to be protected or helped in some regard. But the personality is very vital to the person, and he doesn't want you to do too much, he does not want you to do it too suddenly. You've got to do it slowly, you've got to do it gradually, and you've got to do it in the order in which he can assimilate it.

(Erickson, 1977b, p. 20)

There is a tremendous need for protecting patients in ordinary psychotherapy. How often is the resistance the result of the therapist's intruding upon intimate memories, intimate ideas? This accounts for a great deal of resistance, and in hypnotherapy one can reach that sort of situation by stating to the patients very definitely your intention to protect them.

(Erickson, 1977b, p. 34)

By emphasizing that she should reveal only what she can share with strangers, I'm keeping her on the surface. I'm protecting her.

(Erickson & Rossi, 1979, p. 373)

> **There is a tremendous need for protecting patients in ordinary psychotherapy... And you should not overlook the possibility that you can unwittingly intrude upon the legitimate privacy of a patient.**
>
> *(Erickson, 1977b, p. 34)*

> **In a situation where one feels seriously damaged, there is an overwhelming need for a compensatory feeling of satisfying goodness. [1958]**
>
> *(In Erickson, 1980, Vol. IV, chap. 15, p. 178)*

Therapists Must Give Freedom to Patients

In order to avoid imposing unwarranted demands upon the patient and to provide the patient with a feeling of comfort and trust, the therapist must give the patient complete freedom, or at least the illusion of complete freedom. Even when purposefully guiding the patient's attention in a particular direction, the therapist must provide a variety of alternative paths toward that end. Patients should not feel the need to do exactly what the therapist wants, but should feel free to respond in whatever manner is most comfortable or natural and should be reassured that their responses are good. The feeling of freedom is one of the most pleasant and comforting of feelings, and the therapist's permissive attitude should convey this feeling continuously.

In some respects, this is simply a restatement of previous propositions regarding the creation of a therapeutic setting. The essential message provided by a general recognition, acceptance, and utilization of whatever the patient presents is one of freedom. Patients should be given permission to be whatever they are and thus the therapist should promote their freedom and provide protection for them. Any therapist who enters therapy with this attitude and who responds to patients in a manner that conveys it, will generate trust and cooperation.

It is desirable to do it indirectly, so that the patient does not feel under attack. It is a way of obviating defenses.

(Erickson & Rossi, 1979, p. 386)

You ought to have your techniques so worded that there are escape routes for all resistances — intellectual, emotional, situational.

(Erickson & Rossi, 1981, p. 221)

Let there be no hint of arbitrary demands, since the patient is resistant and this suggestion is one of freedom of response, even though of an illusory freedom. [1964]

(In Erickson, 1980, Vol. I, chap. 13, p. 306)

The common mistake in psychotherapy is to give a patient directions without recognizing there have to be doubts.

(Erickson, Rossi & Rossi, 1976, p. 216)

And so when a patient comes to me, I have all the doubts, I doubt in the right directions. The patient doubts in the wrong direction.

(Zeig, 1980, p. 46)

And nobody can control you, you can defy me any time you want to, or anybody else. You are a free citizen, and be free with yourself.

(Erickson & Rossi, 1979, p. 232)

In therapy this is often the way you get patients to become more aware of their capabilities. You are essen-

tially giving them the freedom to use themselves. Patients come to you because they don't feel free to use themselves.

(Erickson, Rossi & Rossi, 1976, p. 292)

Yes, you always depontentiate her doubts by giving her many possible modes of response.

(Erickson & Rossi, 1979, p. 413)

Your attitude should be completely permissive [1976–78]

(In Erickson, 1980, Vol. I, chap. 23, p. 486)

You only interfere when they try to destroy themselves.

(Erickson & Rossi, 1981, p. 12)

You see, psychologically one needs to give the patient the opportunity both to accept and reject anything you offer. [1976–78]

(In Erickson, 1980, Vol. I, chap. 23, p. 483)

She has a tremendous amount of freedom to explore all these possibilities in her past — and all this by implication.

(Erickson & Rossi, 1979, p. 413)

I give him a feeling of choice even though I'm determining it.

(Erickson & Rossi, 1981, p. 224)

I'm giving her freedom...

(Erickson & Rossi, 1979, p. 199)

I like to *approach* my psychiatric patients — whether they are neurotic, emotionally disturbed, prepsychotic or even psychotic — in a fashion that lets them *feel free to respond to whatever degree they wish.*

(Erickson & Rossi, 1981, p. 4)

That's right. You create a situation in which they can move and respond freely, comfortably, safely, securely.
(ASCH, 1980, Taped Lecture, 7/16/65)

You don't want your patients to feel as if they are under a great burden, so I carefully give her a chance to give this answer.
(Erickson & Rossi, 1979, p. 383)

The Patient's Welfare is the Only Concern

The conduct and content of therapy should reflect only the needs and personality of the patient because the welfare of that patient, i.e. his or her freedom, benefit, and protection, should be the only considerations in the therapist's office. Other considerations that too often enter into the conduct of therapy and displace an awareness of or a responsiveness to the needs of the patient include: the therapist's concern with his or her own prestige or professional image, social conventions or etiquette, and even common courtesy or social niceties. None of these issues should inhibit therapists from doing whatever is necessary to promote the welfare of their patients. Therapists must be willing to look foolish at times, to behave "inappropriately" at others and, in general, to ignore or overlook a "what-will-people-think" attitude.

Erickson had only one concern, the welfare of his patients, and he said or did whatever he judged to be necessary to maximize that welfare without regard for other concerns. By refusing to allow irrelevancies to inhibit his therapeutic style, he was able to create a totally new concept of the therapy process. He put the patient's unique concerns and needs in the central spotlight and he kept them there from the beginning to the end of therapy. His willingness and ability to do this were based upon his recognition of the necessity for doing it, and his recognition of the necessity for doing it gave form and substance to his entire therapeutic strategy. He used what the patient brought into the office and he did not demand or expect more than the patient had to offer or could accomplish.

On the other hand, his concern with his patients' welfare did not prevent him from doing things that were embarrassing or upsetting to them if that was what was necessary to motivate them to use their potentials and understand their experiences. He was concerned with his patients' welfare, but not with being liked or respected by them. He comforted his patients, but not when their welfare required otherwise. The patient's protection and welfare supersede all other general considerations, which makes specific rules of therapy difficult. In a sense, almost anything goes as long as patients are protected and their welfare is promoted. This maxim could be used to justify some pretty strange or totally inappropriate activities, but it does not apply unless patients actually derive benefit from those activities and unless the therapist actually has the patients' protection and welfare at heart. It may seem cruel to intentionally frustrate a brain-damaged patient, but Erickson did so in order to motivate compensatory learning. It may seem inappropriate to have an embarrassed young woman strip, point to and name every part of her body, but Erickson did so to break through her devastating inhibitions and rigidities. In every situation, however, he ensured that the rights and personalities of his patients were completely protected in some obvious manner. He did what he had to do *for their benefit*. He let them react to him in whatever way they needed to *for their benefit*. He even let them pay what they needed to *for their benefit*. The patient's welfare, not the therapist's, was his primary concern.

I think you ought always to recognize your patient as a totality, as a person, as a person with a personality, as a person that thinks and feels and believes and wants, and who understands certain things to a certain degree, and that your task is to communicate with him in a way that gives him the ideas and the understandings that he wants and needs, and to ask him to do some thinking on his own so that he can correct any misunderstandings. That he should participate with you in achieving a goal in common. His welfare, not your welfare, not the establishment of your professional eminence or anything of that sort, but his *welfare*. And your orientation to the patient as a person whose welfare you are interested in is the important thing.

(ASCH, 1980, Taped Lecture, 7/16/65)

Her welfare was the governing purpose of the therapy devised—not sympathy, consideration, or even common courtesy. [1964]

(In Erickson, 1980, Vol. IV, chap. 30, p. 310)

They were all deliberately and intentionally controlled and directed *toward the evoking of whatever capacities for all kinds of responses which she might have or could develop*, without regard for courtesies or social niceties, *but only for whatever responsive behavior might be conducive to restoration of previous patterns of normal behavior.* [1964]

(In Erickson, 1980, Vol. IV, chap. 30, p. 310)

The kind of therapy warranted should be that which is considered clinically to meet the patient's needs and to offer the best possible therapeutic results without regard for social niceties or questions of etiquette. There should be only one ruling principle — the patient's welfare.

(Erickson, 1980, Vol. 4, p. xxi)

Yet medical problems, whatever they are, should be faced, and patients' needs should be met without regard for irrelevant social teachings.

(Erickson, 1980, Vol. IV, p. xxii)

One's professional dignity is not involved but one's professional competence is. [1965]

(In Erickson, 1980, Vol. IV, chap. 30, p. 213)

You see, I think the important thing in working with a patient is do the thing that is going to help the patient. As for my dignity ... the hell with my dignity. (Laughs) I will get along all right in this world. I don't have to be dignified, professional. I do the thing that stirs the patient into doing the right thing.

(Zeig, 1980, p. 143)

Therapy is going to be socially oriented, that the emotional and social needs will be the prime consideration, and that while I may be seemingly offensive, there is a worthy principle involved.

(Erickson & Rossi, 1979, p. 276)

I don't like these physicians who wear a high silk hat and a starched front to their shirt and a fresh suit to the office and very, very professional manner and all that sort of thing. The office is where two human beings meet to solve a problem and I think that you can be a human being and abide by professional ethics and professional courtesy in every way and still be human, so that they know you are and so that they can confide in you. I think that's one of the most important things.

(ASCH, 1980, Taped Lecture, 7/16/65)

My approach is very casual even with this difficult material, and that makes it easier for her. It's hard to say "no" to a casual easygoing approach.

(Erickson & Rossi, 1979, p. 322)

You keep things informal so you give the patient the privilege of concealing just how important some of these things are.

(Erickson & Rossi, 1979, p. 371)

Now, that letting loose — why did she? I set an example of relaxation, of comfort, of actually enjoying her presence no matter how rigid she was, until she had a feeling of comfort out of the situation.

(ASCH, 1980, Taped Lecture, 7/16/65)

I always sprawl out in my chair because I like to be comfortable. In fact I have to be comfortable. And so I sprawl out.

(ASCH, 1980, Taped Lecture, 7/16/65)

In teaching, in therapy, you are very careful to use humor, because patients bring in enough grief, and they don't need all that grief and sorrow. You better get them in a better frame of mind right away.

(Zeig, 1980, p. 71)

In presenting therapeutic understandings a little roughage, as in the diet, is essential. Therapists who insist that everything they present is good and acceptable — and must be accepted because it is always tendered in courteous language and manner — are in error.

(Erickson & Rossi, 1979, p. 436)

However farcical the above procedure may seem in itself, it possessed the remarkable and rare virtue of being satisfying to the patient as a person and meeting his symptomatic needs adequately.

(Erickson, 1954d, p. 111)

This thinking led to extensive experimentation by deliberately making out-of-character, irrelevant, nonsequitur remarks in groups and to single persons. [1964]

(In Erickson, 1980, Vol. I, chap. 10, p. 261)

When you seem to be doing damn fool things, it takes your patient's mind off his pain.

(Zeig, 1980, p. 292)

The primary task in the therapy of various psychopathological conditions may be dependent upon an approach seemingly unrelated to the actual problem. [1943]

(In Erickson, 1980, Vol. II, chap. 14, p. 156)

The goal sought is often infinitely more apparent than the apparent logic of the procedure. [1952]

(In Erickson, 1980, Vol. I, chap. 6, p. 144)

She looked at me as though she thought I ought to have my head examined.

(Erickson, 1977b, p. 31)

I asked him to repeat my name until he wondered who was the patient.

(Erickson, 1977b, p. 22)

There's iron under my velvet gloves.

(Rossi, 1973, p. 14)

Summary

Erickson created an environment wherein patients were encouraged to use their experiences to grow and to develop in whatever manner was suitable for them. As a consequence, they were able to accept the responsibility for change and to feel comfortable enough to risk changing. The creation of such a setting is what being a therapist is all about from Erickson's perspective. Therapists must turn their attention away from themselves, away from their own needs, their own expectations, their professional images, and their evaluation by others. They must direct their attention solely and totally toward the patient because it is the patient whose cooperation is needed to provide the necessary experiences, understandings, and changes. Because each patient is unique, the form of intervention or the type of change required is unique as well. Only patients themselves can provide the specific information or alterations necessary and they will not be able to do so effectively if the therapist fails to create a therapeutic setting — a setting wherein the patient's needs, thoughts, and deeds are primary and where the patient feels understood, accepted, protected, and willing to cooperate.

CHAPTER SEVEN

INITIATING THERAPEUTIC CHANGE

Although there are times when the mere provision of a therapeutic climate will initiate therapeutic change, this is the exception rather than the rule. More typically, the creation of a therapeutic change can then be initiated by appropriate interventions. A therapeutic climate allows the patient to provide the therapist with useful information and makes the patient more willing and able to act upon or respond to the interventions eventually offered by the therapist. The actual change process itself, however, is usually initiated by an experience that occurs within the context of the therapeutic climate and not by the therapeutic climate *per se.*

Erickson argued that therapy itself is accomplished when patients experience something (preferably as a result of actually doing something themselves to cause that experience) which, in some unknown manner, triggers a reorganization or resynthesis and new applications of previous understandings and responses. Such a change-initiating experience may involve the behavioral or perceptual violation of a previously held false-hood, misperception, or rigid restriction or it may simply involve the presentation of the truth of the matter to the patient in a direct, a metaphoric, or a symbolic manner. In some instances, therapeutic change results when patients are provided with a demonstration of skills or abilities they did not believe they had.

Although this may sound like a fairly simple assignment for the therapist, it must be remembered that patients are people who cannot or will not recognize the truth or utilize their experiences and capacities fully. They have and will continue to resist change. They must be propelled into accepting change somehow, not merely asked to do so.

Erickson was a master at generating such propulsions. He consistently discovered aspects of the patient's unique patterns of interest, thought, emotion, or behavior that could be redirected to create an experience that would undermine the undesirable, inappropriate, or limiting conditions brought into the office by that patient and he did so in ways that the patient could not and would not escape. He challenged one patient to a bicycle race in order to create an experience that would prove her capabilities to her. He had a couple compare their reactions to climbing a mountain in order to force them to recognize their basic personality differences. He taught a boy to read by looking at maps of potential vacation spots with him. He motivated neurologically impaired individuals to relearn how to do things by being impolite, by frustrating them, or even by infuriating them. He grabbed hold of whatever unique interests or primary qualities a person brought into the office and he utilized them in ways that would enable his patients to accomplish their purposes.

Erickson's focus upon the unique qualities of each patient

and his remarkable ability to utilize whatever unique attributes he observed in order to stimulate therapeutic change are the central considerations of this chapter. The purpose of the following material is to convey the basic attitude underlying his utilization approach. However, a genuine appreciation for the mechanics of Erickson's utilization techniques will probably not be possible until the reader has also reviewed several of his case examples in detail. Thus, the summary of a number of his therapy cases by Jay Haley (*Uncommon Therapy,* W.W. Norton & Company, 1973) is recommended as a useful clarifying supplement to the content of this chapter.

Unique People Require Unique Interventions

Therapists cannot afford the lazy luxury of allowing their own needs, ideas, or preferences to determine the therapy process. The patient's potentials, knowledge, needs, and emotions are unique and therapists must have the conceptual and behavioral flexibility necessary to respect, to respond to, to utilize, or to redirect that uniqueness. Theoretical considerations, classifications, and constructs should not be allowed to define or to limit what the therapist sees or does nor should the therapist's needs or personality be allowed to do so. The therapist's personality should enter the situation only to the extent necessary to ensure that contact is made with the patient and to ensure that the strategies or techniques eventually employed by the therapist are genuine expressions of informed concern and not mere rote imitation or mechanical reproduction.

The therapist also must be dedicated enough to the welfare

of the patient to spend whatever time or energy is necessary to devise an appropriate strategy for each patient. Erickson did not rely upon short cuts or pat answers, which may be why his interventions were so effective. He often spent hours devising the specific wording he would use with a patient or considering the behavioral assignments he would give. His interventions did not spring magically from thin air but were usually the products of long periods of problem solving.

I think that true psychotherapy is knowing that each patient is an individual, unique and different.

(Zeig, 1980, p. 226)

You're going to find a tremendous divergence in your patients. Why not? People are different, understandings are different.

(ASCH, 1980, Taped Lecture, 7/16/65)

Each patient's problem needs individual scrutiny and the structuring of the therapeutic approach to meet the individuality of the problem. [1966]

(In Erickson, 1980, Vol. IV, chap. 18, p. 192)

I think that psychotherapy is an individual procedure.

(Zeig, 1980, p. 104)

You individualize your therapy to meet the needs of the individual patient.

(Zeig, 1980, p. 113)

In every psychiatric case, you have to take the individual personality into consideration.

(Erickson, 1977b, p. 32)

Any therapy used should always be in accordance with the needs of the patient, whatever they may be, and not based in any way upon arbitrary classifications. [1958]

(In Erickson, 1980, Vol. IV, chap. 15, p. 174)

But the important thing is: Deal with your patient and don't substitute your ideas.

(Zeig, 1980, p. 130)

I think that in hypnotherapy and in experimental work with subjects, you have no right to express a preference; that it is a cooperative venture of some sort, and that the personality of the subject or the patient is the thing of primary importance.

(Erickson, 1977a, p. 14)

I think the textbooks on therapy try to impress upon you a great number of concepts. Concepts that you should take from your patients, not from books, because books teach you you should do things in a certain way.

(Zeig, 1980, p. 226)

This matter of concepts of advanced psychotherapy should include this; That you ought to rely upon the capacity of the individual patient to furnish you the cues, the information by which to organize your psychotherapy because the patient can find a way if you give him an opportunity.

(ASCH, 1980, Taped Lecture, 8/14/66)

One should look upon his adult patient or his childish patient as possessing understandings that are available if you are willing to respect that patient and willing to give that patient the opportunity to make use of his capacities to function and to react to the therapeutic situation.

(ASCH, 1980, Taped Lecture, 8/14/66)

Nor does he [Erickson] know of anybody who has ever really understood the variety and purposes of any one patient's multiple symptoms despite the tendency of many psychiatrists to hypothecate, to their own satisfaction, towering structures of explanation often as elaborate and bizarre as the patient's symptomatology. [1966]

(In Erickson, 1980, Vol. IV, chap. 18, p. 202)

No person can really understand the individual patterns of learning and response of another. [1952]

(In Erickson, 1980, Vol. I, chap. 6, p. 154)

In psychotherapy, you ought to know that your patient knows more about his past learnings than you can ever know.

(Zeig, 1980, p. 46)

The ego, as far as I know, is a helpful and convenient concept, but that is all that it is. [1962]

(In Erickson, 1980, Vol. II, chap. 33, p. 340)

Now too much has been written and said and done about the re-education of the neurotic and the psychotic and the maladjusted personality as if anybody could really tell any one person how to think and how to feel and how to react in any given situation. Everybody reacts differently according to his own particular patterns, his own background of personal experience. What pleases me can displease my wife.

(ASCH, 1980, Taped Lecture, 8/14/66)

Such re-education is, of course, necessarily in terms of the patient's life experiences, his understandings, memories, attitudes, and ideas; it cannot be in terms of the therapist's ideas and opinions. [1948]

(In Erickson, 1980, Vol. IV, chap. 4, p. 39)

You need those divergent understandings. There is no exactly right or absolutely wrong approach. We know too little about human nature and human personality and human potentials to ever say "this" and only "this" is right. We need to take an inquiring, a curious, an interested, a pleasingly interested attitude toward our patients, wondering just how they are going to utilize those countless billions of brain cells they all possess, most of which they'll never be called upon in life to utilize, but which, should certain circumstances arise, they may use another few million that they never expected to use.

(ASCH, 1980, Taped Lecture, 7/16/65)

Properly, it [therapy] is not a matter of advancing particular schools of thought or of attempting to substantiate interpretative psychological theories, but simply a task of appraising a patient's problem or problems in terms of the reality in which the patient lives and in the terms of the realities of the patient's continuing future as he or she may reasonably hope for it to be. [circa 1930's]

(In Erickson, 1980, Vol. IV, chap. 54, p. 482)

The leading of the patient into this more satisfying method of living and of expressing the self is a rightful goal greatly to be desired. ... The achievement of the goal while primary, is not the only consideration. Also worthy of evaluation, planning and thought by the therapist are the matters of time spent, of effective utilization of effort, and above all of the fullest possible utilization of the functional capacities and abilities and the experiential and acquisitional learnings of the patient. These should take precedence over the teachings of new ways of living which are developed from the therapist's possibly incomplete understanding of what may be right and serviceable to the individual concerned. [1965]

(In Erickson, 1980, Vol. I, chap. 29, p. 540)

The importance in therapy of doing what appears to be most important to the patient, that which constitutes an expression of the distorted thoughts and emotions of the patient. The therapist's task should not be a proselytizing of the patient with his own beliefs and understandings. No patient can really understand the understandings of his therapist nor does he need them. What is needed is the development of a therapeutic situation permitting the patient to use his own thinking, his own understandings, his own emotions in the way that best fits him in his scheme of life. [1965]

(In Erickson, 1980, Vol. IV, chap. 20, p. 223)

She is using some material I offered, and what she uses is a function of her personality, not mine.

(Erickson & Rossi, 1979, p. 416)

Yes, I'm emphasizing her own natural memory patterns — rather than having her rely on some way of remembering she was artificially taught.

(Erickson & Rossi, 1979, p. 283)

I think she will probably put into practice the teaching she has had throughout her lifetime.

(Zeig, 1980, p. 246)

She is right about the fact that she should not let me get in the way of her using herself.

(Erickson & Rossi, 1979, p. 212)

I emphasize a patient's own functioning and feelings as a unique personality. With a series of suggestions like this you can focus the patient's attention more and more onto their own inner experiences. [1976–1978]

(In Erickson, 1980, Vol. I, chap. 23, p. 479)

I don't know the kind of thinking you ought to do. But I think you ought to enjoy doing your own thinking in terms of your own field of competence.

(ASCH, 1980, Taped Lecture, 7/18/65)

In any psychotherapeutic situation, whatever the school of thought which predominated, there must be recognized over and above the formalized structure of thinking, the importance of the patient himself as a sentient being with needs, capabilities, experiences, and a separateness as an individual, with his own background of experiential and acquisitional learning. He is not properly to be squeezed into any ritualistic traditional method of procedure, nor limited by teachings governed by predetermined rules and formulae. [1965]

(In Erickson, 1980, Vol. I, chap. 29, pp. 541–542)

And I do wish that Rogerian therapists, Gestalt therapists, transactional analysts, group analysts, and all the other offspring of various theories would recognize that not one of them really recognizes that psychotherapy for person #1 is not psychotherapy for person #2.

(Zeig, 1980, p. 104)

And all the rules of Gestalt therapy, psychoanalysis and transactional analysis, ...many theorists write them down in books as if every person was like every other person.

(Zeig, 1980, p. 220)

Be willing to avoid following any *one* teaching or any *one* technique.

(Haley, 1976, p. 535)

It [Hypnotic Corrective Emotional Experience] is, as is illustrated in the instances cited, best "played by ear" with no elaborate plans formulated, but with a multitude of possibilities floating freely in one's mind ready for adaptation to each new development presented by the patient. [1965]

(In Erickson, 1980, Vol. IV, chap. 58, p. 524)

I've treated many conditions, and I always invent a new treatment in accord with the individual personality. I know that when I take guests out to dinner, I let the guest choose what to eat, because I don't *know* what they like. I think people should dress the way they *want* to.

(Zieg, 1980, p. 104)

The variability of subjects, the individuality of their general and immediate needs, their differences in time and situation requirements, the uniqueness of their personalities and capabilities, together with the demands made by the projected work, render impossible any absolutely rigid procedure. [1952]

(In Erickson, 1980, Vol. I, chap. 6, p. 144)

Hence, to a significant degree, psychotherapy must necessarily be experimental in character since there can be no foreknowledge of the procedures exactly applicable to any one patient.

(Erickson, 1954c, p. 261)

I know that in the situation of dealing with patients I often wish I knew exactly what I was doing and why, instead of feeling, as I know I did with both patients that I was acting blindly and intuitively to elicit an as yet undetermined response with which, whatever it was, I would deal. [1966]

(In Erickson, 1980, Vol. II, chap. 34, p. 353)

One must modify his own behavior; that is, the therapist actually must be fairly fluid in his behavior, because if he is rigid he is going to elicit certain types of rigid behavior in his patient. In turn, his patient's rigid behavior is unfamiliar to him, and he is not going to be able to handle him properly. Therefore, the more fluidity in the hypnotherapist, the more easily you can actually approach the patient.

(Erickson, 1977b, p. 22)

He [the patient] wants to know if you have the right kind of strength and that means a fight. Are you meek and mild as you should be, or are you strong and combative as you should be?

(Zeig, 1980, p. 342)

You accept that prestige and enhance it indirectly because he needs it. You keep it by being very modest about it.

(Erickson & Rossi, 1981, p. 229)

A therapist should have flexibility in his schedule to accommodate the patient's needs.

(Erickson & Rossi, 1979, p. 382)

Then to meet the child's emotional needs further, I proceeded to talk to her, telling interesting things, boring things, exciting things, mildly offensive things, ridiculous things, highly intriguing things.

(Erickson & Rossi, 1979, p. 271)

Much speculative thought was given to the content of her limited understandings to devise some kind of therapeutic approach. [1965]

(In Erickson, 1980, Vol. IV, chap. 20, p. 220)

Three days of intensive thinking of what to do with an obviously brain-damaged patient...[1963]
(In Erickson, 1980, Vol. IV, chap. 30, p. 288)

Use Whatever the Patient Presents

Erickson referred to his therapeutic style as a naturalistic or utilization approach. The basic principle of his utilization approach is to *use whatever dominant beliefs, values, attitudes, emotions or behaviors the patient presents in order to develop an experience that will initiate or facilitate therapeutic change.* Although some contemporaries referred to his style as intuitive or magical, he emphasized that his approach is based upon a simple recognition of conditions as they are and a utilization of those conditions to accomplish the desired ends. Whatever the patient wants, does, or is must by accepted and utilized, according to Erickson. He offered patients what was compatible with their interests, their personalities, their understandings, and their desires and his patients responded to these offerings in the only way that they could, by accepting them and reacting to them in ways that would initiate therapeutic change.

Erickson welcomed anything the patient did or said because he viewed the patient's responses as a gift. Patients give therapists the solution to their situation if only therapists are observant enough to notice, open enough to accept, and flexible enough to utilize what the patient offers. What the patient is and what the patient does are markers indicating the easiest and perhaps the only route to therapeutic change. From Erickson's perspective, all paths do lead to Rome. The only trick is to figure out how to get to Rome on the path the patient presents.

Initially, this requires the adoption of the patient's perspective or frame of reference. When the goal of therapy is viewed from that perspective the roadblocks and open pathways may become more obvious. When the therapist operates from within the patient's perspective, the patient both feels understood and understands the therapist. In addition, when the therapist views the patient from that perspective, what the patient is willing and able to do will become more obvious and the language and behaviors necessary to move the patient in that direction will also become more apparent.

> **And you pick whatever lock is presented to you. And once one lock is picked, all the other locks become vulnerable.**
>
> *(Rossi, 1973, p. 16)*

> **In therapeutic approaches, one must always take into consideration the actual personality of the individual. One must give thought to how they express their behavior.**
> **Are they over-friendly, hostile, defiant, extroverted, introverted, so on?**
>
> *(Erickson, 1977b, p. 22)*

> **The purpose of psychotherapy should be the helping of the patient in that fashion most adequate, available and acceptable. In rendering the patient aid, there should be full respect for and utilization of whatever the patient presents.**
>
> *(Erickson, 1954d, p. 127)*

> *My learning over the years was that I tried to direct the patient too much. It took a long time to let things develop and make use of things as they developed.*
>
> *(Erickson, Rossi & Rossi, p. 265)*

The purpose and procedures of psychotherapy should involve the acceptance of what the patient represents and presents. These should be utilized to give the patient impetus and momentum so as to make his present and future become absorbing, constructive and satisfying.

(Erickson, 1954d, pp. 127–128)

You ought to start simply and let patients elaborate in accord with their own personality needs — not in accord with your concepts of what is useful to them.

(Erickson & Rossi, 1981, p. 12)

Both experimental and clinical subjects often have definite preferences which should be respected. [1964]

(In Erickson, 1980, Vol. I, chap. 10, p. 283)

In brief, whatever the behavior manifested by the subjects, it should be accepted and regarded as grist for the mill. [1952]

(In Erickson, 1980, Vol. I, chap. 6, p. 158)

Whatever the patient presents to you in the office, you really ought to use.

(Erickson & Rossi, 1981, p. 16)

One always tries to use whatever the patient brings into the office. If they bring in resistance, be grateful for that resistance. Heap it up in whatever fashion they want you to — really pile it up.

(Erickson & Rossi, 1981, p. 16)

In other words, you try to accept the patient's ideas no matter what they are, and then you can try to direct (sic — we now prefer *utilize*) them.

(Erickson & Rossi, 1981, p. 13)

If it is their way of functioning, you'd better go along with it.

(Erickson, Rossi & Rossi, 1976, p. 263)

If he wanted that type of behavior, let him have it. But I really ought to be willing to use it.

(Erickson & Rossi, 1981, p. 17)

Therapists wishing to help their patients should never scorn, condemn or reject any part of a patient's conduct because it is obstructive, unreasonable, or even irrational. The patient's behavior is a part of the problem brought into the office; it constitutes the personal environment within which therapy must take effect; it may constitute the dominant force in the total doctor-patient relationship. Since whatever patients bring into the office is in some way both a part of them and a part of their problem, the patient should be viewed with a sympathetic eye appraising the totality which confronts the therapist. [1965]

(In Erickson, 1980, Vol. IV, chap. 20, p. 213)

By naturalistic approach is meant the acceptance and utilization of the situation encountered without endeavoring to psychologically restructure it. In so doing, the presenting behavior of the patient becomes a definite aid and an actual part in inducing a trance, rather than a possible hindrance. [1958]

(In Erickson, 1980, Vol. I, chap. 7, p. 168)

There is an imperative need to accept and to utilize those psychological states, understandings and attitudes that the patient brings into the situation. ...The acceptance and utilization of those factors ... promotes more rapid trance induction, the development of more profound trance states, the more ready acceptance of therapy, and greater ease for the handling of the total therapeutic situation. [1958]

(In Erickson, 1980, Vol. I, chap. 7, p. 175-176)

My mental set in approaching the task was that of discovering what I could understand of the patient's behavior and what I could do about it or with it. [1966]

(In Erickson, 1980, Vol. II, chap. 34, p. 351)

By using the patient's own patterns of response and behavior, including those of their actual illness, one may effect therapy more promptly and satisfactorily, with resistance to therapy greatly obviated and acceptance of therapy facilitated. [1973]

(In Erickson, 1980, Vol. IV, chap. 38, p. 348)

All that I hope to know in most such experimental situations that I devise is the possible general variety of psychological processes and reactions I would like to elicit but do not know if I shall succeed in so doing, nor in what manner this will occur. Then, as the subjects respond in their own fashion, I promptly utilize that response. [1964]

(In Erickson, 1980, Vol. I, chap. 15, p. 347)

Such recognition and concession to the needs of the subjects and the utilization of their behavior do not constitute, as some authors have declared, "unorthodox techniques," based upon "clinical intuition," instead they constitute a simple recognition of existing conditions, based upon full respect for subjects as functioning personalities. [1952]

(In Erickson, 1980, Vol. I, chap. 6, p. 155)

Sometimes — in fact, many more times than is realized — therapy can be firmly established on a sound basis only by the utilization of silly, absurd, irrational, and contradictory manifestations. One's professional dignity is not involved, but one's professional competence is. [1965]

(In Erickson, 1980, Vol. IV, chap. 20, p. 213)

Yes, therapy should always be designed to fit the patient and not the patient to fit the therapy.

(Erickson & Rossi, 1979, p. 415)

I don't argue, I take their frame of reference — in the direction I want it to go. You let your subjects see everything.

(Erickson & Rossi, 1981, p. 251)

Any 52 year-old woman that starts calling me "sonny" has a sense of humor. So I made use of that.

In other words, whatever your patient has, make use of it.

(Zeig, 1980, p. 189)

When you have an intellectual subject, you stick to the intellectual. That is what he will understand and will accept. You have to fit your technique to the patient's frame of reference.

(Erickson & Rossi, 1981, p. 254)

Use the Patient's Desires and Expectations

The desires, wishes, and expectations of a patient can play at least three vital roles in the process of psychotherapy: they can provide permission for the therapist to do something about the problem, they can provide a source of motivation which the therapist can help the patient use to deal with the problem, and they can describe how the therapist should respond to the patient. The desire or need to have something done to alleviate a problem and the expectation that the therapist will do something about it usually are what brings the patient to the therapist's office in the first place. As such, they are sources of motivation that can be used to initiate other responses and they are expressions of the patient's willingness to allow the therapist to help.

However, the patient's desires and expectations often include a specification of how the patient wants or expects to be aided. It seems almost self-evident that if a patient indicates the need or expectation to have therapy conducted in a particular manner then the therapist should conduct therapy in that manner. If a patient expects the therapist to use specific techniques or to behave in particular ways, then that patient probably will be more likely to cooperate and to change if the therapist does so. In this manner the therapist uses the patient's desires and expectations to create an atmosphere and a therapeutic style tailored to that particular patient and in so doing creates a situation that has the greatest likelihood of being maximally effective.

These physically traumatic aspects of the experiences gave rise to an intense wish that these things would not and could not be so, that things would change completely. In response to this great need there developed the psychological processes by which, step by step, there could be utilization of repressions, overemphasis of various elements of the experience and distortion of others, until finally there had been achieved a complete reconstruction of the entire experience in a form which

could meet the compelling needs of the personality. [1938]

> *(In Erickson, 1980, Vol. III, chap. 22, p. 227)*

Effective therapy was based upon the utilization of the personality's need for something to be done in direct relationship to the injury. [1959]

> *(In Erickson, 1980, Vol. I, chap. 8, p. 195)*

She has a very strong desire to do good work. She is strong there, so I'm using that motivation to deal with the place where she is weak — her airplane phobia.

> *(Erickson & Rossi, 1979, p. 333)*

This extremely authoritarian approach was deemed appropriate because it utilized the patient's previous life experience and current expectation that effective guidance always came in an authoritarian form.

> *(Erickson & Rossi, 1979, p. 244)*

These three different case histories are presented to illustrate the importance in therapy of doing what appears to be most important to the patient, that which constitutes an expression of the distorted thoughts and emotions of the patient. [1965]

> *(In Erickson, 1980, Vol. IV, chap. 20, p. 223)*

Use the Patient's Language

All patients have their own unique language and nonverbal behaviors. More often than not, therapists challenge and attempt to revise the language used by patients to discuss therapeutic issues. Analytic patients begin to talk like their analysts, Jungian patients adopt the Jungian vocabulary, and patients of behaviorists discuss their problems in learning-theory terms. As described earlier, however, Erickson revised this process. Rather than altering the patient's language system to suit his style, he altered his own language and behavior patterns to suit the patient's style. He actually used the same words and phrases his patients had used when he presented his thoughts and interventions to those patients.

Aside from the comforting experience of being understood and accepted that this created in his patients, his ability to use the patient's language style enabled him to communicate more effectively with patients about their problems in symbolic or metaphorical terms. If a patient used particular terms to describe a presenting problem or a therapeutic goal, Erickson would use those same terms within the context of metaphors or allegories to provide a new perspective on the problem or on the solution to that problem, sometimes without the patient's direct awareness. The personal impact of a metaphor can be much more intense and its point better understood when couched in personally relevant terms. At the same time, if the patient is not yet ready for such an understanding, the point of the metaphor, because it is not stated directly, may be overlooked for the moment but not dismissed as entirely or permanently as it could have been without the personally meaningful terms. Eventually the therapeutic significance will probably creep through.

Whether presenting metaphors or simple direct statements, Erickson ensured a high level of comprehension and impact by using the linguistic and behavioral style of each patient. Even a simple conversation is easier if both people speak the same language and in the therapeutic setting the patient's language style should be the style of choice.

Transform their own utterances into vitally important suggestions effectively guiding their behavior, although

without such recognition by them at the time. [1964]

(In Erickson, Vol. I, chap. 13, p. 300)

You are using his own words to alter the patient's access to his various frames of reference.

(Erickson & Rossi, 1981, p. 255)

The patient had told his story, and note had been taken of the patterning of his behavior as was revealed by that story. Then came the problem of devising a therapeutic procedure employing symbolic language expressive of his story. [1973]

(In Erickson, 1980, Vol. IV, chap. 38, p. 349)

It [repeating the patient's utterances] serves to comfort them with a conviction that they are secure, that nothing is being done to them or being imposed upon them, and they feel that they can comfortably be aware of every step of the procedure. Consequently they are able to give full cooperation, which would be difficult to secure if they were to feel that a pattern of behavior was being forcibly imposed upon them [1959]

(In Erickson, 1980, Vol. I, chap. 8, p. 183)

This acceptance of a patient's declaration and turning it back upon him in the form of posthypnotic suggestions is often a most effective therapeutic procedure. It gives the patient a feeling of being committed to his own intentions and wishes, and intensifies his ability to act accordingly, without a feeling that he is being forced to accept proferred help. [1954]

(In Erickson, 1980, Vol. IV, chap. 23, p. 234)

Use the Patient's Emotions

The typical emotional tendencies or actual expressions of emotion that a patient brings into the office should be considered to be a valuable potential source of motivation. The elicitation of such typical emotions will initiate behavior that, with some planning, can be directed toward therapeutic goals. Many of Erickson's patients were stirred into effective action by their angers, fears, or frustrations. If patients are willing to overcome their problems to spite their therapists but not to please them, then therapists should be willing to stimulate their spite and indignation. If other patients are motivated by guilt, then therapists should consider using that quality to motivate the desired change in thought or behavior. Therapists must work with what they have, and if what they have is an angry person, they must use that person's anger effectively. The same holds true no matter what emotion is available as a motivator.

Again, there are no secret formulae that show therapists how to use patients' emotions to motivate therapeutic change; therapists must develop this skill by doing it. Trying to stimulate the motivating emotions or interests of others and re-directing those motivations into particular actions can be a fascinating and productive daily game. Most therapists want to do more than wait for patients to decide to change or rationally debate the need for change with them. Utilization of existing motivators can provide a useful alternative.

Underlying the entire procedure was the utilization of the patient's emotions. Each new measure in some manner elicited emotional reactions, attitudes and states — sometimes pleasant, but more often of special personal

displeasure — and these were employed to intensify and promote her learnings and to stimulate her to greater effort. [1964]

(In Erickson, 1980, Vol. IV, chap. 31, p. 312

Then one should bear in mind that these patients are highly motivated, that their disinterest, antagonism, belligerence, and disbelief are actually allies in bringing about the eventual results, nor does this author ever hesitate to utilize what is offered. [1964]

(In Erickson, 1980, Vol. I, Chap. 10, p. 286

I just stirred up *his* anger and let him realize — gently — that I stirred up his anger and was stimulating him into activity. And as soon as he really understood that and really saw what he could do, his anger evaporated.

(ASCH, 1980, Taped Lecture, 7/16/65)

Anne's aggression was instantly transformed into a totally different kind of thing that offered not an opportunity for aggressive retaliative attack but a joyous participation by all others in the transformation of the aggression. Yet, Anne was, in essence, left unscathed as a person, since there still remained with her the control of the aggression.

(Erickson & Rossi, 1979, p. 360)

Her repressed and guilty resentments and hostilities toward her son and his misbehavior were utilized. Every effort was made to redirect them into an anticipation of a satisfying, calculated, deliberate watchfulness in the frustrating of her son's attempts to confirm his sense of insecurity and to prove her ineffectual. [1962]

(In Erickson, 1980, vol. IV, chap. 57, p. 511)

The rationale of the author's decision was that the patient had a well-developed pattern of frustration and despair which, properly employed, could be used constructively as a motivational force in eliciting responses with a strong and probably compelling emotional force and tone leading to actual new learnings of self-expression. [1963]

(In Erickson, 1980, Vol. IV, chap. 30, p. 289)

Capitalizing upon her frustration and despair by employing measures which might conceivably make use of resulting strong emotional drives as a basis of evoking a great variety of response patterns and of motivating learning. [1963]

(In Erickson, 1980, Vol. IV, chap. 30, p. 311)

Frustration was used deliberately to prevent despair by compelling the patient, in self-protection, to strive to secure some satisfaction of ordinary, reasonable and legitimate desires. [1963]

(In Erickson, 1980, Vol. IV, chap. 30, p. 309)

This type of cavalier offer to help him utilized his need for inferiority even in the therapeutic situation and actually pleased him. [1937–38]

(In Erickson, 1980, Vol. IV, chap. 55, p. 492)

Use the Patient's Resistance

One of Erickson's most noteworthy attributes as a professional was his ability to work effectively with highly resistant patients. Most therapists are completely frustrated by a total lack of cooperation, but Erickson accepted resistance and utilized it to effect therapeutic progress. He had no magical powers for doing this; he simply acknowledged the patient's right to resist and then arranged circumstances in such a manner that in order to resist, patients had to respond in a therapeutically beneficial way. He permitted their resistance, even encouraged it, because he knew he could redirect it to suit the patient's therapeutic needs.

> **Since negativity was the dominant mental set, it was the most effective one to achieve the desired results.**
>
> *(Erickson & Rossi, 1979, p. 363)*

> **Such resistance should be openly accepted, in fact, graciously accepted, since it is a vitally important communication of a part of their problems and often can be used as an opening into their defenses. This is something that the patients do not realize. [1964]**
>
> *(In Erickson, 1980, Vol. I, chap. 13, p. 299)*

> **Resistances constituting a part of the problem can be utilized by enhancing them and thereby permitting the patient to discover, under guidance, new ways of behavior favorable to recovery. [1948]**
>
> *(In Erickson, 1980, Vol. IV, chap. 4, p. 48)*

> **The therapist who is aware of this, particularly if well skilled in hypnotherapy, can easily and often quickly transform these overt, seemingly uncooperative forms of behavior into a good rapport, a feeling of being understood, and an attitude of hopeful expectancy of successfully achieving the goals being sought. [1964]**
>
> *(In Erickson, 1980, Vol. I, chap. 13, p. 299)*

> **His hostile manner and attitude suggested the inadvisability of attempting any routine traditional technique. [1936]**
>
> *(In Erickson, 1980, Vol. IV, chap. 26, p. 253)*

Why shouldn't I give her something to reject? I think whenever you have a patient who is rejecting, who is antagonistic, who is resisting, you ought to appreciate the fact that they are antagonistic. And you ought to be able to mention antagonism and resentment in such a fashion that they can take the initiative in rejecting that antagonism, in rejecting that resistance and in achieving the relaxation that you want them to achieve.

(ASCH, 1980, Taped Lecture, 2/2/66)

Use the Patient's Symptoms

Like all other aspects of patients' response styles, their symptomatology can be therapeutic ammunition. Symptoms often can be used to initiate therapeutic change or can be transformed into useful or more manageable responses. Anxieties, phobias, delusions, and all other symptoms constitute important and compelling features of the individual's experiential life. Rather than attacking them or overlooking them, the therapist may be able to utilize them therapeutically. The psychological, emotional, and behavioral energy underlying these symptoms can become a beneficial source of impetus for change if used creatively. Even pathological symptoms must be accepted at times as a necessary feature of that particular individual's personality. Rather than expending the inordinate amount of time and energy it might take to reorganize the person's personality to the extent necessary to eliminate the sympton, it may be wise to transform the expression of the underlying pathology into less disruptive behaviors. For example, replacing an hysterical paralysis of the right arm with an hysterical paralysis of the third joint of the left little finger may be a satisfactory solution for everyone involved. Hating the therapist may be a satisfactory alternative to hating everybody. Transformation of a pathological thought, emotion or behavior into an insignificant manifestation often is the most pragmatic solution.

A short summary of Erickson's attitude is that *anything that occurs in the therapy session can be used to initiate therapeutic movement,* be it resistance, anger, a preferred topic of conversation, a behavior, or even an error on the part of the therapist. No matter what happens, therapists should be ready to twist it in a direction that will turn it into a therapeutic occurrence.

> This author has repeatedly stressed the importance of utilizing patients' symptoms and general patterns of behavior in psychotherapy. Such utilization renders unnecessary any effort to alter or transform symptomatology as a preliminary measure to the reeducation of patients in relation to the crucial problems confronting them in their illness. Such problems cause a distortion of their thinking, feeling, and patterns of living, thereby causing them to seek therapy. [1973]
>
> *(In Erickson, 1980, Vol. IV, chap. 38, p. 348)*

> Therapy had to be based upon an apparently complete acceptance of the symptoms, and it was achieved by ameliorating the symptoms.
>
> *(Erickson, 1954d, p. 117)*

> Consequently, the therapeutic task becomes a problem of intentionally utilizing neurotic symptomatology to meet the unique needs of the patient. Such utilization must satisfy the compelling desire for neurotic handicaps, the limitations imposed upon therapy by external forces, and, above all, provide adequately for constructive adjustments aided rather than handicapped by the continuance of neuroticisms.
>
> *(Erickson, 1954d, p. 109)*

There is a utilization of neurotic behavior by a transformation of the personality purposes it serves without an attack upon the symptomatology itself.

(Erickson, 1954d, p. 112)

Therefore, as therapy, there was substituted for the existing neurotic disability another, comparable in kind, nonincapacitating in character, and symptomatically satisfying to them as constructively functioning personalities.

(Erickson, 1954d, p. 112)

Utilizing the patient's own neurotic irrationality to affirm and confirm a simple extension of his neurotic fixation relieved him of all unrecognized unconscious needs to defend his neuroticism against all assaults. [1965]

(In Erickson, 1980, Vol. IV, chap. 20, p. 218)

For both patients, the utilization of anxiety by a continuance and a transformation of it provided for a therapeutic resolution into a normal emotion permitting a normal adjustment.

(Erickson, 1954d, p. 116)

Therapy was accomplished by systematically utilizing this anxiety through a process of redirecting and transforming it.

(Erickson, 1954d, p. 116)

One tries to make it possible for the patient to exercise his own ambivalence for your benefit and for his benefit.

(Erickson & Rossi, 1981, p. 4)

Use Your Own Observations

Therapists should enter the therapy situation with a backlog of observations about people. There are some general patterns of stimuli and response that will hold true across populations and that thus will apply to each patient. This knowledge should be used by the therapist whenever possible to elicit generally predictable responses that will promote or represent therapeutic change for that particular patient.

Therapists must observe each patient carefully but they must also observe carefully the everyday behavior of people in order to discover the common reactions to various situations, events, and words. This generalized knowledge can be used later to initiate desired therapeutic responses or to guide the patient's attention and experience in the necessary directions. Erickson's observations about people in Section I can serve as a starting point for the further accumulation of useful observations by each therapist. Much of the data in the psychological research literature can serve a similar purpose. Ultimately, however, therapists must assume personal responsibility for observing carefully and accumulating general information that will be meaningful and useful to them. Similar observations, of course, must be made rapidly and efficiently about each patient.

Stimulating therapeutic change in an Ericksonian manner actually involves the application of rather mechanical skills. They are admittedly complex skills requiring an extensive background of observation and experience, but all therapy really amounts to is pushing the perceptual, emotional, intellectual, and behavioral buttons that the therapist is already reasonably sure will cause the desired therapeutic reactions and experiential learnings on the part of the patient. The therapist simply becomes so familiar with the general operation of people and with the peculiar motivations and response patterns of each patient that by word and deed, the therapist can push the buttons that experience and observation have taught will generate the needed reactions.

> **In every attempt at psychotherapy there is always the need to utilize the common experiences and understandings that permeate the pattern of daily living, and to adapt such utilization to the unique needs of the individual patient.**
>
> *(Erickson, 1954c, p. 261)*

> **Suggesting eight hours of rest also utilizes what we experience in everyday life. You frequently sleep on something in order to deal with it.**
>
> *(Erickson & Rossi, 1979, p. 325)*

> **Now, there is nothing magical about what I did — *it was a recognition of the thinking Cathy would do*... the thinking and the understanding that would derive out of Cathy's ordinary life. A woman who grew up in this culture, in this age, would have certain learnings as a result of just being alive.**
>
> *(Erickson & Rossi, 1979, p. 137)*

Summary

The problem confronting therapists is how to say or to do something that will initiate an experience from which the patient can benefit. The goal may be to confront patients with their unused or misused capacities, to force them into a reevaluation of their beliefs or assumptions or to alter their inappropriate behaviors but, no matter what aspect of reality requires a more objective appraisal or response, it remains the therapist's job to provide an experience that will move patients in a behavioral, emotional, or intellectual direction they have been unable or unwilling to move in previously.

Erickson's solution to this problem consisted entirely of his willingness to accept and to utilize whatever responses were typical or normal for the patient. He tried to use whatever attitudes, interests, emotions, or symptoms the patient brought into his office. If anger was the patient's predominant characteristic, he used that anger. If the patient's pride was noticeable, he used that. If his patients were interested in gardening or travel, he used that. He even adopted and used the language style of his patients. He allowed his patients to determine the dominant characteristics of the therapeutic context and then used those characteristics to initiate or trigger a therapeutic experience.

The creativity involved in transforming or redirecting whatever the patient presents into a therapeutic response should not be underestimated. In fact, the conceptual problem involved is the same type of problem frequently encountered in tests of creativity, i.e., "Given these tools, how do you accomplish that task?" Careful observation to notice the primary motives, needs, attitudes, etc. of other people and considerable conceptual flexibility to adopt their perspectives and language patterns are also necessary. Therapeutic intervention requires a combination of all these abilities: creativity, observation, and flexibility as well as practice and a willingness to take risks.

Effective teachers seem to be especially adept at presenting information within a context that has some personal significance or importance to their students. They allow their students to experience things that demonstrate the truth of what they are saying in a direct and undeniable fashion. Good teachers can make any topic personally relevant and can package any material in an appealing and motivating manner. The parallels seem obvious and may account for Erickson's tendency to focus upon the therapist's role as teacher. His patients learned things that were therapeutic; they were not "cured" by him. He always spoke of the therapy process as a learning process. Perhaps as we begin to think of ourselves as teachers, the utilization technique and the general set of attitudes underlying it will become more comprehensible and usable.

SECTION III
HYPNOSIS AND HYPNOTHERAPY

SECTION III
HYPNOSIS AND HYPNOTHERAPY

The vast majority of Erickson's lectures, demonstrations, and publications dealt exclusively with the topics of hypnosis and hypnotherapy. Almost all of the quotations employed in the previous sections of this book occurred originally within the context of discussions about the hypnotherapeutic process where they apparently were presented in order to establish a perspective within which the phenomenon of hypnosis could be discussed and understood.

Erickson recognized that hypnosis and hypnotherapy are topics that cannot be studied apart from the careful study of the basic nature of people or the processes of psychotherapy. He viewed hypnosis as a natural, albeit fascinating, expression or redirection of normal human functioning and emphasized that a comprehension of hypnosis and hypnotic techniques depends upon a comprehension of normal and abnormal human behavior. Furthermore, he maintained that hypnosis is only a tool of therapy, a means of accomplishing desired therapeutic results more rapidly, more efficiently, or more comfortably than might be possible otherwise. Hypnosis can be used to create a therapeutic atmosphere and it can be used to tap unconscious knowledge or potentials. It can be used in a variety of ways to initiate important learning experiences and to enhance a person's ability to profit from those experiences. Essentially, however, hypnosis is only another way to do what therapists should be attempting to do throughout the therapy process. Thus, a thorough understanding of Erickson's principles and goals of psychotherapy is a prerequisite to an effective use of hypnosis in therapy. Unless these overriding principles and goals are followed, there can be no Ericksonian form of hypnotherapy and there can be no understanding of what Erickson said about it.

The material presented in the final section of this book was not designed to provide training in or a thorough review of hypnotherapeutic skills and techniques. A careful reading of this material should allow people who are already familiar with the use of hypnosis to refine their hypnotherapeutic approaches and should provide an understanding of hypnosis that will allow a more rapid accumulation of hypnotic skills by novices in a workshop setting.

The primary purpose of the following, however, is to convey Erickson's description of the hypnotic state and his general recommendations for an effective elicitation and utilization of that state. Specific techniques and phrasings are given minimal emphasis or coverage. As was the case in the discussion of psychotherapy, the focus of attention here is on the development of the mental set or perspective required of anyone who would understand or use hypnosis in an Ericksonian manner.

CHAPTER EIGHT

UNDERSTANDING HYPNOSIS

Before therapists can learn how to induce the hypnotic state effectively or how to utilize hypnotic phenomena therapeutically, they must first develop some comprehension of what hypnosis is. Without such an understanding there would be nothing to guide their behavior except rote imitation of standardized inductions.

Erickson's understanding of hypnosis was purely descriptive. He offered no elaborate theoretical definitions and avoided physiological or psychological explanations. In fact, he explicitly stated that a scientific explanation was not yet possible. The material in this chapter, therefore, offers descriptions of the hypnotic process and of hypnotized subjects, not general theories of hypnosis. Erickson's apparent purpose in providing these descriptions was simply to differentiate the hypnotic condition from the normal, everyday condition of awareness. An understanding of the phenomenon of hypnosis, based on

Erickson's observations, provides the basis for effective use of hypnosis, including effective inductions, therapeutic interventions, and even direct personal experience of it.

Trance Involves Focused Attention

Unlike ordinary awareness, which involves a constantly changing focus of attention, the hypnotic condition involves a focusing of attention and an elimination of distractions. It is not a condition of oblivion or cognitive unresponsiveness, such as sleep, but a state of consciousness wherein the normal "hyperactivity" of awareness has been reduced and attention has been directed toward a selected set or category of stimuli.

> **All hypnosis is, is a loss of the multiplicity of the foci of attention.**
>
> *(Erickson & Rossi, 1981, p. 187)*

> **It [hypnosis] is a lack of response to irrelevant external stimuli.**
>
> *(Erickson & Rossi, 1981, p. 188)*

> **Trance is a focusing on one thing...dropping all the peripheral foci and narrowing it down to one focus.**
>
> *(Erickson & Rossi, 1979, p. 369)*

> **Therapeutic trance is focused attention in the best manner to achieve the patient's goals.**
>
> *(Erickson & Rossi, 1979, p. 130)*

> **I don't let the conversation jump to anything else. Yes, trance is a focusing on one thing. Watkins has written a paper describing trance as dropping all the peripheral foci and narrowing it down to one focus. I agree with that.**
>
> *(Erickson & Rossi, 1979, p. 369)*

When hypnotized, or in the hypnotic trance, the subject can think, act and behave in relationship to either ideas or reality objects as adequately as, and usually better than, he can in the ordinary state of awareness. In all probability this ability derives from intensity and restriction of attention to the task in hand, and the consequent freedom from the ordinary conscious tendency to orient constantly to distracting, even irrelevant, reality considerations.

(Erickson, 1970, p. 995)

Subjects spontaneously volunteered the information that going into hypnosis was "exactly like introspection and concentration." [1964]

(In Erickson, 1980, Vol. I, chap. 1, p. 10)

It's [loss of multiple foci of attention] an altered state of consciousness in the same sense as you experience in everyday life when you are reading a book and your wife speaks to you and you make no immediate response.

(Erickson & Rossi, 1981, p. 188)

As one subject aptly declared, "It is not a question of being unaware of stimuli but, rather, a giving of all attention to certain stimuli or to certain aspects of a stimulus complex without other stimuli entering into the situation." [1944]

(In Erickson, 1980, Vol. II, chap. 4, p. 34)

I told them any hypnotic subject can work as well in a trance state as he can in a waking state, and probably do it much better because there are fewer distractions.

(Zeig, 1980, p. 227)

If I were having my chauffeur drive me in dangerous traffic, I would put him in a deep trance. I would want him to pay attention to the traffic problem... I wouldn't want anything outside the car to distract him — anything, outside of driving problems, to distract him.

(Zeig, 1980, pp. 227–228)

It [hypnosis] is a state of consciousness — not unconsciousness or sleep — a state of consciousness or awareness in which there is a marked receptiveness to ideas and understandings and an increased willingness to respond either positively or negatively to those ideas. [circa 1950's]

(In Erickson, 1980, Vol. IV, chap. 21, p. 224)

Physiologically, there is much more resemblance between the hypnotic and the waking states than with physiological sleep. [1944]

(In Erickson, 1980, Vol. IV, chap. 2, p. 16)

The hypnotic state is essentially a psychological phenomenon, unrelated to physiological sleep, and dependent entirely upon full cooperation between hypnotist and subject.

(Erickson, 1941, p. 14)

Hypnosis is a state of awareness, a very definite state of awareness with special types of awareness. Hypnotic subjects are not unconscious in any sense of the word. Rather they are exceedingly aware of a great number of things and yet able to be unaware of an equally great number of things. The can direct and redirect their attention in remarkable ways ordinarily not possible in the waking state but possible in the nighttime dream state, which is a form of cerebration. They can do the same sort of things that they do in the ordinary waking state, but often in a more intentional, controlled and directed manner. [1962]

(In Erickson, 1980, Vol. II, chap. 33, p. 347)

Reality is Less Important in Trance

Perception and response are normally directed toward the maintenance of a reality orientation. Everyday conscious awareness is conducted within the constraints and demands of external reality and is a means of adaptation and survival. As subjects move into a hypnotic condition, however, they pay less and less attention to external reality and make fewer efforts to monitor or interpret external events. Staying in touch with external events simply becomes less and less important or necessary. Eventually they give up the effort it takes to keep in touch, and enter a "deeper" trance.

> **In the lighter stages of hypnosis external reality seemed to remain constant, but "less important,"..."not so real." ... As the trance depth progressed from the very light stage to the deeper and deeper levels, external realities became increasingly "unreal," "not there," or "I forgot them." [1967]**
>
> *(In Erickson, 1980, Vol. I, chap. 2, p. 62)*

> **And it isn't necessary for you to waste mental energy on the realities, the external realities.**
>
> *(Erickson, Rossi & Rossi, 1976, p. 243)*

> **Going into trance is like "going away" because you are going distant from external reality.**
>
> *(Erickson, Rossi & Rossi, 1976, p. 97)*

> **A slight pause in the subject's immediate activity, a facial expression of distraction and detachment, a peculiar glassiness of the eyes with a dilation of the pupils and failure to focus, a condition of catalepsy, a fixity and narrowing of attention, an intentness of pur-**

pose, a marked loss of contact with the general environment, and an unresponsiveness to any external stimulus. [1941]

(In Erickson, 1980, Vol. I, chap. 19, p. 390)

It isn't just a *monoidea*, but all the multiple foci of attention; the desk, the birds, the bus, have all been eliminated.

(Erickson & Rossi, 1981, p. 187)

As patients learn to be more comfortable with these spontaneous alterations, they can allow themselves to go deeper into trance. They learn to give up more and more of this generalized reality orientation (Shor, 1959).

(Erickson & Rossi, 1979, p. 133)

Attention Turns Inward During Trance

During the time that external reality events are decreasing in importance and are being given less attention, awareness is increasingly directed toward internal events such as imagery, sensations, thoughts, etc. Absorption with such internal experiences is a predominant characteristic of the trance state. Eventually the subject's awareness may become completely absorbed by particular internal events, with external events fading from conscious attention entirely unless the hypnotist directs the subject's now highly focused attention to them.

They are comparable in some degree to those common spontaneous limited restrictions of awareness seen in states of intense concentration, abstraction and reverie or in the failure to perceive something obvious because of a state of expectation of something quite different. [1944]

(In Erickson, 1980, Vol. II, chap. 4, p. 49)

You are oblivious to the external lecture and your surroundings as you tune into inner realities. Everyone has had that experience.

(Erickson, Rossi & Rossi, 1979, p. 47)

Their attention was not directed away from their own inner world of experience to the author but remained fixated upon their own inner processes. [1964]

(In Erickson, 1980, Vol. I chap. 13, p. 329)

My voice in the background is where I want it to be. It's in the background of *her* experience. Her own experience is in the focus of attention.

(Erickson & Rossi, 1979, p. 291)

You can call it anything you want. I call it hypnosis, relaxation, various terms. I like to call it comfortable self-awareness. I like to teach my patients a comfortable self-awareness. And I'd like to have all of you from time to time become comfortably aware, aware in an inward sort of way of yourself.

(ASCH, 1980, Taped Lecture, 7/16/65)

But meditation is thinking for the self, by the self, and thinking freely and easily, just wondering about what the self has to offer for the self.

(Erickson & Lustig, 1975, Vol. 2, p. 5)

It [light trance] is, he [Huxley] explained, "a simple withdrawal of interest from the outside to the inside." That is, one gives less attention to externalities and directs more and more attention to inner subjective sensations. Externalities become increasingly fainter and more obscure, inner subjective feelings more satisfying until a state of balance exists. In this state of balance, he had the feeling that, with motivation, he could "reach out and seize upon reality," that there is a definite retention of a grasp upon external reality but with no motivation to deal with it. [1965]

(In Erickson, 1980, Vol. 1, chap. 3, p. 90)

The field of consciousness narrows and external stimuli, except those given by the hypnotist, lose their significance. Ultimately, the subject loses contact with the external world except for the operator.

(Erickson, 1934, p. 612)

Subjects Respond to Internal Realities

As subjects successfully give up their old orientation within external reality and begin to focus on internal stimuli, they naturally become less and less dependent upon the parameters of their external reality context to provide meaning and structure to their perceptions or responses. Ordinary reality considerations tend to be replaced by the rules of an internally constructed definition of what is real. This internal construction can be developed by the hypnotist via specific suggestions or implications and/or it may be constructed by subjects in response to their own idiosyncratic concepts of what hypnosis is. In essence, a new context for thought, experience, and behavior is developed in hypnosis and subsequent events will enter awareness and be responded to only within the parameters of that context. What is real for the subject and what occurs within that reality is specified internally and not by actual external events or circumstances. It is as if hypnotized subjects enter a new world, one in which the ordinary rules and events of reality no longer apply but are replaced by internally based ones.

Hypnotic responsiveness is, however, of quite another character. The reality situation in which hypnosis occurs is, in itself, essentially an "extrapolated reality" sometimes deriving only from experiential processes within the subject and having little or no relationship to objective reality. [1958]

(In Erickson, 1980, Vol. II, chap. 19, p. 192)

People in the nontrance state do not lose complete general awareness of the immediate reality surroundings nor of the general context of thinking and speaking; and should they do so in partial fashion, they "come to" with a start, explaining (Usually without a request to do so), "For a moment or two there I absentmindedly forgot everything except what I was thinking," reorienting themselves as they so speak to their general environment. But it is to the actual reality that they orient themselves.

This is not so with deeply hypnotized somnambulistic subjects, even though it may be their first experience with hypnosis, and eyes may have been continuously wide open, and they may have been hypnotized by some ritualistic verbalized technique of suggestions, or by any other method that had been written out in full or recorded and that could then be examined for hidden or implied meanings of the words employed. ... All sensory intake apparently has lost its value except the awareness of the presence of the experimenter as a part of the hypnotic situation, and the reality stimuli have been replaced in the subjects' experiential behavior responses by memory images unrelated to his actual reality situation. [1967]

(In Erickson, 1980, Vol. I, chap. 2, pp. 40–41)

In the hypnotic state subjects take one look at the hypnotic situation and they have established their orientation. They do not need to keep returning, verifying and reverifying their reality situation. They know the situation, and they are aware that, should any change in that reality orientation occur, they would be able to make the modifications. [1960]

(In Erickson, 1980, Vol. II, chap. 31, p. 321)

She was apparently totally unable to respond to anything not belonging strictly to the hypnotic situation. [1941]

(In Erickson, 1980, Vol. I, chap. 19, p. 402)

The author does not know how to measure and how to define what happens to the physical realities that the hypnotic subject can see as clearly as the waking subject and yet make responses in terms of hypnotic realities. [1967]

(In Erickson, 1980, Vol. I, chap. 2, p. 50)

The fashion in which the patients made their fantasies a part of their reality life was in keeping with the ordinary natural evolution of spontaneous behavior responses to reality. It was not in compliance with therapeutic suggestions nor did it seem to derive even indirectly from anything other than the patients' responses to their realities. Furthermore, their behavior was experienced by them as arising within them and in relation to their needs in their immediate life situation.

(Erickson, 1954c, p. 283)

There existed the type of reality one encounters in vivid dreams, a reality that one does not question. Instead, one accepts such reality completely without intellectual questioning, and there are no conflicting contrasts nor judgemental comparisons nor contradictions, so that whatever is subjectively experienced is unquestioningly accepted as both subjectively and objectively genuine and in keeping with all else. [1965]

(In Erickson, 1980, Vol. I, chap. 3, p. 102)

Responses could be limited to the immediate stimuli of the hypnotic situation, uninfluenced by their usual associative and habitual modes of reaction. [1938]

(In Erickson, 1980, Vol. II, chap. 10, p. 82)

They become so absorbed and automatic in their performance and so limited in their responses to their general environment, that there is little possibility of, no need for, the retention of conscious attitudes and patterns of behavior. Instead, there is effected a dissociation from the immediate circumstances. [1941]

(In Erickson, 1980, Vol. I, chap. 19, p. 403)

In the trance state a new and different reality developed. [1967]

(In Erickson, 1980, Vol. I, chap. 2, p. 59)

They had in some manner left the reality world in which they could be identified as members of the audience and had entered another world of reality belonging only to their own personal life experiences. [1967]

(In Erickson, 1980, Vol. I, chap. 2, p. 76)

The replies received were invariably couched in the subject's apparent *trance understandings* or apprehension of the physical reality, which was definitely not in accord with their ordinary understandings of reality. In fact, the subjects' reality apprehension appeared definitely to be another type of experience than that of their waking state. [1967]

(In Erickson, 1980, Vol. I, chap. 2, p. 56)

Hypnotized people have perceived their reality surroundings in a manner entirely foreign to actualities but
most real to themselves. [1967]

(In Erickson, 1980, Vol. I, chap. 2, p. 76)

This hypnotic reality situation is limited by and
restricted to the subject's understandings of what is required in the hypnotic situation with an exclusion of, or
unresponsiveness to, objective realities that may be
regarded as irrelevant, coincidental, or merely concommi-
tant. [1958]

(In Erickson, 1980, Vol. II, chap. 19, p. 192)

Hypnosis can so alter a person's consciousness of his
environment that, in his reactions, he can call upon past
experiences and learnings to utilize and accomplish equally phenomenal changes. [1970]

(In Erickson, 1980, Vol. IV, chap 6, p. 75)

Hypnosis Facilitates Rapport

During hypnosis the subject's attention is turned primarily
inward with virtually the only contact with external reality being an awareness of the hypnotist's voice. This tendency to be
responsive only to the hypnotist, who, as a result, can direct
the subject's attention almost anywhere, is called *rapport*.

Usually the subject responds spontaneously only to
stimuli from the hypnotist who may limit or direct the
subject's state of awareness as he wishes. [1954]

(In Erickson, 1980, Vol. III, chap. 3, p. 22)

Rapport, a condition in which the subject responds only to the hypnotist and is seemingly incapable of hearing,

seeing, sensing or responding to anything else unless so instructed by the hypnotist. It is in effect a concentration of the subject's attention upon, and awareness only of, the hypnotist and those things the hypnotist wishes included in the trance situation, and it has the effect of dissociating the subject from all other things. [1944]

(In Erickson, 1980, Vol. IV, chap. 2, p. 19)

The author regarded the trance state as colored by what is called "rapport" and as marked by such rigidities of behavior as those deriving from catalepsy and other alterations of physical behavior and by the reality detachment, dissociation, and ideomotor and ideosensory manifestations that appear to be important, but which are not always consistently present, characteristics of the somnambulistic state. Also characteristic of the trance state are the subjects' apparent unawareness of items of reality and stimuli which are not pertinent to their trance or to the potentiation of other mental frames of reference. [1967]

(In Erickson, 1980, Vol. 1, chap. II, pp. 37–38)

Hypnosis Facilitates Responsiveness

The hypnotic state creates a condition of passivity and rapport which can be used to enhance a subject's responsiveness or suggestibility. As the subject develops a sense of trust and confidence in the hypnotist, responsivity will tend to develop automatically and this tendency should be carefully cultivated or encouraged. An increased responsiveness to the ideas or suggestions presented by the hypnotist is desirable because it is what enables the hypnotist to guide the subject's use of memories and previously unused or misused capacities in ways that eventually will generate the hypnotic experiences and phenomena sought.

> **In the state of hypnosis, as in the state of conscious awareness, you give your attention but you give your attention to selected ideas. Your mind is open to these ideas.... In the hypnotic state the subject is susceptible to ideas and accepts them. [1959]**
>
> *(In Erickson, 1980, Vol. III, chap. 4, p. 28)*

> **Hypnosis is primarily a state in which there is increased responsiveness to ideas of all sorts.**
>
> *(Erickson & Rossi, 1981, p. 3)*

> **The hypnotic trance may be defined, for purposes of conceptualization, as a state of increased awareness and responsiveness to ideas. [1958]**
>
> *(In Erickson, 1980, Vol. IV, chap. 15, p. 174)*

> **Functioning at this special level of awareness is characterized by a state of receptiveness and responsiveness in which inner experiential learnings and understandings can be accorded values comparable with or even the same as those ordinarily given only to external reality stimuli.**
>
> *(Erickson, 1970, p. 995)*

> **He becomes much more responsive to ideas and is able to accept suggestions and to act upon them more readily than in his ordinary state of awareness. [1957]**
>
> *(In Erickson, 1980, Vol. IV, chap. 5, p. 49)*

> **The induction of a clinically satisfactory trance leads to the development of a peculiar psychic state of passive responsiveness in which the subject automatically accepts**

and acts upon any suggestion given as a purely responsive form of behavior. [circa 1960]

(In Erickson, 1980, Vol. II, chap. 29, p. 301)

Rather, there should be recognition of the fact that the general tendency of the hypnotic subject to be passive and receptive is simply expressive of the suggestibility of the hypnotic subject and hence a direct result of the suggestions employed to induce hypnosis and not a function of the hypnotic state. [1944]

(In Erickson, 1980, Vol. II, chap. 4, p. 35)

A further and much more difficult step lies in the utilization of the subject's passive responsiveness to secure a spontaneous development of a pattern of behavior merely initiated by the suggestions given. [circa 1960]

(In Erickson, 1980, Vol. 2, chap. 29, p. 302)

Hypnosis can be employed to elicit purely responsive behavior, which apparently constitutes a remarkable and vivid portrayal of memories, experiences, and understandings in a fashion adequate to permit a general comprehensive survey of the various forms of hypnotic behavior, or that it may be employed to initiate by suggestion spontaneously developed forms of behavior comparable to those evoked by outer realities. [circa 1960]

(In Erickson, 1980, Vol. II, chap. 29, p. 303–304)

Suggestibility is, of course, a primary feature of hypnosis, and is necessarily present. However, there is always a need, if serious and satisfactory purposes are to be achieved, to give suggestions in accord with the subject's understandings and desires, although in the type of hypnosis practiced on the vaudeville stage, ridiculous and undignified suggestions can be given.

(Erickson, 1941, p. 15)

Subjects Create Internal Realities
Via Vivification

As mentioned previously, when attention has been highly focused and turned inward, subjects naturally become absorbed by internal events and begin to experience and respond almost exclusively to the reality generated by these internal events. Internal thoughts and images become so absorbing and convincing that they are subjectively indistinguishable from the experience of ordinary reality. These internally derived definitions and experiences of reality are responded to as if they were reality, while the ordinary definitions and events of reality are momentarily displaced or ignored.

Erickson referred to this bringing to life of memories, ideas, emotions, and previously hidden capacities as vivification. A memory, an imagined event, or a mere notion about what is happening can be experienced so vividly that it seems real. This vivification process is what is responsible for most of the phenomena which can be elicited by hypnosis and, thus, it is important for the hypnotist to be able to influence it. The carefully nurtured increases in responsiveness or suggestibility described earlier make it possible for the hypnotist to guide awareness in specific ways or to create internal events which can be vivified into "real" hypnotic experiences for the subjects. Past events may be relived, current events may be perceived and thought about in a totally new manner, and all sensations or perceptions may be amplified, distorted, reduced, eliminated, or replaced by an awareness of those derived entirely from internal events. Such utilization of the natural patterns of memory, thought, and response to stimulate the experience of an alternate or hypnotic reality is characteristic of most Ericksonian hypnotherapeutic interventions.

The process is essentially the vivification of memories, ideas, and understandings so effectively that they are subjectively experienced as external events rather than as internal processes, with a consequent endowment of them as reality experiences.

(Erickson, 1954b, p. 23)

The psychological processes involved are essentially those of vivification of memories, ideas, understandings, emotions — indeed, any type of experiential acquisition — so that they are experienced subjectively as deriving from external events rather than from internal processes.

(Erickson, 1970, p. 996)

They explained with varying degrees of clarity how they withdrew from objective reality and created out of the memories and ideas an "experiential reality." [1958]

(In Erickson, 1980, Vol. II, chap. 19, p. 194)

Understanding of this projection of memories is important to the understanding of hypnosis. This particular phenomenon can be defined as a state of ordinary awareness, but it is devoted primarily to the consideration of ideas in themselves, with full attentiveness to the idea. This differs from our conscious attention, which is directed only to reality. [1959]

(In Erickson, 1980, Vol. III, chap. 4, p. 28)

They identified it with actual past experiences, and thus endowed it definitely with a subjective validity. [1938]

(In Erickson, 1980, Vol. II, chap. 10, p. 97)

Hypnosis is a special but normal type of behavior, encountered when attention and the thinking processes are directed to the body of experiential learnings acquired from or achieved in, the experiences of living. [1970]

(In Erickson, 1980, Vol. IV, chap. 6, p. 54)

Then out of their own past experiential learnings and conditionings, they "created a reality" that permitted a responsive functioning in accord with the demands of the experiment. [1958]

(In Erickson, 1980, Vol. II, chap. 19, p. 195)

Hypnosis Offers Access To Unused Potentials

Hypnotized subjects are open to a more effective utilization of their experientially acquired understandings and previously unused potentials of response. Basically, they are in contact and able to draw upon the vast reservoir and potential of their unconscious. The role of the hypnotist in such a situation is to provide a series of communications (verbal or nonverbal) that will automatically focus attention upon or elicit these unconscious abilities and capacities, hence generating "hypnotic responses." The systematic or goal-oriented elicitation and vivification of these underlying, unrecognized capacities can be observed with curiosity and amazement by subjects who may become more aware of and more able to utilize their own potentials as a result.

[In hypnosis] there is an interchangeable use of reality stimuli and remembered experiences, visual memories, auditory memories, kinesthetic memories, etc. It is out of the use of these understandings, learnings, and memories in the mind that hypnotic subjects develop their behavior. In this state of special awareness, or special consciousness the operator (the hypnotist) plays a role in communicating ideas to the subjects, of orienting the subjects to that unique, individual hypnotic situation in which each particular subject finds himself. [1960]

(In Erickson, 1980, Vol. II, chap. 31, p. 313)

Hypnosis is essentially a communication of ideas and understandings to a patient in such a fashion that he will be most receptive to the presented ideas and thereby motivated to the explore his own body potentials for the control of his psychological and physiological responses and behavior. [1967]

(In Erickson, 1980, Vol. IV, chap. 24, p. 237)

Hypnosis is a technique of communication whereby you make available the vast store of learnings that have been acquired, the usefulness of which lies primarily in the way of automatic responses. In hypnosis we make a direct call on these learnings that have been dropped into the area of automatically available learnings.

(Erickson & Rossi, 1981, p. 100)

Hypnosis is not some mystical procedure, but rather a systematic utilization of experiential learnings — that is, the extensive learnings acquired through the process of living itself. [circa 1950's]

(In Erickson, 1980, Vol. IV, chap. 21, p. 224)

Hypnosis is a state of readiness to utilize learnings. Why should it be viewed as a distortion of reality instead of some kind of readiness to use abilities normally? [1962]

(In Erickson, 1980, Vol. II, chap. 33, p. 340)

All of us have a tremendous number of these generally unrecognized psychological and somatic learnings and

conditionings, and it is the intelligent use of these that constitutes an effectual use of hypnosis. [circa 1950's]
(In Erickson, 1980, Vol. IV, chap. 21, p. 224)

In other words, the hypnotic technique serves only to induce a favorable setting in which to instruct patients in a more advantageous use of their own potentials of behavior. [1966]
(In Erickson, 1980, Vol. IV, chap. 28, p. 262)

Hypnosis Does Not Create New Abilities

Erickson refused to accept that the abilities demonstrated by hypnotized subjects are unique to the hypnotic condition. On the contrary, he vehemently insisted that all hypnotic alterations in behavior or experience are merely the intensified manifestations of ordinary behavior. Hypnosis itself neither adds to nor detracts from the subject's capacities and personality; the person remains the same individual. Hypnosis merely provides an opportunity for that individual to utilize normal learnings and capacities in a more directed manner.

This insistence that hypnotic phenomena are examples of normal capacities, many of which are used in everyday life without conscious awareness, was an extremely important element in Erickson's whole approach to hypnosis and hypnotherapy. Most hypnotic phenomena or hypnotic responses were elicited by Erickson using the same kinds of communications that would generate similar responses from non-hypnotized subjects. The hypnotic condition evidently allows the response to be more intense and more noticeable to the subject, but hypnosis is not itself responsible for the behavior. The subject's experiential background and normal capacities are responsible for the behavior. Erickson's observations enabled him to predict that people in general or that one subject in particular would automatically respond to a specific communication in the manner he desired. He then used that knowledge with his subjects to help them learn the extent of their capacities.

A serious misconception of hypnosis frequently encountered even among those who have had extensive experience... is that hypnosis in some peculiar, undefined fashion necessarily deprives subjects of their natural abilities for responsive, self-expressive, and aggressive behavior, and limits and restricts them to the role of purely passive and receptive instruments of the hypnotist. [1944]

(In Erickson, 1980, Vol. II, chap. 4, p. 35)

The hypnotized person remains an individual, and only certain limited general relationships and behavior are temporarily altered by hypnosis. [1944]

(In Erickson, 1980, Vol. III, chap. 21, p. 207)

I believe that the hypnotic subject can do in a trance state the same sort of things he can do in the waking state. [1960]

(In Erickson, 1980, Vol. II, chap. 31, p. 334)

I think that hypnotic behavior is a normal, controlled, directed behavior useful to the individual. .. In hypnosis you have the right behavior, in the right place, doing the right thing, at the right time. [1960]

(In Erickson, 1980, Vol. II, chap. 31, p. 326)

When you produce in hypnosis tremendous alterations in the subject's behavior, is it not possible that processes comparable to those which sometimes occur under ordi-

nary or pathological conditions are set into action in a limited, but controlled and instructive fashion? [1962]

(In Erickson, 1980, Vol. II, chap. 33, p. 343)

Why not assume that the same forces that condition people in ordinary life can be as effective in hypnosis? The people are the same, they still possess their innate abilities, and we all know that a single starry-eyed look can initiate generations of events. Why assume that hypnosis negates the possibility of sudden effective conditioning? [1962]

(In Erickson, 1980, Vol. II, chap. 33, p. 344)

The hypnotized person remains the same person. His or her behavior only is altered by the trance state, but even so, that altered behavior derives from the life experience of the patient and not from the therapist. At the most the therapist can influence only the manner of self-expression. [1948]

(In Erickson, 1980, Vol. IV, chap. 4, p. 38)

In the special state of awareness called hypnosis the various forms of behavior of everyday life may be found — differing in relationships and degrees, but always within normal limits. [1970]

(In Erickson, 1980, Vol. IV, chap. 6, p. 54)

In the author's experience there can be developed in a person a special state of awareness that is termed, for the sake of convenience and historical considerations, *hypnosis* or *trance*. This state is characterized by the subject's ability to retain the same capacities possessed in the waking state and to manifest these capacities in ways possibly, though not necessarily, dissimilar to the usual actions of conscious awareness. *Trance permits the operator to evoke in a controlled manner the same mental mechanisms that are operative spontaneously in everyday life.* [circa 1960's]

(In Erickson, 1980, Vol. III, chap. 8, p. 61)

There seems to be no valid reason to expect hypnotized subjects to lose their capacities for spontaneous, expressive and capable behavior or to expect them to become simply an instrument of the hypnotist. [1944]

(In Erickson, 1980, Vol. II, chap. 4, p. 50)

The fact that the subject's psychological state of awareness has been altered constitutes no logical barrier to any form of self-expressive behavior within that general frame of reference; and experience discloses that, in addition to their usual abilities, hypnotic subjects are often capable of behavior ordinarily impossible for them. [1944]

(In Erickson, 1980, Vol. II, chap. 4, p. 35)

These studies [Milgram, 1963, 1964, 1965] are studies that should be read most thoughtfully by whomever undertakes either laboratory or clinical hypnosis, since they are indicative of the stresses a person in the waking state will endure and thereby, by inference, indicating that situations, motivations, obedience, and personality factors are highly significant in human behavior and response in a manner not yet understood in the waking state of a subject, much less in hypnotic states or other states of altered awareness. [1967]

(In Erickson, 1980, Vol. II, chap. 30, p. 312)

Hypnotized Subjects Are Not Automatons

Although a hypnotic state will enable subjects to respond more effectively to suggestions, it does not guarantee that they will do so. Suggestions must be presented in an appropriate manner, one that is meaningful and useful to the individual subjects, given their unique personalities, experiential backgrounds, and needs; otherwise the subjects will be unable or unwilling to comply. Furthermore, the suggested experience or response must be one that is acceptable to the subjects or they will refuse to comply and may become upset with and unresponsive to the hypnotist. Hypnosis does not create automatons who will automatically understand or obey the hypnotist's every command. Subjects remain true to themselves, no matter how deeply hypnotized, and will comply with requests only if they understand how to comply and decide that they actually want to comply.

Because subjects remain the same people when hypnotized, their tendency to protect themselves remains operative as well. For this reason, hypnosis cannot usually be used for destructive or harmful purposes with normal individuals, even unintentionally. There are notable exceptions to this statement, however, especially with regard to individuals who have particular areas of pathological vulnerability, and it is always the hypnotist's responsibility to guarantee proper protections for the patient.

> **Any suggestion not objectionable to the subject will be accepted and acted upon. [1934]**
> *(In Erickson, 1980, Vol. III, chap. 1, p. 9)*

> **Suggestibility plays another role after the trance is induced, in that any desired behavior can be suggested to**

the subject and an adequate performance can be secured, provided that the suggestions are not offensive to the subject. [1944]

(In Erickson, 1980, Vol. IV, chap. 2, p. 20)

The subjects need not necessarily accept anything the operator suggests. The subjects tend to respond in accord with patterns unique to each. [1960]

(In Erickson, 1980, Vol. II, chap. 31, p. 313)

Suggestions must be acceptable to the subject, and rejection of them can be based upon whims as easily as upon sound reasons.

(Erickson, 1954b, p. 23)

Suggestions unacceptable to their total personalities lead either to a rejection of the suggestions or to a transformation of them so that they can be satisfied by pretense behavior. [1952]

(In Erickson, 1980, Vol. I, chap. 6, p. 146)

In the hypnotic state subjects are open to ideas. *They like to examine ideas in terms of their memories, their conditionings and all of the various experiential learnings of life.* They take your suggestion and translate that into their own body learnings. [1960]

(In Erickson, 1980, Vol. II, chap. 31, p. 318)

Also, they emphasized that invariably they scrutinized carefully every suggestion offered, primarily as a measure of understanding it fully to permit complete obedience and not for the purpose of taking exception to it, and that, if they were at all uncertain of it, their hypnotic state would force them to await either more adequate instruction or a better understanding by a direct, thoughtful, and critical consideration of the command.

(Erickson, 1939a, p. 394)

The process of becoming hypnotized is perceived by the subject as a peculiar alteration of his control over the self, necessitating compensatory measures in relationship to any occurrence seeming to imply a threat to the control of the self.

(Erickson, 1939a, p. 401)

One has the feeling that, as a result of their hypnotic state, they sensed a certain feeling of helplessness reflected in intensifed self-protection.

(Erickson, 1939a, p. 402)

It is of interest to note that certain subjects actually inflicted punishment and humiliation upon the experimenter in retaliation for his objectionable commands.

(Erickson, 1939a, p. 393)

In this instance, at least, the subject was more capable of resisting the experimenter's commands in the trance state or by unconscious measures than she was in the waking state.

(Erickson, 1939a, p. 403)

Not only did the subjects resist suggestions for acts actually acceptable under ordinary waking conditions, but they carried over into the trance state the normal waking tendency to reject instrumentalization by another.

(Erickson, 1939a, p. 403)

The findings disclosed consistently the failure of all experimental measures to induce hypnotic subjects, in response to hypnotic suggestion, to perform acts of an objectionable character, even though many of the suggested acts were acceptable to them under circumstances of waking consciousness.

(Erickson, 1939a, p. 414)

Apparently, in attempting to induce felonious behavior by hypnosis, the danger lies not in the possibility of success, but in the risk to the hypnotist himself.

(Erickson, 1939a, p. 411)

The subjects demonstrated a full capacity and ability for self-protection, ready and complete understanding with critical judgement, avoidance, evasion, or complete rejection to instrumentalization by the hypnotist, and for aggression and retaliation, direct and immediate, against the hypnotist for his objectionable suggestions and commands.

(Erickson, 1939a, p. 414)

Neither is it [hypnosis] injurious or detrimental to the subject in any way, nor can it be used for anti-social or criminal purposes.

(Erickson, 1941b, p. 14)

Briefly, there are no injurious or *detrimental effects* upon the subject other than those that can develop in any other normal interpersonal relationship; hypnosis cannot be used for *anti-social* or criminal purposes. [1944]

(In Erickson, 1980, Vol. IV, chap. 2, p. 16)

In over 30 years of experimental and clinical work with hypnosis I have not been able to discover any harmful effects. ... [circa 1950's]

(In Erickson, 1980, Vol. IV, chap. 21, p. 226)

Trance is Manifested in a Variety of Ways

There are no clear-cut indicators of the development of a hypnotic state. Trance is a gradually increasing phenomenon, that varies in depth from subject to subject and even from moment to moment within any one subject. Every subject seems to experience different patterns of alteration as the depth of hypnosis increases, although there are some typical trends. Usually there is a gradual loss of ideomotor movements and an increase in physical and physiological relaxation. Catalepsy may be noticed if it is checked for in the way one tests for waxy flexibility in the catatonic patient. Amnesia for trance events is a frequent occurrence, as is dilation of the pupils. Finally, a gradual loss of contact with external reality, frequently including an apparent unresponsiveness to extraneous stimuli such as outside distractions or sudden, unexpected noises, is also characteristic of the trance state.

Hypnosis is a phenomenon of degrees, ranging from light to profound trance states but with no fixed constancy.

(Erickson, 1970, p. 996)

To judge trance depths and hypnotic responses, consideration must be given not only to average responses but to the various deviations from the average that may be manifested by the individual. [1952]

(In Erickson, 1980, Vol. I, chap. 6, p. 139)

She is evidencing here her own pattern of trance behavior. There is no such thing as pure trance behavior.

(Erickson & Rossi, 1979, p. 365)

Patients all have their own patterns of experiencing hypnotic phenomenon in a segmental manner.

(Erickson, Rossi & Rossi, 1976, p. 103)

R: And that body stillness can be taken as a reliable indicator of trance.

E: Yes.

(Erickson, Rossi & Rossi, 1976, p. 177)

One of the important trance manifestations occurring in nearly every well-hypnotized subject is catalepsy. [1939]

(In Erickson, 1980, Vol. IV, chap. 1, p. 7)

Another hypnotic phenomenon which has a direct bearing upon psychiatric problems is the amenesia which develops for all trance events following profound hypnosis. [1939]

(In Erickson, 1980, Vol. IV, chap. 1, p. 7)

The pupils were noted to be widely dilated, as is frequently the finding in deep hypnosis. [1956]

(In Erickson, 1980, Vol. IV, chap. 49, p. 440)

Many hypnotic subjects manifest altered pupillary behavior in the trance state. Most frequently this is a dilation of the pupils particularly in the somnambulistic state and the pupillary size changes when visual hallucinations are suggested at various distances. There are also pupillary changes that accompany suggestions of fear and anger states, and of the experience of pain. [1965]

(In Erickson, 1980, Vol. II, chap. 9, p. 78)

Deep Trance Involves the Unconscious

Movement from a light trance to a deep or stuporous trance involves a gradual loss of conscious awareness of the external environment. Eventually, as the subject enters a *deep* trance, the confines, biases, concerns, and patterns of the externally defined conscious mind may disappear altogether, leaving the unconscious mind in full control. The subject does not become unconscious, does not lose awareness of ongoing events. Rather, the subject remains aware but that awareness is of the perceptions, understandings, and patterns of response of the unconscious mind. Awareness is no longer directed through or by the conscious mind, but by the unconscious mind alone. This is an immensely important aspect of the deep trance. An accurate grasp of the involvement of the unconscious in deep trance is absolutely necessary to an understanding of Erickson's use of hypnosis in therapy.

When in a deep trance, patients hear and respond to the hypnotherapist with only the unconscious mind. What people in a deep trance hear, see, know or do, is a function of the perceptions, knowledge, and response patterns of their unconscious minds. They experience and respond from within a new frame of reference, a new perspective; that is, from within their unconscious minds. For the time being, all of the concerns, fears, beliefs, values, learnings, and response tendencies of their ordinary conscious minds become irrelevant and inoperative. Deep hypnosis frees subjects from the constrictions of the conscious model of reality and places them in direct contact with their unconscious knowledge, experiential learning histories, and abilities, all of which may be vivified into new experiential understandings.

Those in a light trance found it difficult to maintain a trance state if they opened their eyes and performed a

task in relation to external reality....Those in a medium trance were also disinclined to cooperate, and questioning revealed as their reason that the opening of the eyes and the doing something not in relationship to themselves would disturb them and tend to awaken them; they were willing to do things that affected them as persons, but they felt that any manipulation of external objects by them placed an undue burden on them. [1967]

(In Erickson, 1980, Vol. I, chap. 2, p. 49)

At the lighter levels, there is an admixture of conscious understandings and expectations and a certain amount of conscious participation. In the deeper stages, functioning is more properly at an unconscious level of awareness. [1952]

(In Erickson, 1980, Vol. I, chap. 6, p. 145)

Subjects in a deep trance function in accord with unconscious understandings, independently of the forces to which their conscious mind ordinarily responds; they behave in accordance with the realities which exist in the given hypnotic situation for their unconscious mind. Conceptions, memories, and ideas constitute their reality world while they are in deep trance. The actual external environmental reality with which they are surrounded is relevant only insofar as it is utilized in the hypnotic situation. Hence, external reality does not necessarily constitute concrete objective matter possessed of intrinsic value. [1952]

(In Erickson, 1980, Vol. I, chap. 6, p. 146)

The reality of the deep trance must necessarily be in accord with the fundamental needs and structure of the total personality. Thus it is that profoundly neurotic persons in the deep trance can, in that situation, be freed from their otherwise overwhelming neurotic behavior, and thereby a foundation laid for their therapeutic reeducation in accord with each fundamental personality. The overlay of neuroticism, however extensive, does not distort the central core of the personality, though it may disguise and cripple the manifestations of it. [1952]

(In Erickson, 1980, Vol. I, chap. 6, p. 146)

You frequently find that patients say being in trance is being in a different part of themselves: "You know you are you, but you are in a different you."

(Erickson & Rossi, 1979, p. 372)

Deep hypnosis is that level of hypnosis that permits subjects to function adequately and directly at an unconscious level of awareness without interference by the conscious mind. [1952]

(In Erickson, 1980, Vol. I, chap. 6, p. 146)

Hypnosis is the ceasing to use your conscious awareness; in hypnosis you begin to use your unconscious awareness. Because unconsciously you know as much and a lot more than you do consciously.

(Zeig, 1980, p. 39)

It is a technique based upon an immediate direct eliciting of meaningful, unconsciously executed behavior which is separate and apart from consciously directed activity, except that of interested attention. [1959]

(In Erickson, 1980, Vol. I, chap. 8, p. 184)

Essentially, the "consciousness" is in a state of sleep, while the "subconsciousness" is left in control and in rapport with the hypnotist. This rapport, which constitutes a fixed phenomenon of hypnotic trances, may be defined as a state of harmony between the subject and hypnotist, with a dependence of the former upon the latter for motivating and guiding stimuli, and is somewhat similar to the "transference" of the psychoanalytic situation. It enables the hypnotist to remain in full contact with his subject while to the rest of the world the hypnotized person remains an unresponsive object.

(Erickson, 1934, p. 612)

An effective technique is one based upon repeated, long-continued hypnotic trances in which the subject reaches a stuporous state. In this trance stupor the subject is taught, by slow degrees, to obey suggestions and to react to situations in an integrated fashion. Only in this way can there be secured an extensive dissociation of the conscious from the subconscious elements of the personality which will permit a satisfactory manipulation of those parts of the personality under study. [1939]

(In Erickson, 1980, Vol. IV, chap. 1, p. 7)

The stuporous trance is characterized primarily by passive responsive behavior, marked by both psychological and physiological retardation. Spontaneous behavior and initiative, so characteristic of the somnambulistic state if allowed to develop, are lacking. There is likely to be a marked perseveration of incomplete responsive behavior, and there is a definite loss of ability to appreciate the self...the stuporous trance is difficult to obtain in many subjects, apparently because of their objection to losing awareness of themselves as persons. [1952]

(In Erickson, 1980, Vol. I, chap. 6, p. 147)

What hypnosis actually is can be explained as yet only in descriptive terms. Thus it may be defined as an artificially enhanced state of suggestibility resembling sleep wherein there appears to be a normal, time-limited and stimulus-limited dissociation of the "conscious" from the "subconscious" elements of the psyche. This dissociation is manifested by a quiescence of the "consciousness" simulating normal sleep and a delegation of the subjective control of the individual functions, ordinarily conscious, to the "subconsciousness." But any understanding of hypnosis beyond the descriptive phrase is purely speculative.

(Erickson, 1934, p. 611)

I carefully separate the conscious and unconscious and keep them separate.

(Erickson & Rossi, 1979, p. 290)

Well-trained subjects are not those laboriously taught to behave in a certain way, but rather those trained to rely completely upon their own unconscious patterns of response and behavior. [1952]

(In Erickson, 1980, Vol. I, chap. 6, p. 146)

The conscious mind is to give full cooperation to the unconscious. You're feeding it to the unconscious.

(Erickson, Rossi & Rossi, 1976, p. 89)

Without proper differentiation, patients will utilize both conscious and unconscious behavior in the trance instead of relying primarily upon unconscious patterns of behavior. This leads to inadequate, faulty task performance. [1948]

(In Erickson, 1980, Vol. IV, chap. 4, p. 37)

Only by building up in each subject a capacity to function in an organized, integrated fashion while in the trance state can extensive complicated therapeutic or experimental work be done. [1939]

(In Erickson, 1980, Vol. IV, chap. 1, p. 6)

> **R:** *Trance is actually an active process wherein the unconscious is active but not directed by the conscious mind.* **Is that right?**
> **E: That's right.**
>
> *(Erickson, Rossi & Rossi, 1976, p. 138)*

Subjects Become Childlike and Literal in Deep Trance

A tendency to respond to the hypnotist in childlike, simple, and literal ways is a typical unconscious form of response and, as such, it is a good indicator that a deep trance condition has been established. Effective hypnotists recognize this shift in response style and adjust their own patterns of speech and response accordingly. In fact, they usually shift into a simpler, more literal or straightforward pattern of speech before the subject moves into this deep trance state because doing so seems to facilitate the subject's achievement of it. In this way the hypnotist anticipates the shift into an unconscious level of awareness, creates the expectation of it in the subject and actually elicits it.

It is interesting to note that this literalism of deeply hypnotized subjects is comparable to what has been termed "trance logic" in the relevant research. Research by Erickson and others has demonstrated consistently that a manifestation of "trance logic" is the only valid means of differentiating hypnotized subjects from persons instructed to simulate hypnosis. Evidently, it is a genuine demonstration of a fundamental shift in the mode of thought, perception and response of the subject. In Erickson's terms, it demonstrates the subject's use of and the availability of the natural literalism of the unconscious.

Regression, or a return to earlier and simpler patterns of behavior, characterizes all trances and can be utilized and enhanced to a remarkable degree. In the ordinary trance there tends to occur a significant literalness of a childlike character in the subject's understandings, the handwriting and other motor activities are childlike, and emotional attitudes reflect those of an earlier age.

(Erickson, 1954b, p. 23)

Her contention, with which I came to agree strongly, was that every hypnotic suggestion should be given in language permitting "ready and simplistic interpretation," explaining that the hypnotic state tended to limit the spoken word to its literal meaning. She further contended that precision and conciseness of instruction allowed subjects to respond in terms of their own understandings, free from added enforced implications of social adjustments. [1964]

(In Erickson, 1980, Vol. I, chap. 18, p. 374)

Hypnotic subjects do regress to simpler forms of thinking, feeling, and behavior. Simpler, more youthful, less complicated forms.

(Erickson, Rossi & Rossi, 1976, p. 175)

When you have a patient in a trance, the patient thinks like a child and reaches for an understanding.

(Erickson, Rossi & Rossi, 1976, p. 255)

It's [trance] a regression to a more simple mode of functioning, less complicated.

(Erickson, Rossi & Rossi, 1976, p. 257)

This literalness and this peculiar restriction of awareness to those items of reality constituting the

precise hypnotic situation is highly definitive of a satisfactory somnambulistic hypnotic trance. [1965]
(In Erickson, 1980, Vol. I, chap. 3, p. 95

Ordinarily, all trance behavior is characterized by a simplicity, a directness and a literalness of understanding, action and emotional response suggestive of childhood.
(Erickson, 1970, p. 996)

R: In the trance it's harder to think?
E: Yes.
(Erickson, Rossi & Rossi, 1976, p. 56)

The experiment was based originally upon the observed literalness of hypnotic subjects when responding to instructions, questions, or suggestions. Such literalness of response is decidedly infrequent in everyday living — when it does occur then is suspect of being a deliberate play, as it often is. [circa 1940's]
(In Erickson, 1980, Vol. III, chap. 10, p. 92)

The *literalness* of the trance state causes the patient to have a new pattern of listening. He listens to the words in a trance state rather then to the ideas. [1973]
(In Erickson, 1980, Vol. III, chap 11, p. 100)

Trance is a simpler and uncomplicated way of functioning.
(Erickson, Rossi & Rossi, 1976, p. 252)

You see, hypnotic behavior at all levels is much more uncomplicated than adult behavior. Your walking's different, your writing is different, your speech is different. Your replies to things are much less complicated and your emotional reactions are much simpler. Now that's covered up with a veneer of adult culture.
(ASCH, 1980, Taped Lecture, 8/8/64)

> **I like to joke with my patients in the trance state,
> rather simple jokes, rather childish jokes.**
>
> *(ASCH, 1980, Taped Lecture, 2/2/66)*

Somnambulism and Post-Hypnotic Suggestions

The deep trance state can be utilized to secure other forms of hypnosis. Subjects can be instructed to act as if they were in their normal state, but to remain deeply hypnotized all the while they are doing so. The result is termed *somnambulism.* Although this is an interesting phenomenon, it is not necessary in order to elicit most hypnotic responses. Its primary therapeutic value lies in its potential to enable a subject to conduct routine business for several hours or days while remaining deeply hypnotized. Such extended hypnosis may enable the subject to utilize previously unavailable unconscious material to solve problems and to learn new patterns of response.

Post-hypnotic responses provide a similar opportunity to extend the hypnotic experience beyond the boundaries of the immediate hypnotic situation. An instruction or suggestion can be provided to the subject which will trigger the reappearance of the trance condition later on in a situation where it may be useful. How or why this can occur is unknown, but it remains a useful tool nonetheless.

> **A striking phenomenon of the profound trance is somnambulism. This is a state of deep hypnosis in which the subject can present the outward appearance and behavior of ordinary awareness but is able to manifest readily and often spontaneously any type of hypnotic behavior within his personal capabilities.**
>
> *(Erickson, 1970, p. 996)*

Finally, there can be induced in trances by means of posthypnotic suggestions a state of somnambulism wherein the subject appears to be normally awake. ... In appearance and nature this somnambulistic state is an experimental equivalent to the state of dissociation in dual personalities met in psychiatric practice. It differs only in being benign, time-limited and wholly dependent upon definite suggestions from the hypnotist.

(Erickson, 1934, p. 612)

This author feels that a somnambulistic hypnotic subject spontaneously apprehends the surrounding environment of realities differently than does a subject in the ordinary state of waking consciousness, and that the one type of reality apprehension does not preclude the other type of reality apprehension. [1967]

(In Erickson, 1980, vol. I, chap. 2, p. 82)

The author was [in 1920's] much interested in the nature and wording of suggestions that would be most effective and was very much under the mistaken impression that all hypnotic phenomena depended upon the induction of a somnambulistic state. [1967]

(In Erickson, 1980, Vol. I, chap. 2, p. 18)

The post-hypnotic performance and its associated spontaneous trance constitute dissociation phenomena, since they break into the ordinary stream of conscious activity as interpolations, and since they do not become integrated with the ordinary course of conscious activity. [1941]

(In Erickson, 1980, Vol. I, chap. 19, p. 411)

[The fact is disregarded] that there must necessarily be some state of mind which permits a coming forth into consciousness, or partial consciousness, of the post-hypnotic suggestion, of which, quite frequently, no awareness can be detected in the subject until after the proper cue is given. Even then that awareness is of a peculiar, limited, and restricted character, not comparable to ordinary conscious awareness. [1941]
(In Erickson, 1980, Vol. I, chap. 19, p. 386)

Physiological and Perceptual Alterations

Hypnosis can be used to alter physiological and perceptual processes in various ways. Accomplishment of such alterations by hypnotic suggestion seems to require a recognition of the fact that subjects are restricted to their own experiential histories in generating such responses and of the fact that such alterations do not occur in isolation, they must occur within the total psychological/physiological context of the person.

To initiate the desired alterations, the hypnotist may have to assist subjects to discover a past experience that they can use to create the desired result. Subjects do not automatically know how to induce such negative hallucinations as deafness, color-blindness, anesthesias, or other alterations in perception; they may not even know that they can do so. The hypnotist must use their experiential histories to teach them. Furthermore, an alteration in one perceptual or physiological system may be correlated with alterations in other perceptual or motor systems. The exact pattern of alterations associated with a particular shift in one system varies from subject to subject, but an awareness of these correlations may help the hypnotist to discover which, if any, alterations in other systems will facilitate the desired change.

Finally, although alterations in physiological functions are possible and may be useful, hypnosis is seldom able to provide the immediate and profound improvements a patient would like. There are limits to the degree of improvement in physiological functioning that hypnosis can initiate. It is not, as many patients hope it will be, a miracle cure.

While a negative hallucination could be achieved readily in a deep trance, it would be most difficult in a light or medium trance, because negative hallucinations were most destructive of reality values, even those of the hypnotic situation. [1965]

(In Erickson, 1980, Vol. I, chap. 3, p. 98)

If such subjects are given adequate time to reorganize their neuro and psychophysiological processes, negative hallucinations can be developed which will withstand searching test procedures. [1952]

(In Erickson, 1980, Vol. I, chap. 6, p. 142)

Direct suggestions of color blindness were ineffectual since they were at absolute variance with the subject's intellectual grasp of reality and thus in utter conflict with the established products of past learnings and experience. [1939]

(In Erickson, 1980, Vol. II, chap. 3, p. 26)

You give them the idea of a particular sensory state because, you see, all hypnotic phenomena derive from learnings that you experience in everyday life. [1959]

(In Erickson, 1980, Vol. III, chap. 4, p. 31)

The suggestion to see a specific color would serve to establish a certain "mental set," leading to the various preliminary psychophysiological processes upon which

could be based the initiation of the actual activity of color vision, and which would be derived from the psychophysiological activities based upon past learnings. [1938]

(In Erickson, 1980, Vol. II, chap. 1, pp. 8-9)

First is the effect of the instruction to *see*. This instruction itself, even if the subject had his eyes closed, would constitute an actual stimulus serving to arouse into activity various psychophysiological processes preliminary to vision and upon which visual activity could be based. [1938]

(In Erickson, 1980, Vol. II, chap. 1, p. 8)

In addition to the behavior that is suggested, there may also be elicited, as seemingly coincidental manifestations, marked changes in one or another apparently unrelated modality of behavior. [1943]

(In Erickson, 1980, Vol. II, chap. 14, p. 145)

Hypnotic suggestions bearing upon one sphere of behavior may remain ineffective until, as a preliminary measure, definite alterations are first induced hypnotically in an apparently unrelated and independent modality of behavior. [1943]

(In Erickson, 1980, Vol. II, chap. 14, pp. 145-146)

Also it was learned that in these subjects it was not possible to induce deafness unless they were allowed to develop other sensory disturbances. [1938]

(In Erickson, 1980, Vol. II, chap. 10, p. 91)

In brief, the hypnotic induction of disturbances in any chosen modality of behavior is likely to be accompanied by disturbances in other modalities. [1943]

(In Erickson, 1980, Vol. II, chap. 14, p. 153)

Now I think all of you ought to consider this matter of re-educating the physiological responses of the body. If we can do it in one area, we can do it in another...Such an attitude of expectancy is far more conducive to our task of exploration, discovery and healing. [1958]

(In Erickson, 1980, Vol. II, chap. 20, p. 202)

Hence, when I try to induce physiological changes, I try to start at the beginning; that is, as far as I personally can understand the beginning of those things. I try to build it up, and to build it up in such a general fashion that my subject or my patient can translate it into his own experiential life.

(Erickson, 1977a, p. 19)

To produce physiological changes, one ought to go about it with the realization that those physiological changes occur in the total body and in relationship to the total psychological picture that exists at the time.

(Erickson, 1977a, p. 18)

Consequently, efforts to alter the physical state, regardless of the technical skill employed and the excellence of the results obtained, are not appreciated, since the patient's hopeful expectations are not limited to the actual possibilities of the physical realities. [1955]

(In Erickson, 1980, Vol. IV, chap. 56, p. 499)

Summary

Erickson's descriptions of the hypnosis experience emphasize the focusing of attention toward internal events and the loss of interest in or conscious awareness of external realities. Gradually, subjects become aware of and responsive only to these internally generated realities and only the hypnotist remains in rapport with the subject. The subject's passive responsiveness can be enhanced and can enable the hypnotist to stimulate and guide awareness of internal events in ways that elicit the vivification of memories, thoughts, and previously hidden abilities.

Hypnosis, however, does not create new abilities. All hypnotic phenomena depend upon the use of normal capacities in new ways. Similarly, hypnosis does not create automatons who respond unthinkingly to any and all suggestions. Subjects will reject suggestions that they find unacceptable.

Although all subjects respond to the hypnotic process differently and manifest their hypnotized conditions in unique ways, there are some universal indicators of trance development. These are more apparent as subjects enter a deep trance state wherein all awareness and functioning occurs through the unconscious mind and the patterns of the conscious mind are ignored for the time being. This reversal of the ordinary relationship of the conscious and unconscious minds is marked by the appearance of a more literal and childlike pattern of response from the subject and an increased availability of thoughts and memories previously hidden from awareness.

Hypnosis may be used to initiate somnambulism, the performance of waking patterns of activity even though the subject remains in a deep trance condition. It may also be used to establish post-hypnotic responses of various kinds and to modify physiological and perceptual processes, although the effective elicitation of any and all hypnotic responses generally requires some learning on the part of the subject. Finally, the recognition that these responses occur in a larger psychological/physiological context which may require some seemingly extraneous modifications in order for the suggested responses to occur can facilitate matters for both the hypnotist and the subject.

CHAPTER NINE

INDUCING HYPNOSIS: GENERAL CONSIDERATIONS

Before attempting an hypnotic induction, there are several general principles that must be taken into consideration. These general principles form the context within which the actual induction process should be conducted. Interestingly, these principles bear a striking resemblence to many of the general considerations previously reviewed in the discussion of psychotherapy.

Anyone Can Be Hypnotized

Most contemporary research has indicated that only a small percentage (about 20%) of the general population is highly hypnotizable. The remainder is usually labeled only mildly hypnotizable or not hypnotizable at all. Erickson challenged the accuracy of these findings and attributed them to the faulty or inappropriate hypnotic techniques used to elicit hypnotic responses in the research tradition. To him, hypnosis was a normal and common experience in which virtually anyone can participate given the right circumstances and the right hypnotist. Obviously, no hypnotist can hypnotize everyone, but Erickson maintained that a good hypnotist could hyponotize many more people than the research would suggest.

> **So far as I know, hypnosis as a form of human behavior has been in existence since the beginning of the human race. [1960]**
>
> *(In Erickson, 1980, Vol. II, chap. 33, p. 341)*

> **Trance is a common experience. A football fan watching a game on TV is awake to the game but is not awake to his body sitting in the chair or his wife calling him to dinner.**
>
> *(Erickson, Rossi & Rossi, 1976, p. 47)*

> **In an airport I will notice someone seated, staring into space in what I recognize as the *common everyday trance*.**
>
> *(Erickson & Rossi, 1981, p. 49)*

> **Hypnotic phenomena are universal and must be taken into consideration in all efforts to understand the neuroses. [1939]**
>
> *(In Erickson, 1980, Vol. III, chap. 23, p. 253)*

> **It [hypnosis] is a normal phenomenon of the human mind, fairly explicable, as are all other psychological processes, in our crude concepts of mental mechanisms. [1932]**
>
> *(In Erickson, 1980, Vol. I, chap. 24, p. 493)*

The best hypnotic subjects are normal people of superior intelligence and any really cooperative person can be hypnotized.

(Erickson, 1941b, p. 14)

Any normal person and some abnormal persons can be hypnotized provided there is adequate motivation. [circa 1950's]

(In Erickson, 1980, Vol. IV, chap. 21, p. 226)

One hundred percent of normal people are hypnotizable. It does not necessarily follow that 100 percent are hypnotizable by any one individual. [1959]

(In Erickson, 1980, Vol. III, chap. 4, p. 29)

The eidetic imagery of children, their readiness, eagerness and actual need for new learnings, their desire to understand and to share in the activities of the world about them, and the opportunities offered by "pretend" and imitation games all serve to enable children to respond competently and well to hypnotic suggestions. [1958]

(In Erickson, 1980, Vol. IV, chap. 15, p. 180)

Practically all normal people can be hypnotized, though not necessarily by the same person, and practically all people can learn to be hypnotists. [1944]

(In Erickson, 1980, Vol. IV, chap. 2, p. 17)

Hypnosis Requires the Right Atmosphere

Because hypnosis is a cooperative endeavor, it requires almost exactly the same atmosphere as psychotherapy. If the interpersonal communication of ideas necessary for hypnosis is to be accomplished, the hypnotist must create a situation wherein the subject experiences a confident expectation of success, a casual freedom, a considerate protection, and an appreciative acceptance by the hypnotist.

One needs the respect, confidence, and trust of a subject.

(Erickson, 1941b, p. 15)

I learned that when you give suggestions, therapeutically or experimentally, you try to give them in a way that is going to permit the patient or the subject to handle them in a fashion that does not arouse too much difficulty.

(Erickson, 1977b, p. 21)

You must be careful to protect the integrity of the personality and not exploit the trance state.

(Erickson, Rossi & Rossi, 1976, p. 13)

A systematic effort is made to demonstrate to the subjects that they are in a fully protected situation. Measures to this end are relatively simple and seemingly absurdly inadequate. Nevertheless, personality reactions make them effective. [1952]

(In Erickson, 1980, Vol. I, chap. 6, p. 150)

In any hypnotic work careful attention must be given to the full protection of the subjects' ego by meeting readily their needs as individuals. [1952]

(In Erickson, 1980, Vol. I, chap. 6, p. 151)

In addition she was made aware at a deep level that she, as a personality, was fully protected, that her functioning rather than the hypnotist's was the primary consideration in trance induction, and that utilization of one

process of behavior could be made a stepping-stone to development of a similar but more complex form. [1952]
(In Erickson, 1980, Vol. I, chap. 6, p. 157)

This protection should properly be given subjects in both the waking and the trance states. It is best given in an indirect way in the waking state and more directly in the trance state. [1952]
(In Erickson, 1980, Vol. I, chap. 6, p. 149)

Appreciation must be definitely expressed in some manner, preferably first in the trance state and later in the ordinary waking state. [1952]
(In Erickson, 1980, Vol. I, chap. 6, p. 151)

You always give praise to the unconscious.
(Erickson & Rossi, 1979, p. 183)

She was always adequately praised for her cooperation in both the trance and waking states. [1960]
(In Erickson, 1980, Vol. IV, chap. 16, p. 185)

I make this clear to patients in the waking state as well as in the trance state, because you are dealing with a person that has a conscious mind and an unconscious mind.
(Erickson & Rossi, 1981, p. 6)

The simpler and more permissive and unobtrusive is the technique, the more effective it has proved to be. [1964]
(In Erickson, 1980, Vol. I, chap. 1, p. 15)

The more casually hypnotic work can be done, the easier it is for subjects to adapt to it. Casualness permits ready utilization of the behavioral developments of the total hypnotic situation. [1952]
(In Erickson, 1980, Vol. I, chap. 6, p. 166)

An essential consideration in this technique, however, is an attitude on the part of the operator of utter expectancy, casualness, and simplicity, which places the responsibility for any developments entirely upon the subject. [1959]

(In Erickson, 1980, Vol. I, chap. 8, p. 186)

In brief, hypnosis is a cooperative experience depending upon a communication of ideas by whatever means available, and verbalized ritualistic, traditional rote-memory techniques for the induction of hypnosis are no more than one means of beginning to learn how to communicate ideas and understandings in a joint task in which one person voluntarily seeks aid or understandings from another. [1964]

(In Erickson, 1980, Vol. I, chap. 14, p. 336)

Long overdue is the fulfillment of the need to recognize that meaningful communication should replace repetitious verbigerations, direct suggestions, and authoritarian commands.

(Bandler & Grinder, 1975, p. ix)

Now in hypnotizing the psychiatric patient I think one of the important things to do first is to establish a good conscious rapport. Let him know that you are definitely interested in him and his problems, and definitely interested in using hypnosis if in your judgement you think it will help.

(Erickson & Rossi, 1981, p. 5)

Hypnosis Depends Upon Cooperation

The hypnotist is totally dependent upon the cooperation of the subject to secure good results. Anything the hypnotist does to enhance cooperation is an important element in the induction process and any circumstance that may inhibit cooperation should be eliminated.

Any really *cooperative* subject may be [hypnotized] regardless of whether he is a normal person, a hysterical neurotic, or a psychotic schizophrenic patient. [1939]
(In Erickson, 1980, Vol. 4, chap. 1, p. 5)

Hypnosis depends primarily upon cooperation by the subject. [1944]
(In Erickson, 1980, Vol. IV, chap. 2, p. 16)

Since hypnosis is dependent fundamentally upon the subject's cooperativeness and his willingness to be hypnotized, any technique eliciting the necessary cooperation is adequate to this highly specialized interpersonal relationship. [1945]
(In Erickson, 1980, Vol. IV, chap. 3, p. 28)

Actually, the important consideration in inducing hypnosis is that the subject be willing, cooperative and interested in learning a new experience.
(Erickson, 1970, p. 995)

The *hypnotist-subject relationship* is entirely one of voluntary cooperation, and no subject can be hypnotized against his will or without his cooperation. [1944]
(In Erickson, 1980, Vol. IV, chap. 2, p. 16)

And bear this in mind, that you cannot hypnotize any patient who is unconsciously unwilling to be hypnotized.
(ASCH, 1980, Taped Lecture, 2/2/66)

Any unwillingness on the part of the subjects will cause them to become unresponsive and to awaken. [1941]
(In Erickson, 1980, Vol. I, chap. 19, p. 403)

Actually, of course, hypnosis depends upon full cooperation between hypnotist and subject, and without willing cooperation there can be no hypnosis. Furthermore, the hypnotic subject can be both hypnotist and subject, and more than one hypnotist has been hypnotized in turn by his own subjects to further the development of experimental work.

(Erickson, 1941b, p. 14)

No hypnotist knows for a certainly whether or not he is going to succeed with a particular subject at a given time or whether his technique for the occasion will be sufficient for the maintenance of the trance.

(Erickson, 1934, p. 612)

The presence of a certain mood may facilitate or hinder hypnotic responses. [1952]

(In Erickson, 1980, Vol. I, chap. 6, p. 142)

Experience since medical school days has progressively emphasized to the author that personal needs are strongly correlated with the intensity of the hypnotic state development. [1967]

(In Erickson, 1980, Vol. I, chap. 2, p. 70)

Since hypnosis is dependent upon cooperation in a common purpose, a feeling of goodness and adequacy is desirable for both participants. [1958]

(In Erickson, 1980, Vol. IV, chap. 15, p. 175)

Ordinarily trance induction is based upon securing from the patients some form of initial acceptance and cooperation with the operator. [1959]

(In Erickson, 1980, Vol. I, chap. 8, p. 178)

Hence, any technique that permits the hypnotist to secure adequate and ready cooperation in this highly

specialized interpersonal relationship of hypnosis constitutes a good technique. [1944]

(In Erickson, 1980, Vol. IV, chap. 2, p. 17)

It [subject's behavior] was an expression of an actual willingness to cooperate in a way fitting to her needs. It needed to be utilized as such rather than to be overcome or abolished as resistance. [1952]

(In Erickson, 1980, Vol. I, chap. 6, p. 153)

I'm the teacher, therefore I really want her to do these things because I as the teacher can help her to learn the things that she really wants to learn. So it becomes a cooperative venture. [1965]

(In Erickson, 1980, Vol. I, chap. 9, p. 214)

Subjects Create Hypnosis

The hypnotist, like the teacher of any skill, merely provides instruction, advice, and an appropriate setting within which learning can occur. What, if anything, subjects learn and how they use that learning ultimately is up to them. Hypnotists do not induce trance; they help their subjects learn how to induce trances in themselves. The subject is the most important element of the hypnotic process and the hypnotist must remain mindful of that fact. Everything that happens during a hypnosis session is dependent primarily upon the subject's willingness and ability to learn the requisite responses and only secondarily upon the hypnotist's ability to assist in that process. The hypnotist creates an appropriate atmosphere, guides attention in particular directions, and offers stimuli in order to elicit helpful responses. Whether or not those efforts have any impact is purely up to the subject.

Actually, the development of a trance state is an intra-psychic phenomenon, dependent upon internal processes, and the activity of the hypnotist serves only to create a favorable situation. [1952]

(In Erickson, 1980, Vol. I, chap. 6, p. 151)

The proper use of hypnosis lies in the development of a situation favorable to responses reflecting the subject's own learnings, understandings, capabilities and experiences. This can then give the operator the opportunity to determine the proper approach for responsive behavior by the subject.

(Erickson, 1973, p. 105)

Thus the subjects discover by actual experience that they are not helpless automatons, that they can actually enjoy cooperating with the hypnotist, that they can succeed in executing hypnotic suggestions, and that it is their behavior rather than the hypnotist's that leads to success. [1952]

(In Erickson, 1980, Vol. I, chap. 6, p. 151)

There should be a constant minimization of the role of the hypnotist and a constant enlargement of the subject's role. [1952]

(In Erickson, 1980, Vol. I, chap. 6, p. 152)

The hypnotic state is not really induced by me but by yourselves.

(Erickson, Rossi & Rossi, 1976, p. 137)

The basic approach is to orient all hypnotic techniques about the subjects, who are the responsive components of the situation. [circa 1940's]

(In Erickson, 1980, Vol. I, chap. 11, p. 292)

Hypnosis becomes a vital personality experience in which the hypnotist plays primarily the role of an instrument, merely guiding or directing processes developing within the subject. [1945]
(In Erickson, 1980, Vol. IV, chap. 3, p. 33)

At best operators can only offer intelligent guidance and then intelligently accept their subjects' behaviors. [1964]
(In Erickson, 1980, Vol. I, chap. 1, p. 17)

Deep hypnosis is a joint endeavor in which the subject does the work and the hypnotist tries to stimulate the subject to make the necessary effort.
(Erickson & Rossi, 1979, p. 61)

Hence the hypnotic trance belongs only to the subject — the operator can do no more than learn how to proffer stimuli and suggestions that evoke responsive behavior based upon the subject's own experiential past. [1967]
(In Erickson, 1980, Vol. I, chap. 2, pp. 42–43)

It (hypnosis) derives from processes and functionings within the patient. The operator is merely someone who can offer intelligent advice and instruction to the patient and thus elicit from the patient the behavioral responses best fitted to the situation. [circa 1950's]
(In Erickson, 1980, Vol. IV, chap. 21, p. 224)

The operators or experimenters are unimportant in determining hypnotic results regardless of their understandings and intentions. It is what the subjects understand and what the subjects do, not the operators' wishes, that determine what shall be the hypnotic

phenomena manifested. [1964]
(In Erickson, 1980, Vol. I, chap. 1, pp. 16–17)

They should bear ever in mind that the role of the operator is no more than that of a source of intelligent guidance while the hypnotic subjects proceed with the work that demonstrates hypnotic phenomena, insofar as is permitted by the subjects' own endowment of capacities to behave in various ways. **[1964]**
(In Erickson, 1980, Vol. I, chap. 1, p. 15)

The less the operator does and *the more he confidently and expectantly allows the subjects to do*, the easier and more effectively will the hypnotic state and hypnotic phenomena be elicited in accord with the subjects' own capabilities and uncolored by efforts to please the operator. **[1964]**
(In Erickson, 1980, Vol. I, chap. 1, p. 15)

Whatever the part played by the hypnotist may be, the role of the subjects involves the greater amount of active functioning — functioning which derives from the capabilities, learnings, and experiential history of their total personalities. Hypnotists can only guide, direct, supervise, and provide the opportunity for subjects to do the productive work. To accomplish this, hypnotists must understand the situation and its needs, protect the subjects fully and be able to recognize the work accomplished. They must accept and utilize the behavior that develops and be able to create opportunities and situations favorable for adequate functioning of their subjects. **[1952]**
(In Erickson, 1980, Vol. I, chap. 6, p. 167)

> It (hypnosis) is not a matter of the operator *doing*
> something to subjects or *compelling* them to do things or
> even *telling them what to do and how to do it.* When
> trances are so elicited, they are still the result of ideas,
> associations, mental processes and understandings
> already existing and merely aroused within the subjects
> themselves. Yet too many investigators working in the
> field regard *their activities* and *their intentions and
> desires* as the effective forces; and they actually un-
> critically believe that their own utterances to the subject
> elicit, evoke or initiate specific responses without seeming
> to realize that what they say or do only serves as a means
> to stimulate and arouse in the subjects past learnings,
> understandings, and experiential acquisitions, some con-
> sciously, some unconsciously, acquired. [1964]
>
> *(In Erickson, 1980, Vol. I, chap. 13, p. 326)*

Hypnosis Must Be Tailored

Because the cooperative participation of the subject is such
a crucial aspect of effective hypnosis, it is logical to conclude
that the hypnotic technique used should be tailored to fit the
needs, attitudes, and expectations of the subject. It is the subject, not the hypnotist, who defines effective hypnotic technique. Hypnotists must be observant and flexible enough to
adapt their style to those needs and attitudes. There is no right
way to do hypnosis, except whatever way will work with each
unique collection of each subject's needs and beliefs.

Erickson's emphasis upon the necessity for tailoring the
hypnotic approach to suit both the needs of each subject and
the dynamics of the situation conveys the essence of his
criticism of the standardized approaches and of the research

results obtained using these approaches. He argued that the use of any standardized approach, especially an authoritarian one, was a totally inadequate way to determine the hypnotizability of a subject or to measure hypnotic phenomena in any respect. The results obtained using standardized approaches, especially the low hypnotic responsiveness of the general population, were viewed by Erickson as inadvertent measures of the relative ineffectiveness of such approaches. His vehemence on this topic should be enough to dissuade any prospective hypnotist from trying to become a hypnotist by memorizing a set of phrases. If it does not, the ineffectiveness of such an approach probably will.

Adaptation of hypnotic techniques to the patient and his needs, rather than vice versa, leads readily and easily to effective therapeutic results. [1958]

(In Haley, 1967, p. 430)

Regardless of a hypnotist's experiences and ability, a paramount consideration in inducing deep trances and securing valid responses is a recognition of each subject as a personality, the meeting of their needs, and an awareness and a recognition of their patterns of unconscious functioning. The hypnotists, not the subjects, should be made to fit themselves into the hypnotic situation. [1952]

(In Erickson, 1980, Vol. I, chap. 6, p. 161)

Concerning the technique of the induction of hypnotic trances, this is a relatively simple matter requiring primarily time, patience, and careful attention to and consideration for the subject, his personality, and his emotional attitudes and reactions.

(Erickson, 1941b, p. 14)

A good hypnotic technique is one that offers to the patients, whether child or adult, the opportunity to have their needs of the moment met adequately, the opportunity to respond to stimuli and ideas, and also the opportunity to experience the satisfactions of new learnings and achievements. [1958]

(In Erickson, 1980, Vol. IV, chap. 15, p. 180)

No set, rigid technique can be followed with good success since, in medical hypnosis, the personality needs of the individual subject must be met, and such is the purpose of hypnosis rather than the mere induction of a trance. [1945]

(In Erickson, 1980, Vol. IV, chap. 3, p. 30)

Too often, the effort is made to fit the patients to an accepted formal technique of suggestion, rather than adopting the technique to the patients in accord with their actual personality situation. [1958]

(In Erickson, 1980, Vol. I, chap. 7, p. 175)

It must be borne in mind that subjects differ as personalities, and that hypnotic techniques must be tailored to fit the individual needs and the needs of the specific situation. [1964]

(In Erickson, 1980, Vol. I, chap. 1, p. 15)

One of the reasons for the decision not to publish at that time was the author's dubiousness concerning Hull's strong conviction that the operator, through what he said and did to the subject, was much more important than any inner behavioral processes of the subject. This view Hull carried over into his work at Yale, one instance of which was his endeavor to establish a "standardized technique" for induction. By this term he meant the use of the same words, the same length of time, the same tone of voice, etc., which finally eventuated in an attempt to elicit comparable trance states by playing "induction phonograph records" without regard for individual differences in subjects, and for their varying degrees of interest, of different motivations, and of variations in the capacity to learn. Hull seemed thus to disregard subjects as persons, putting them on a par with inanimate laboratory apparatus despite his awareness of such differences among subjects that could be demonstrated by tachistoscopic experiments. [1964]

(In Erickson, 1980, Vol. I, chap. 1, p. 4)

In other words the "standardized technique," or the giving of identical suggestions to different subjects described by Hull (1933), is not, as he appears to believe, a controlled method for eliciting the same degree or type of response, but merely a measure of demonstrating the general limitations of such a technique. [1941]

(In Erickson, 1980, Vol. I, chap. 19, p. 399)

Adequate use of hypnosis is not dependent upon patter, verbiage, what the operator knows, understands, expects, hopes for, wants to do, or the offering of instruction in accord with the operator's understandings, hopes, and desires. On the contrary, the proper use of hypnosis lies in the development of a situation favorable to responses reflecting the subject's own learnings, understandings, capabilities, and experiences. This can give the operator the opportunity to determine the proper approach for responsive behavior by the subject. These considerations have been increasingly recognized by the author during the past 20 years as basic requisites in the development of hypnotic techniques and of psychotherapy. Subject behavior should reflect only the subject himself and not the teachings, hopes, beliefs, or expectations of the operator. [1973]

(In Erickson, 1980, Vol. II, chap. 13, p. 137)

One of the most absurd of these endeavors, illustrative of a frequent tendency to disregard hypnosis as a phenomenon in favor of an induction technique as a rigidly controllable process apart from the subject's behavior, was the making of phonograph records. This was done on the assumption that identical suggestions would induce identical hypnotic responses in different subjects and at different times. There was a complete oversight of the individuality of subjects, their varying capacities to learn and to respond, and their differing attitudes, frames of reference, and purposes for engaging in hypnotic work. There was oversight of the importance of *interpersonal relationships* and of the fact that these are both contingent and dependent upon the *intrapsychic* or *intrapersonal relationships* of the subject. [1952]

(In Erickson, 1980, Vol. I, chap. 6, p. 140)

In his comments he [Erickson] spoke adversely about the direct, emphatic and authoritative suggestions that had been employed and indicated that no real effort had been made to meet the subject's seeming uneasiness and self-consciousness in being before an audience or his possible resentments or resistances toward the autocratic way in which he had been handled. The author stressed the importance of *gentle, permissive,* and *indirect* suggestions, emphasizing that *direct* suggestions may give rise to resistances.

The author's comments were somewhat resented by the speaker. [1964]

(In Erickson, 1980, Vol. I, chap. 15, p. 352)

In the light of present day knowledge hypnotism is looked upon in intelligent circles as a normal though unusual and little understood phenomenon of the human mind, dependent wholly upon the cooperation of the subject, and which can be practiced by anybody willing to

learn the psychological principles and technique involved. [1932]

(In Erickson, 1980, Vol. I, chap. 24, p. 495)

Use Whatever the Subject Presents

Utilization of whatever behaviors, attitudes or emotions the subject displays throughout the hypnosis process is a fundamental principle of Erickson's approach to hypnosis just as it is fundamental to his approach to psychotherapy. Anything the subject does, thinks or feels, can be used to facilitate an hypnotic experience. Resistance can be encouraged and resistant responses can be directed toward an hypnotic induction. Resistance, hostility, constant movement, uncontrollable giggling, anxiety, etc., are only problems if the hypnotist believes that there is a right way to enter hypnosis. If subjects have agreed to participate in hypnosis, even if they have simply entered a hypnotist's office, then anything they do is just fine and should be reacted to as such by the hypnotist. Their actions and reactions can be viewed as their demonstration of the routes they have to take to get into hypnosis from where they are and they should be accepted gratefully and utilized creatively to gradually or rapidly move the person into an hypnotic state.

Whatever the behavior offered by the subjects, it should be accepted and utilized to develop further responsive behavior. Any attempt to "correct" or alter the subjects' behavior, or to force them to do things they are not interested in, militates against trance induction and certainly deep trance experience. [1952]

(In Erickson, 1980, Vol. I, chap. 6, p. 155)

The Confusion Technique alters the situation from a contest between two people and transforms it into a therapeutic situation in which there is joint cooperation and participation in the mutual task centering properly about the patient's welfare and not about a contest between individuals, an item clinically to be avoided in favor of the therapeutic goal. [1964]

(In Erickson, 1980, Vol. I, chap. 10, p. 288)

Don't do what so many of us do and that's try to deal with what "should" be. Deal with what *is*. Deal with the patient as he is there.

(Beahrs, 1977, p. 60)

In Techniques of Utilization the usual procedure is reversed to an initial acceptance of, and ready cooperation with, the patient's presenting behavior by the operator, however seemingly adverse the presenting behaviors appear to be in the clinical situation. [1959]

(In Erickson, 1980, Vol. I, chap. 8, p. 178)

The value of this type of Utilization Technique probably lies in its effective demonstration to the patients that they are completely acceptable and that the therapist can deal effectively with them regardless of their behavior. *It meets both the patients' presenting needs and it employs as the significant part of the induction procedure the very behavior that dominates the patients.* [1959]

(In Erickson, 1980, Vol. I, chap. 8, pp. 181–182)

Another essential element in technique — for either investigative or therapeutic work — is the utilization of the subject's own patterns of learning and response, rather than an attempt to force upon him by suggestion the hypnotist's limited comprehension of what constitutes experiential validity for the subject.

(Erickson, 1970, p. 995)

Unfortunately lack of critical observation or inexperience sometimes leads to the inference that the subjects are unresponsive rather than the realization that they are most responsive in a more complex fashion than was intended. [1964]

(In Erickson, 1980, Vol. I, chap. 1, p. 13)

Such persons remain seemingly unhypnotizable, often despite an obvious capacity for responsiveness, until their special individual needs are met in a manner satisfying to them. [1959]

(In Erickson, 1980, Vol. I, chap. 8, p. 188)

Many times, the apparently active resistance encountered in subjects is no more than an unconscious measure of testing the hypnotist's willingness to meet them halfway instead of trying to force them to act entirely in accord with his ideas.

(Erickson & Rossi, 1979, p. 67)

In general teaching about hypnosis, they tell you to avoid resistance. ... Use it.

(Zeig, 1980, p. 338)

You can always yield and come out on top.

(Zeig, 1980, p. 322)

There are patients who prove unresponsive and resistant to the usual induction techniques, who are actually readily amenable to hypnosis.....These patients are those who are unwilling to accept any suggested behavior until after their own resistant, contradictory or opposing, behavior has first been met by the operator. [1959]

(In Erickson, 1980, Vol. I, chap. 8, p. 177)

One often reads in the literature about subject resistance and the techniques employed to circumvent or overcome it. In the author's experience the most satisfactory procedure is that of accepting and utilizing the resistance as well as any other type of behavior, since properly used, they can all favor the development of hypnosis. [1952]

(In Erickson, 1980, Vol. I, chap. 6, p. 154)

Thus a situation is created in which the subjects can express their resistance in a constructive, cooperative fashion; manifestation of resistance by subjects is best utilized by developing a situation in which resistance serves a purpose. [1952]

(In Erickson, 1980, Vol. I, chap. 6, p. 154)

I'm taking control of any rebellion by telling him how to rebel.

(Erickson & Rossi, 1981, p. 183)

You don't dispute with patients when you see them responding...Too many people who use hypnosis try to argue with skepticism. I don't bother. That is part of my prestige — I just don't argue.

(Erickson & Rossi, 1981, p. 250)

As she entered the office, she remarked that she would probably be hypnotized by a single glance from the writer and that she most likely would not even know she was in a trance. No effort was made to disillusion her. [1955]

(In Erickson, 1980, Vol. IV, chap 56, p. 500)

The author then simply, deliberately, *utilized* their own state of irrational thinking to effect a favorable outcome by the use of a hypnotic technique of the presentation of ideas in a fashion conducive to acceptance.

(Erickson & Rossi, 1979, p. 363)

Thus his distressing feeling of weakness and his dull, throbbing ache were utilized to secure a redirection and a reorientation of his attentiveness and responsiveness to his somatic sensations and to secure a new and acceptable perception of them. [1959]

(In Erickson, 1980, Vol. IV, chap. 27, p. 259)

Now here is a trained man, skeptical! I had to meet him at that level. I had to give my suggestions in a way that would meet his needs for scientific understanding. I had to phrase what I said in ways that would appeal to his unconscious mind...ways he would not be able to analyze.

(Erickson & Rossi, 1981, p. 181)

Use Language to Elicit Responses

The hypnotist is heavily dependent upon the use of language to elicit the desired reactions and internal responses. The natural tendency in this circumstance is simply to tell subjects what to do. However, this direct authoritarian approach does nothing to help the subject learn how to respond and may lead to frustration and failure unless the subject is especially amenable to such directives *and* is capable of executing them.

Effective hypnotists avoid the unnecessary creation of an opportunity to fail by giving direct suggestions only for experiences that are inevitable in the natural course of events and that, thus, will happen no matter what the subject does or does not do. They also tend to rely almost exclusively upon indirect, even unnoticeable, suggestions. These indirect suggestions consist of statements, phrases, words, etc., that they know from past experience will initiate the desired shifts in awareness, patterns of thought, or internal response. In addition, suggestions are given in the broadest or most permissive manner possible or in double-bind fashion so that any response by the subject will seem to be a compliant response and they will become even more convinced and trusting of their own hypnotic capacities.

As mentioned previously, Erickson was fascinated by the unconscious impacts and idiosyncratic meanings of words. He used words that had one literal meaning and different associative meanings or connotations to communicate indirect messages. In this fashion he was able to initiate or elicit responses from subjects automatically and indirectly. Perhaps the most familiar example of this approach in our daily lives is the use of the sexual double-entendre when discussing a nonsexual topic with a member of the opposite sex. Although usually too blatant to be classifiable as an indirect communication, the similarity between this form of exchange and the indirect suggestion frequently used by Erickson is unmistakable. Even the typical shift in tone of voice to convey sexual intent is comparable to Erickson's use of the tone of his voice to convey his message of relaxation and comfort. These and other aspects of his linguistic skills are reflected in the following quotations and in the quotations presented in the next section of this chapter.

In speaking to patients, I always try to speak in the simplest kind of language that fits them as individuals.
(ASCH, 1980, Taped Lecture, 7/18/65)

The type of suggestions you give to a patient depends upon the attitude of that patient toward you and the therapeutic process.
(Erickson & Rossi, 1981, p. 14)

Suggestions are always given in a form that the patient can accept easily. Suggestions are statements that the patient cannot possibly argue with.

(Erickson, Rossi & Rossi, 1976, p. 7)

It is an inevitability and thus a safe suggestion that cannot be rejected. [1976–78]

(In Erickson, 1980, Vol. I, Chapter 23, p. 482)

It is always safe to suggest behavior that is inevitable in the natural course of things.

(Erickson, Rossi & Rossi, 1976, p. 29)

R: You make a lot of statements to patients that evoke certain *natural associative responses* within them. It is these responses *within them* that are the essence of hypnotic suggestion.
E: That is the hypnotic stuff, yes!

(Erickson & Rossi, 1981, p. 28)

However, regardless of the suggestibility of the subject, there is frequently a primary need to give suggestions indirectly rather than directly and dogmatically.

(Erickson, 1941b, p. 15)

In the induction of an hypnotic trance, one induces suggestions and primarily gives the suggestions in an indirect fashion. You should try to avoid as much as possible commanding or dictating to your patient. If you wish to use hypnosis with the greatest possible success, you present your idea to patients so that they can accept and examine it for its inherent value. [1959]

(In Erickson, 1980, Vol. III, chap. 4, p. 33)

Much of hypnotic psychotherapy can be accomplished indirectly.

(Erickson & Rossi, 1981, p. 12)

I may mispronounce a potent word because that is the word I want the patients to hear. I want that word to echo in their own minds correctly. If I mispronounce it slightly, they mentally correct it, but they are the ones that are saying it, they are making the suggestion to themselves. [1976–78]

(In Erickson, 1980, Vol. I, chap. 23, p. 489)

No one can predict with utter certainty just how a subject is going to use such stimuli. One names or indicates possible ways, the subjects behave in accord with their learnings. Hence the importance of loosely organized, comprehensive, permissive suggestions. [1964]

(In Erickson, 1980, Vol. I, chap. 13, p. 327)

We use words that have both a general and a very specific personal significance.

(Erickson, Rossi & Rossi, 1976, p. 93)

Because I can't always be certain just exactly where I am. But, I know how to play it. There are multiple meanings of words.

(Zeig, 1980, p. 312)

I'm amazed how long experience has taught me to cover many possibilities of response whenever I'm exploring a patient's inner life.

(Erickson & Rossi, 1979, p. 414)

You make general statements that a person can apply to specifics within his own life. [1973]

(In Erickson, 1980, Vol. III, chap. 11, p. 101)

But I learned thoroughly how to graduate my suggestions, and how to lead from one suggestion to another. When one does that sort of thing, *one learns how to follow the leads given by his patient.*

(Erickson & Rossi, 1981, p. 3)

You always use the patient's own words and experience as much as possible for trance induction and suggestion.

(Erickson, Rossi & Rossi, 1976, p. 29)

"Other experiences, other feelings" is a very inclusive generalization. It includes the possibility of utilizing trance feelings from everyday life that we all commonly experience when we are "absorbed" or in deep "reverie," concentrating very deeply on something. The patient does not recognize, however, that in accepting "other experiences, other feelings" he is actually including this possibility of trance experience from everyday life when he was similarly focused on a few inner feelings. [1976–78]

(In Erickson, 1980, Vol. I, chap. 23, p. 480)

It is very pleasant to wait also has sexual connotations. You just keep in mind all these ploys from everyday experience.

(Erickson & Rossi, 1979, p. 156)

R: You use words that have connotations, associations and patterns of meaning that have multiple applications for the person's interests and individuality. Is that the basic principle you use in your indirect approach to hypnotic communication?

E: Yes.

(Erickson & Rossi, 1981, p. 27)

"Perhaps" means you're not ordering, you're not instructing. [1976–78]

(In Erickson, 1980, Vol. I, chap. 23, p. 480)

How do you merge your voice with a patient's inner experience? You use words that ordinary life has taught you: "the whispering wind."

(Erickson, Rossi & Rossi, 1976, p. 91)

This sort of seemingly casual conversation loaded with minimal cues has many times been practiced by the author and his oldest son, sometimes on each other, more frequently upon others as a definite game or means of entertainment by enjoying intellectual ingenuity. [1964]
(In Erickson, 1980, Vol. I, chap. 15, p. 356)

The art of suggestion depends upon the use of words and the varied meaning of words. I've spent a great deal of time reading dictionaries. When you read the various definitions the same word can have, it changes entirely your conception of that word and how language may be used.
(Erickson & Rossi, 1981, p. 26)

There are *charged* words and you select words that carry a wealth of affective meaning and you select them with the greatest of care.
(ASCH, 1980, Taped Lecture, 7/16/65)

You have to be aware of the possible double-meaning words like "sun" that could be "son." I may have my ideas about what it means but I'm not going to ask her to betray it.
(Erickson & Rossi, 1979, p. 410)

He has a big itch! Never forget folk language! You should always recognize how the folk language is related to symptom formation.
(Erickson & Rossi, 1979, p. 277)

From my childhood on, I practiced talking on two or three levels.
(Erickson & Rossi, 1981, p. 27)

I think it's awfully important if you want to deal with patients with organic illness or psychogenic illness, that you know what you say and what the implications of what you say are. How they extend into the future and how they reach into the past and how they modify the present and how they convey understandings by the natural elaboration in terms of their own thinking that occurs when you speak.

(ASCH, 1980, Taped Lecture, 7/16/65)

If I want you to talk about your family, the easiest approach and the one least likely to arouse your resistance is for me to first talk about my family.

(Erickson & Rossi, 1979, p.386)

I can get any one of you to think about your school by saying "University of Wisconsin." I can tell you I was born in the Sierra Nevada Mountains, and all of you will know where you were born. You think about that. I speak about my sisters, and you think about yours if you have some — or think about not having sisters, if you don't have sisters. We respond to the spoken word in terms of our own learnings. Therapists ought to keep that in mind.

(Zeig, 1980, p. 70)

You need the practice of repeatedly attempting to get a patient to talk about something in ordinary everyday life.

(Erickson & Rossi, 1981, p. 8)

Essentially, the task, as worked out, was comparable to that of composing music intended to produce a certain effect upon the listener. Words and ideas, rather than notes of music, were employed in selected sequences, patterns, rhythms, and other relationships, and by this composition it was hoped to evoke profound responses in the subject, not only in terms of what the story could mean but which would be in accord with the established pat-

terns of behavior deriving from his experiential past.
[1944]

(In Erickson, Vol. III, chap. 29, p. 338)

Communication With the Unconscious

Erickson's use of indirect forms of communication was designed to do more than elicit responses in a reflex sort of way. Many, if not all, of his indirect communications also were designed to bypass the conscious mind and to contact the unconscious mind instead. By directing his communications to the unconscious mind he was able to initiate a deep trance state and to solicit the assistance of the unconscious mind in the accomplishment of hypnotic or therapeutic purposes.

Erickson accepted the ability of the unconscious mind to detect and to respond to indirect forms of communication that the conscious mind would miss or overlook. His acceptance and utilization of this fact led him to an emphasis upon the more subtle forms of communication such as tone of voice, inflection, breathing patterns, pauses, and body language, in addition to the linguistic indirect forms of communication mentioned previously. His constant endeavor was to communicate with and to elicit responses from the subject's unconscious mind whether or not the other person was in a trance state. Hypnosis was intriguing to him primarily because it facilitated this communication process, it made the subject's unconscious more available and responsive.

> **I wanted those ideas to soak into his unconscious.**
>
> *(Erickson, 1977b, p. 26)*

> **I set her up to place unconscious understandings on whatever I say.** *They* **will be her unconscious understandings.**
>
> *(Erickson & Rossi, 1979, p. 172)*

The more of my communications that are in her unconscious, the better she will be as a hypnotic subject.
                                    (Erickson & Rossi, 1981, p. 102)

They are not paying attention to what I say consciously. They are paying attention unconsciously, so there is no interference from consciousness.
                                    (Erickson, Rossi & Rossi, 1976, p. 9)

Semantics are important, but communication is basic. Hypnosis needs to be recognized as a science of intercommunication. [1970]
                                    (In Erickson, 1980, Vol. IV, chap. 6, p. 70)

You see, communication is not just words, it isn't just ideas. It is vocal stimulation, auditory stimulation and it is apparently leading somewhere (e.g. dangling phrases, repetition and then a complete sentence) causing the patient to reach out.
                                    (Erickson & Rossi, 1981, p. 104)

Use your voice — inflections, intonations, pauses, hesitations — in every possible way to convey your meaning.
                                    (ASCH, 1980, Taped Lecture, 7/16/65)

In therapeutic work I use intonations to influence more adequate personal responses by the patient. [1965]
                                    (In Erickson, 1980, Vol. I, chap. 3, pp. 94–95)

We are usually unaware of all the automatic responses we make on the basis of the locus of sound and the inflections of voice (Erickson, 1973). Thus such vocal cues are indirect forms of suggestion because they tend to facilitate automatic responses that can bypass conscious intentionality. [1976–78]
                                    (In Erickson, 1980, Vol. I, chap. 23, p. 481)

But you talk to the patient and you space your words and you alter intonations so that their unconscious mind separates out the various phrases that you want them to apply to themselves.

(ASCH, 1980, Taped Lecture, 2/2/66)

I use one tone of voice to speak to the conscious mind and another to speak to the unconscious. When you use one tone of voice that pertains to conscious thinking and another tone of voice that expresses other ideas which you intend for the unconscious, you are establishing a duality.

(Erickson & Rossi, 1976, p. 159)

Their mere presence within hearing distance of you allows their unconscious mind to work satisfactorily.

(Erickson & Rossi, 1981, p. 18)

When I am talking to a person at the conscious level, I expect him to be listening to me at an unconscious level, as well as consciously. And therefore I am not very greatly concerned about the depth of the trance the patient is in because I find that one can do extensive and deep psychotherapy in the light trance as well as in the deeper medium trance. One merely needs to know how to talk to a patient in order to secure therapeutic results.

(Erickson & Rossi, 1981, p. 3)

Now when you want to deal with patients, I think all of you ought to write out your speculating, theoretical suggestions. I think you ought to analyze them for the content and meanings of the individual words, content and meanings of the individual phrases and the sentences. And I think you recognize how to put into a phrase or word, a pause or a sentence, a meaning that is quite opposite to its apparent overt meaning.

(ASCH, 1980, Taped Lecture, 2/2/66)

This general difference between waking and hypnotized persons in the meaningfulness of communications has been noted in many other regards and has led to the general admonition to offer suggestions to the hypnotic subject with clarity and meaningfulness. Operators must be aware of what they are actually saying. [circa 1940's]
(In Erickson, 1980, Vol. III, chap. 10, p. 99)

Therapeutic trance enables patients to receive multiple levels of communication more easily.
(Erickson & Rossi, 1981, p. 27)

All of us are responsive, often unwittingly so, to a minimal change in the spoken voice when the head is changed to a different position and the voice thereby given a new direction. [1964]
(In Erickson, 1980, Vol. I, chap. 10, p. 267)

Altered tone of voice can constitute an actual vocabulary of transformation of verbal communications, as can body language.
(Bandler & Grinder, 1975, p. viii)

The body has learned how to follow minimal cues. You utilize that learning. You give your patient minimal cues. As he starts responding to those minimal cues, he gives more attention to any further cues you offer him.
(Erickson & Rossi, 1981, p. 44)

When you deal with patients you put the great big headlines on your face if their eyes are open, you put the great big headlines in your voice. But you use certain words for those headlines. And their unconscious is just as intelligent at age fifty as it was at age six months.
(ASCH, 1980, Taped Lecture, 2/2/66)

When you give a suggestion to a patient, feel it, sense it and mean it. Mean it with every bit of sincerity within you. Enter into it.

(ASCH, 1980, Taped Lecture, 7/16/65)

If you want a patient to feel relaxed, express it in your voice.

(ASCH, 1980, Taped Lecture, 7/16/65)

Summary

Erickson noted that anyone can be hypnotized, although he was quick to add that hypnosis is something subjects must do to themselves. Only subjects who are comfortable enough to cooperate will be able to learn to enter a hypnotic trance and even they must be allowed and even encouraged to enter the state in their own way and in accord with their own needs. Hypnotists must accept and utilize whatever qualities the subject presents and must carefully consider the form of their own verbalizations. Instead of rote memorization of a standardized technique, Erickson recommended that hypnotists utilize indirect suggestions and unconscious communications which are tailored to meet the subject's needs. Essentially, Erickson's general comments regarding the attitudes and roles of hypnotists are indistinguishable from his comments regarding the attitudes and roles of psychotherapists. Given that they are derived from the same background of observation and orientation toward people, this is not surprising.

CHAPTER TEN

INDUCING HYPNOSIS: SPECIFIC TECHNIQUES

The first question most students ask is, "What exactly do you say to induce hypnosis?" It should be apparent by now that there is no single or best thing to say; there is no universal script. If hypnotists know in general what is supposed to happen and have a clear understanding of their role in the process, then they will automatically do pretty much the right thing. Naturally, like any new teacher they will be nervous, awkward, and somewhat ineffectual at first, but given the right background and feedback during a series of practice sessions they will eventually begin to master the process in their own way.

The Ericksonian technique of inducing a trance, or, more properly, of helping people allow themselves to experience a trance, is a product of Erickson's descriptions of the hypnosis process and of his attitudes toward the respective roles of hypnotist and subject. The material contained in this chapter provides a view of the synthesis of these two components of Erickson's hypnotic technique. It is not a prescription for what to say or do but rather a broad description of the variety of things that can be done to facilitate or elicit the different phases of hypnotic induction.

Keep Your Role and Goal in Mind

The following section of quotations is a rather eclectic mix of general advice and guidelines. It is presented here to answer some typical questions about the induction process, to refute common misunderstandings and mistakes, and to re-emphasize the appropriate roles and goals of the hypnotist. The orientation outlined here should be reviewed carefully prior to the beginning of a hypnosis session and held firmly in mind throughout.

> **In all the experimental work that I've done my feeling is that drugs of any sort are a handicap, cause then you have to deal with the patient *and* the drug effects, and you're handicapping yourself. The only drug I favor is an ounce of whiskey half an hour before the patient arrives — *you* take it.**
>
> *(ASCH, 1980, Taped Lecture, 8/8/64)*

> **In hypnosis what you want your patient to do is respond to an idea. It is your task, your responsibility, to learn how to address the patient, how to speak to the patient, how to secure his attention, and how to leave him wide open to the acceptance of an idea that fits into the situation.**
>
> *(Erickson & Rossi, 1981, p. 42)*

I do not like this matter of telling a patient, "I want you to get tired and sleepy, and to get tired and sleepier." That is an effort to force your wishes upon the patient. That is an effort to dominate the patient. It is much better to suggest that they *can* get tired, that they *can* get sleepy, that they *can* go into a trance.

(Erickson & Rossi, 1981, p. 4)

Hypnosis does not come from mere repetition. It comes from facilitating your patient's ability to accept an idea and to respond to that idea.

(Erickson & Rossi, 1981, p. 43)

Avoid a repetitious belaboring of the obvious. Once the patients and the therapist have a clear understanding of what is to be done, only fatigue is to be expected from further reiteration. [1958]

(In Erickson, 1980, Vol. I, chap. 7, p. 176)

Hypnosis, whether for adults or children, should derive from a willing utilization of the simple, good, and pleasing stimuli that serve in everyday life to elicit normal behavior pleasing to all concerned. [1958]

(In Erickson, 1980, Vol. IV, chap. 15, p. 175)

Hypnotic technique is giving stimuli that can be resolved by the subject into the hypnotic experience you wish her to have.

(Erickson & Rossi, 1979, p. 183)

Now here you are merely taking the learnings that the person already has and applying them in other ways.

(Erickson, Rossi & Rossi, 1976, p. 7)

It is the fashion in which you present the suggestion to the patient that is important.

(Erickson & Rossi, 1981, p. 3)

> **You don't have to know hypnosis. All you have to know is how people think this way and that way. You say this, and they absolutely are conditioned to think in a certain way.**
>
> *(Erickson & Rossi, 1981, p. 217)*

Fixate Attention

Ordinary conscious attention or awareness constantly flits from one thing to another and is focused in many different directions at once. Hypnosis, on the other hand, is characterized by focused awareness. The first task of the hypnotist, therefore, is to do or say something that will, in one way or another, fixate or capture the subject's attention or interest. There is no best way of doing this, it all depends upon the nature of the subject and of the situation. Some subjects can focus their attention reasonably well when simply asked to do so, but most will find it impossible to cease or quiet their constantly shifting awareness even when told to stare at a particular thing. We all know from personal experience and from routine observation of others that there are specific kinds of events that will capture and fixate attention even when there are many other potentially distracting events going on. Erickson employed an amazing array of such attention-catching devices in his inductions. The following examples may be used as guidelines, but obviously each hypnotist must develop individual repertoires of attention-compelling stimuli and must be willing to observe potential subjects closely to see what events normally capture their attention. Then, as a first step in the induction process, the hypnotist does or says things that will focus the subject's attention purely upon the hypnotist.

In the therapeutic use of hypnosis, one primarily meets the patients' needs on the terms they themselves propose; and then one fixates the patients' attention, through adequate respect for and utilization of their method of presenting their problem, to their own inner processes of mental functioning. This is accomplished by casual but obviously earnest and sincere remarks, seemingly explanatory but intended solely to stimulate a wealth of the patients' own patterns of psychological functioning so that they meet their problems by use of their learnings already acquired or that will develop as they continue their progress. [1964]

(In Erickson, 1980, Vol. I, chap. 13, p. 330)

He is verbalizing the forces that interfere with his discovering more about trance. There are so many forces: foci of attention.

(Erickson & Rossi, 1981, p. 238)

The induction procedure provides a setting, only a setting, in which hypnosis may develop; it offers a period of time during which it develops; it offers various distractions to absorb the attention of the subject while hypnosis occurs. [1962]

(In Erickson, 1980, Vol. II, chap. 33, p. 349)

As for research on hypnotic techniques, one should never forget that these are only a means of attracting the subject's attention, and we should not lose sight of the purpose of these techniques because of fascination with the variations which can be employed. [1960]

(In Erickson, 1980, Vol. II, chap. 31, p. 325)

The technique employed so successfully upon such diverse patients was essentially a rigid arresting and fixation of their attention and then placing them in a situation of extracting from the author's words certain meanings and significances that would fit into the patterns of their own thinking and understanding, their own emotions and wishes, their own memories, ideas, understandings, learnings, conditionings, associational and experiential acquisitions, and into their own pattern of response to stimuli. The author did not really instruct them. [1964]

(In Erickson, 1980, Vol. I, chap. 13, p. 329)

Therefore, keeping well and clearly in mind his actual wishes, the author casually and permissively (or apparently permissively) presents a wealth of seemingly related ideas in a manner carefully calculated to hold or to fixate the subject's attention rather than the subject's eyes or to induce a special muscle state. [1964]

(In Erickson, 1980, Vol. I, chap. 13, p. 328)

Therefore, it would be part of my responsibilities to be as aware as possible of the patient's various emotional states, to direct and to utilize them in such a fashion that the patient's attention and interest would be directed to me rather than elsewere. [1966]

(In Erickson, 1980, Vol. II, chap. 34, p. 351)

His interest was maintained at a high pitch and his attention was rigidly fixated

(Erickson & Rossi, 1975, p. 146)

With his attention and understandings thus fixated and centered, a hypnotic technique was used. [1964]

(In Erickson, 1980, Vol. I, chap. 13, p. 300)

Often it has been used to secure, to fixate and to hold the attention of difficult patients and to distract them from creating difficulties that would impede therapy. [1966]

(In Erickson, 1980, Vol. IV, chap. 28, p. 262)

Hypnosis began with the first statement to him and became apparent when he gave his full and undivided interested and pleased attention to each of the succeeding events that constituted the medical handling of his problem. [1958]

(In Erickson, 1980, Vol. IV, chap. 15, p. 179)

When you speak to a person, you let them know, "I'm speaking to *you!*" You can speak directly with your eyes or your voice or with a gesture. You have to have the person's attention.

(Erickson & Rossi, 1981, p. 208)

I use a soft voice because that compels attention.

(Erickson & Rossi, 1981, p. 208)

The use of the word "hell" arrested her attention completely. [1958]

(In Erickson, 1980, Vol. I, chap. 7, p. 174)

It is the continuity of the experience that is of importance — it is not just a single touch or pat or caress, but a continuity of stimulation that allows the child, however short its span of attention, to give a continued response to the stimulus. So it is in hypnosis, whether with adults or children....There is a need for a continuum of response-eliciting stimuli directed toward a common purpose. [1958]

(In Erickson, 1980, Vol. IV, chap. 15, p. 175)

She was told emphatically that she could do exactly as she wished, and this was followed by repeated, carefully worded suggestions given to her in a gentle, insistent and attention-compelling fashion, which served to induce the passively receptive state that marks initiation of a light hypnotic trance. [1938]

(In Erickson, 1980, Vol. III, chap. 17, p. 160)

Elaborate instruction was given to him to insure a calm, comfortable feeling and to induce an overwhelming interest in whatever the writer might have to say.

(Erickson, 1954c, p. 268)

R: You find an interest area of the person. An area where there are strong programs built into the person, and you focus on that to induce trance.

E: That's all!

R: But why do your subjects become so absorbed in their interest areas that trance behavior is evident?

E: Because I stick to that one thing!

(Erickson & Rossi, 1979, p. 369)

They are going to be *interested* in what makes me think they can be put into a trance. So I merely make use of their interest and keep away from a formal trance induction.

(Erickson & Rossi, 1979, p. 367)

R: How do you make use of their interest? You direct it to the inner parts of their own world?

E: Yes. And then I stay with them.

(Erickson & Rossi, 1979, p. 368)

I am willing to attract attention and then allow patients to be in mental doubt as to what they should think and do in that particular situation. This makes the patients amenable to any suggestion that fits the immediate situation.

(Erickson & Rossi, 1981, p. 42)

They are questions; they fixate attention and call upon thoughts and associations that are inevitable in her future.
(Erickson & Rossi, 1979, p. 194)

"How did you" is a question that gets him inside his own thoughts.
(Erickson & Rossi, 1981, p. 185)

I'm shifting her focus of attention with this question.
(Erickson & Rossi, 1976, p. 153)

When you hypnotize patients you are asking them to pay attention to ideas or to any parts of reality pertinent to the situation. The patients then narrow their attention down to the task at hand and give their attention to you. [1959]
(In Erickson, 1980, Vol. III, chap. 4, p. 29)

Each would cooperate in going into a deep trance by assessing, appraising, evaluating, and examining the validity and genuineness of each item of reality and of each item of subjective experience that was mentioned... In this manner there was effected for each woman a progressive narrowing of the field of awareness and a corresponding increase in a dependency upon, and a responsiveness to, the writer. [1959]
(In Erickson, 1980, Vol. I, chap. 8, p. 187)

Direct Attention Away From Reality

Once attention has been focused it must be directed toward the hypnotist (if the focusing stimulus was not the hypnotist in the first place) and away from the external events of reality. The hypnotist's actions or voice are the only external stimuli that should enter the subject's awareness at this point. Subjects may need to be reassured that they *can* continue to pay attention to the things happening around them but that there is *no need to try* to make the effort to do so for the time being. Their loss of contact with externalities may create a certain uneasiness or anxiety and cause an effort to re-establish reality contact unless the subject is reassured in this manner. Because the prior creation of an appropriate atmosphere of trust and cooperation facilitates this letting-go, it should actually be considered the first step in most induction situations.

Generally speaking, if subjects focus their attention entirely upon one thing, their perception of all other reality events will diminish or cease quite automatically. Recognition of this necessary product of highly focused attention can speed up the induction process considerably by eliminating the need to say or do anything extra to diminish the subject's perception of reality. The stimulus condition that was used to focus attention can be used at the same time to direct that focused attention away from other reality events. The hypnotist can merely point out this loss of reality contact as an indicator of trance without ever having directly suggested a loss of reality contact. This can be an impressively convincing demonstration to the subject that a trance induction is happening.

> **And it isn't necessary for you to waste mental energy on realities, the external realities.**
>> *(Erickson, Rossi & Rossi, 1976, p. 243)*

> **And I want your attention just on me.**
>> *(Erickson & Lustig, 1975, Vol. I, p. 5)*

> **So far as I was concerned, she was in outer space *sensing* only my voice.**
>> *(Zeig, 1980, p. 182)*

Repeated experimentation disclosed that carefully worded suggestions serving to emphasize the availability of external reality and to enhance subjective comfort could serve to deepen the trance. [1965]

(In Erickson, 1980, Vol. I, chap. 3, p. 91)

I altered the intonation of my voice there and I leaned toward her and that attracted her attention to my voice... So no matter where I was, she could go deeper and deeper and further and further away from me and yet be close to me... She would go deeper into trance and then move away from me. An external reality. So I get myself very close to her and she can leave reality and still be close to me.

(Zeig, 1980, p. 305)

You are asking patients to lose a certain amount of their reality contact. You are asking them to alter it.

(Erickson & Rossi, 1979, p. 132)

If they will sit down in a comfortable chair and close their eyes and just direct their hearing toward me, their vision is not going to distract them.

(ASCH, 1980, Taped Lecture, 7/16/65)

Most workers in hypnosis do not know that as the subject closes the eyes, the subject is cutting off the visual field and is really losing something but he doesn't know what he is losing. He thinks he is just closing his eyes.

(Erickson, Rossi & Rossi, 1976, p. 107)

Direct Attention Internally

An hypnotic trance develops as awareness is focused, directed away from a monitoring of external events, and then is moved toward a focus upon particular internal experiences. It evidently makes little difference whether this is accomplished in a step-by-step fashion or in a more direct one-step leap to an internally focused attentiveness. The initiation of an internal experience that will capture attention seems to accomplish the same end as the more gradual movement from a captivating external event to a comfortable refocusing upon an internal event. It simply does it more rapidly and easily.

As noted earlier, most people move in and out of light trances or reverie states several times a day. Some internal sensation, thought, memory, or mental image captures and holds their attention for a time and the events of the surrounding world fade from awareness. Hypnosis is induced by using this natural mental process. Thus, the hypnotist should be interested in helping the subject become focused upon an internal event of some sort; whether a physical sensation, a memory, an emotion, a thought, or an internal image. The hypnotist may say or do something to generate or elicit the captivating internal event, knowing beforehand that it will automatically fixate the subject's attention, or subjects may be asked to pay close attention to an internal event that they have initiated themselves or that is a natural outgrowth of their relaxed state — for example, heaviness, drowsiness, etc.

The use of an internal event as the initial focus of attention speeds the induction process and may even enhance the subject's ability to respond well. Focusing upon an imaginary sound or sight was found by Erickson to be a more effective induction approach then focusing upon an actual sound or an actual visual stimulus. Perhaps for this reason, a majority of Erickson's inductions began with the initiation of an event that focused attention upon internal experience. Most of the material contained in the remainder of this chapter consists of Erickson's comments regarding the various techniques he developed to do just that. Their significance for the aspiring hypnotherapist cannot be over-emphasized, because any technique used to initiate an internally focused awareness for induction purposes can also be used to deepen the trance, to re-direct attention toward important issues once trance has developed and to stimulate hypnotic responses that validate the hypnotic state for subjects and help them learn how to use their own hypnotic potentials more effectively.

Some subjects seem to be able to redirect their awareness internally themselves if simply asked or instructed to do so, which may account for whatever success the standardized, authoritarian induction procedures enjoy. But most people require assistance in this endeavor, and that is the hypnotist's responsibility or purpose.

> **A trusted operator can progressively, persuasively, and repetitiously suggest tiredness, relaxation, eye closure, loss of interest in externalities and an increasingly absorbing interest in inner experiential processes, until the subject can function with increasing adequacy at the level of unconscious awareness.**
>
> *(Erickson, 1970, p. 995)*

> **There are many ways of inducing a trance. What you do is to ask patients primarily to give their attention to one particular idea. You get them to center their attention on their own experiential learning... to direct their attention to processes which are taking place within them. Thus you can induce a trance by directing patients' attention to processes, to memories, to ideas, to concepts that belong to them. All you do is direct the patients' attention to those processes within themselves. [1959]**
>
> *(In Erickson, 1980, Vol. III, chap. 4, p. 29)*

Another type of Utilization Technique is the employment of the patients' inner, as opposed to outer, behavior, that is, using their thoughts and understandings as the basis for the induction procedure. [1959]

(In Erickson, 1980, Vol. I, chap. 8, p. 182)

She didn't recognize that when I told her to attend to the processes within herself that she was being literally asked to go into a hypnotic trance. Because as she attended to the processes within herself she would withdraw from external reality and in withdrawing from external reality she would limit her degree of consciousness, her *field* of conscious awareness.

(ASCH, 1980, Taped Lecture, 2/2/66)

My voice in the background is where I want it to be. It's in the background of *her* experience. Her own experience is in the focus of attention.

(Erickson & Rossi, 1979, p. 291)

All these things are taking place in her body, as I am limting her attention to herself and downgrading all outside distractions. By mentioning her "experiencing" I am referring to her own history. I am now evoking her personal history, and she knows it and cannot dispute it.

(Erickson, Rossi & Rossi, 1976, p. 31)

Primarily, emphasis should be placed upon the intrapsychic behavior of the subjects rather than upon the relationship to externalities. [1952]

(In Erickson, 1980, Vol. I, chap. 6, p. 140)

R: In other words, you want patients to be active in the inner world, not just sitting there passively.
E: That's right.

(Erickson, Rossi & Rossi, 1976, p. 244)

"How do you tell the difference between an upside-down nine and a right-side-up six?" Well, that is intriguing. So he is not going to be thinking about anything else. I am focusing his attention inward to his own experience.

(Erickson & Rossi, 1981, p. 186)

She was trapped. She was forced to think internally.

(Zeig, 1980, p. 327)

"Attend to memories" — that is, not external realities.

(Erickson & Rossi, 1981, p. 200)

The art of deepening the trance is not necessarily yelling at him to go deeper and deeper: it is giving minimal suggestion gently, so the patient pays more and more attention to the processes within himself and thus goes deeper and deeper.

(Erickson & Rossi, 1981, p. 44)

He is going to search his mind, and that is where I want him to be.

(Erickson & Rossi, 1981, p. 184)

The essential point is that they pay attention, not necessarily to me, but to their own thoughts — especially the thoughts that flash through their mind, including the manner and sequence in which those thoughts flash through their mind.

(Erickson & Rossi, 1981, p. 5)

The essential consideration is to evoke visual images related to experiential learnings and thus to initiate within the subjects, apart from externalities, a progressive series of responsive reactions that can develop into a trance. [circa 1940's]

(In Erickson, 1980, Vol. I, chap. 11, p. 292)

> **But it is easier to deal with the images a person has in his mind. There's a large variety of images in his mind, and he can slip easily from one to another without leaving the situation.**
>
> *(Erickson, Rossi & Rossi, 1976, p. 8)*

> **Some external thing has no real value to them, but the images they have within are of value.**
>
> *(Erickson, Rossi & Rossi, 1976, p. 8)*

Use Ideomotor Responses

Attention directed toward an imagined sound, sight, or body is an effective way to focus awareness internally, but the initiation of an involuntary ideomotor response can genuinely capture the subject's interest and attention. People are not used to observing movement in their limbs that was not intentionally initiated, although it occurs all the time. As a result, when the hypnotist creates a situation that elicits these ideomotor responses, subjects are usually puzzled and fascinated by the experience. Aside from focusing their experience internally, the initiation of an ideomotor response can also dispel their doubts and convince them of their own ability to respond to hypnotic suggestions.

Readers interested in learning specific techniques to trigger ideomotor movement and catalepsy are referred to Section II and III of Erickson & Rossi's book, *Experiencing Hypnosis*, Irvington Publishers, 1981, for a lengthy discussion of this issue.

> **Trances could be induced in both naive or experienced subjects by techniques based upon (1) the visualization of a motor activity such as hand levitation or by visualizing**

the self climbing up or down a long stairway, and (2) upon "remembering the body and muscles and joint feeling sensations" of motor activity of many kinds. [1961]
(In Erickson, 1980, Vol. 1, chap. 5, pp. 137-138)

It became apparent that the effectiveness of many supposedly different techniques of trance induction derived only from a basic use of ideomotor activity rather than from variations of procedure, as is sometimes naively believed and reported. [1961]
(In Erickson, 1980, Vol. 1, chap. 5, pp. 135-136)

The elicitation of a single hypnotic phenomenon is often an excellent technique of trance induction and should, for the patient's benefit, be used more often. [1964]
(In Erickson, 1980, Vol. 1, chap. 13, p. 308)

The elicitation of one hypnotic response leads so easily to another, catalepsy, pupillary dilation, and then an all-comprehensive set of suggestions was given to insure a deep trance and its maintenance. [1964]
(In Erickson, 1980, Vol. 1, chap. 10, p. 289)

The development of a trance state is concurrent with the development of levitation, regardless of the significance of the reply. [1961]
(In Erickson, 1980, Vol. 1, chap. 5, p. 138)

The essential consideration in the use of ideomotor techniques lies not in their elaborateness or novelty but simply in the initiation of motor activity, either real of hallucinated, as a means of fixating and focusing the subjects' attention upon inner experiential learnings and capabilities. [1961]
(In Erickson, 1980, Vol. 1, chap. 5, p. 138)

To secure active participation, hand levitation suggestions are given as the first step. [1945]
(In Erickson, 1980, Vol. IV, chap. 3, p. 31)

Once an ideomotor response is made, without further
delay it can be utilized immediately. [1964]
(In Erickson, 1980, Vol. I, chap. 13, p. 309)

The really important thing is not whether your hand
lifts up or presses down or just remains still; rather, it is
your ability to sense fully whatever feelings may develop
in your hand. [1952]
(In Erickson, 1980, Vol. I, chap. 6, p. 154)

The hand is employed for the reason that in the
passively expectant state of the subjects, the idea of
motor activity is easily related to the subject's hand
without disturbing their general physical inactivity. The
subjects have a lifetime of experience of hand movement
while the body is at rest. [circa 1940's]
(In Erickson, 1980, Vol. I, chap. 11, p. 293)

This is a technique [hand levitation] the author has
employed in teaching others, and in teaching autohypnosis to others for some legitimate purpose. [1964]
(In Erickson, 1980, Vol. I, chap. 15, p. 342)

All day long you keep your head in a state of balanced
tonicity... In other parts of your body you are not ac-
customed to balanced tonicity.
(Erickson & Rossi, 1981, p. 198)

I've set up a situation in which his patterns can come
forth. He doesn't know they were called forth, but they
are, so he starts examining them. We all can dissociate

naturally... But we don't know how well we can do it.
(Erickson & Rossi, 1981, p. 235)

It is the subjective sensation of lightness, of free, involuntary, or consciously effortless motor activity that is the primary consideration, not the direction of the movement...it is the subjective sensation of involuntary or consciously effortless movement that is desired. [circa 1940's]
(In Erickson, 1980, Vol. I, chap. 11, p. 293)

His body is in a trance because he no longer has control over it. [1976–78]
(In Erickson, 1980, Vol. I, chap. 23, p. 487)

Subjects become absorbed in sensing their own psychosomatic phenomena as a personal experience in which they are active. Thus the situation is transformed from one of passive responsiveness for the patient to one of active interest, discovery, integration, and participation in these changes produced by hypnosis. [1945]
(In Erickson, 1980, Vol. IV, chap. 3, p. 32)

The subjects should participate. They are not placid, indifferent people when in trance. They should be participating much more than you because you are only offering them a wealth of suggestions, knowing that at best they're going to select this one here, that one there, and still another one over there to act upon. [1976–78]
(In Erickson, 1980, Vol. I, chap. 23, p. 489)

R: You like to use pantomime and nonverbal approaches to trance because they activate and reach more deeply to the simpler levels of functioning.
E: Yes. You thereby bypass the enforced rigid forms

of later conscious acquisitions. You don't have to have things put into words.

(Erickson, Rossi & Rossi, 1976, p. 253)

The therapist needs to practice these movements [lifting hand to create catalepsy] over and over because they are one of the quickest and easiest ways of distracting the conscious mind and securing fixation of the unconscious mind.

(Erickson & Rossi, 1981, p. 44)

Use Demonstrations and Simulations

Hypnotic responses can be elicited by the hypnotist in a very indirect manner. Subjects may be asked to observe the induction of another subject, for example. As they do so, the suggestions and responses they are observing will initiate an automatic tendency to undergo similar internal responses. Just listening to a detailed description of a successful induction will tend to stimulate the described internal experiences. Once internal imitative responses have been initiated, it is relatively simple to direct the subject's attention toward them and to offer additional suggestions that will further enhance the hypnotic internal focus of awareness.

Other indirect approaches for the creation of hypnosis include instructing prospective subjects simply to imagine what it would be like to experience hypnosis or asking them to act as if they were already hypnotized. Subjects may be assisted by descriptions of various possible experiences or they may be left entirely to their own devices. In either case, they are being allowed to give themselves the salient suggestions and are almost forced to focus upon and to monitor internal events in order to do so effectively. The more absorbed they become by their simulation assignments, the more deeply they move into an hypnotic condition and the easier it becomes for the hypnotist to use their condition to initiate a satisfactory trance.

This indirect approach is especially useful with subjects who have experienced trance previously. Recounting or just remembering previous trance experiences in vivid detail almost invariably results in the re-establishment of a trance state.

> **The induction of a trance in the group situation, aside from the exceptional case, decreases the time and effort required and leads to a more rapid and better training of the individual subject. Especially is this true when a trained or unusually capable subject is used as an object lesson for the group. [1945]**
>
> *(In Erickson, 1980, Vol. IV, chap. 3, p. 29)*

> **The procedure is relatively simple. The experimental or therapeutic subjects are either asked or allowed to express freely their thoughts, understandings, and opinions. As they do this, they are encouraged to speculate aloud more and more extensively upon what could be the possible course of their thinking and feeling if they were to develop a trance state. As patients do this, or even if they merely protest the impossibility of such speculation, their utterances are repeated after them in their essence, as if the operator were either earnestly seeking further understanding or were confirming their statements. [1959]**
>
> *(In Erickson, 1980, Vol. I, chap. 8, p. 182)*

> **If a nonhypnotic subject is innocently...asked to perform, at a waking level, the same sort of behavior that can be used to induce a hypnotic trance, although no mention of hypnosis is made, a hypnotic state can unmistakably result. [1964]**
>
> *(In Erickson, 1980, Vol. I, chap. 1, p. 16)*

The inexperienced, unsophisticated subjects simply did not know what to do but could easily learn to go into a trance state by being told how to simulate hypnosis. This has become a technique much used by this author, particularly with resistant subjects and patients who fear hypnotic states. [1967]

(In Erickson, 1980, Vol. I, chap. 2, p. 26)

The better the simulation, the greater would be the actualization. [1967]

(In Erickson, 1980, Vol. 1, chap. 2, p. 23)

The simple measure of seating the patient comfortably and asking him to give a detailed account of a previous successful trance experience results in a trance. [1959]

(In Erickson, 1980, Vol. 1, chap. 8, p. 184)

Trance tends to be revivified when you review any hypnotic phenomenon that has occured in the subjects.

(Erickson, Rossi & Rossi, 1976, p. 172)

Use Boredom or Surprise

Everyday observation can make us aware of situations that will automatically trigger an internal focus of attention. For example, anyone who has surveyed the faces of an audience forced to listen to an incredibly boring speech has seen the blank stare characteristic of hypnotic inner absorption. Similarly, people confronted by a surprising or unexpected incident may become "frozen in their tracks." Given the universality of these phenomena, it seems natural that Erickson would have used both boredom and surprise as effective induction procedures. In the right circumstances they may be the best, most appropriate avenues available into hypnosis, therefore, prospective hypnotists should practice generating them in a variety of settings.

> **The angry belligerent man can strike a blow that hurts his hand and not notice it, the disbeliever loses his mind to exclude a boring dissertation but that excludes the pain too and from this there develops unwittingly in the patients a different state of inner orientation, highly conducive to hypnosis and receptive to any suggestions that meet their needs. [1964]**
>
> *(In Erickson, 1980, Vol. I, chap. 10, p. 286)*

> **Boredom narrows your vision and restricts the freedom of your mind to think.**
>
> *(Erickson, & Rossi, 1979, p. 340)*

> **The simple explaining of the situation, repetitiously, in a boresome fashion, so that she would get rather tired of listening to what I had to say, so that she would withdraw more and more within herself.**
>
> *(ASCH, 1980, Taped Lecture, 2/2/66)*

> **Often with highly sophisticated subjects you resort to uninteresting detail to bore the hell out of them.**
>
> *(Erickson, Rossi & Rossi, 1976, p. 240)*

> **The function of surprise is this. The patient comes to you with a certain mental set, and they expect you to get into that set. If you surprise them, they let loose of their mental set and you can frame another mental set for them.**
>
> *(Erickson, Rossi & Rossi, 1976, p. 128)*

> **Again a Surprise Technique was used by asking a sudden question in a suitable situation, reply to which required an absolute affirmation of a postulated or implied**

**hypnotic phenomenon in order to answer the question.
[1964]**
(In Erickson, 1980, Vol. 1 chap. 15, pp. 349–350)

**Here the child, taken completely by surprise, readily
developed a somnambulistic trance. [1958]**
(In Erickson, 1980, Vol. 1, chap. 7, p. 173)

Use Confusion

Erickson noticed that few things capture attention more effectively than confusion. Perhaps because people are so highly
dependent upon their ability to decipher the meaning of
stimuli in order to decide how to respond appropriately, confusion or a lack of understanding is a startling and disarming
event. When confused, people become dumbfounded and their
awareness withdraws inward in a search for understanding or
escape. This may explain why the single most frequently used
and most effective ingredient in Erickson's repertoire of induction and suggestion techniques was confusion. While other
clinicians, and people in general, were trying to figure out
ways to communicate clearly, Erickson was developing his
ability to communicate in ways that were confusing. He
learned to speak and to move in confusing ways and, paradoxically, he used this knowledge to enable people to enter realms
of awareness that provided increased clarity and understanding. Confusion of conscious awareness forces people to resort
to unconscious patterns of thought and response, a circumstance that can then be emphasized and utilized by observant
hypnotists and willing subjects.

Erickson offered some general guidelines and procedures for
the creation of confusion which are summarized in his statements below. The readers are referred to his transcripts and

articles on hypnosis for specific confusion techniques. Ultimately, however, effective use of this and other Ericksonian approaches must be based upon personal observation and utilization of situations in everyday life that are responsible for confusing outcomes similar to those desired in the hypnotic setting. What worked for Erickson is not necessarily what will be most useful for someone else. All hypnotic techniques must be tailored to fit the personalities and situations involved.

Finally, there may be an urge to explain one's seemingly bizarre and confusing behavior to the subject. Such attempts to maintain one's image as a rational, reasonable professional are understandable, but self-defeating. The less understanding subjects have regarding the rationale for certain hypnotic procedures, the more responsive they will be to them. There is nothing more difficult than trying to help a knowledgeable subject experience an hypnotic response. What occurs is an intellectual analysis of the hypnotist's style instead of an automatic, unthinking response to it. Imagine how difficult it would be to perform magic in front of a group of master magicians in such a way that they would be fooled and you begin to get a sense of the reason for not explaining one's actions to subjects. It merely makes them more difficult to confuse later on and removes some of the desirable mystery or magic from the situation.

Please note that confusion is not the same as misunderstanding or believing that the speaker is not making sense. Confusion or lack of understanding leaves the mind open and searching for the missing meaning, whereas misunderstanding closes the mind upon a wrong meaning. Believing that the speaker is nonsensical also closes off the search for meaning because there no longer seems to be any meaning to find. These points are emphasized to stress the fact that creating confusion by what you do or say is not the same as babbling nonsense or acting inappropriately. It, like all other aspects of an Ericksonian hypnotherapeutic approach, demands skill and a clear sense of purpose. Practice and careful observation are the primary prerequisites for an effective accomplishment of confusion in others, strange as that may sound to those of us who feel that we generate confusion in others quite unwittingly on a daily basis.

I also sometimes tell irrelevant stories and make non sequitur remarks to induce confusion.

(Erickson & Rossi, 1981, p. 166)

The next item in the Confusion Technique is the employment of irrelevancies and non sequiturs, *each of which taken out of context* appears to be a sound and sensible communication. Taken *in context* they are confusing, distracting and inhibiting and lead progressively to the subjects' earnest desire for and an actual need to receive some communication which, in their increasing state of frustration, they can readily comprehend and to which they can easily make a response. [1964]

(In Erickson, 1980, Vol. I, chap. 10, p. 258)

Whenever you do the unexpected you jog a person out of their setting.

(Erickson & Rossi, 1976, p. 154)

These are all ways of disconcerting the subject, ways of making them have doubts about themselves.

(Erickson, Rossi & Rossi, 1976, p. 106)

As they would explain in the trance state, "As soon as I experienced the slightest feeling of confusion, I just dropped into a deep trance." They simply did not like to be confused. [1964]

(In Erickson, 1980, Vol. I, chap. 10, p. 279)

R: You're dislodging the erroneous conscious sets that are giving them problems.
E: Yes. That's also what you do with confusion technique.

> *(Erickson, Rossi & Rossi, 1976, p. 128)*

Yes, it is not a "misunderstanding" but an *absence of understanding* that leaves you dumbfounded and open.

> *(Erickson & Rossi, 1981, p. 246)*

So much of what I do is confusion. You're dealing with patches of conscious awareness along with patterns of unconscious behavior. [1976–78]

> *(In Erickson, 1980, Vol. I, chap. 23, p. 488)*

It [confusion] is the basis of all good techniques.

> *(Erickson, Rossi & Rossi, 1976, p. 107)*

Yes, it is a confusion technique. *In all my techniques, almost all, there is a confusion.* It is a confusion within them.

> *(Erickson, Rossi & Rossi, 1976, p. 85)*

It [confusion technique] is based upon the utilization of everyday experiences familiar to everyone. [1952]

> *(In Erickson, 1980, Vol. I, chap. 6, p. 159)*

As a verbal technique, the Confusion Technique is based upon plays on words. [1964]

> *(In Erickson, 1980, Vol. I, chap. 10, p. 258)*

A primary consideration in the use of a Confusion Technique is the consistent maintenance of a general casual but definitely interested attitude and speaking in a gravely earnest manner expressive of certain, utterly complete, expectation of their understanding of what is being said or done together with an extremely careful shifting of the tenses employed. Also of great importance is a ready flow of language, rapid for the fast thinker, slower for the slow-minded, but always being careful to give a little time for a response but never quite sufficient. Thus the subjects are led almost to begin a response, are frustrated in this by then being presented with the next idea, and the whole process is repeated with a continued development of a state of inhibition, leading to confusion and a growing need to receive a clear-cut comprehensible communication to which they *can make* a ready and full response. [1964]

(In Erickson, 1980, Vol. 1, chap. 10, p. 259)

In summary, if into any simple little situation evocative of simple natural responses, there is introduced just previous to the moment of response a casual simple irrelevancy or non sequitur, confusion results, and there is an inhibition of natural responses. The non sequitur is completely meaningful in itself but has no bearing *except as an interruption* upon the original situation calling for a response. The need experienced to respond to the original situation and the immediate inhibition of that response by a seemingly meaningful communication results in an increased need to do something. [1964]

(In Erickson, 1980, Vol. 1, chap. 10, p. 261)

Finally, a clear-cut, definitive, easily grasped and understood statement is uttered and the striving subject seizes upon it. [1964]

(In Erickson, 1980, Vol. 1, chap. 10, p. 263)

But the slow, impressive, utterly intense, and quietly, softly emphatic way in which these plays on words and the unobtrusive introduction of new ideas, old happy memories, feelings of comfort, ease, and relaxation are presented usually results in an arrest of the patient's attention, rigid fixation of his eyes, the development of physical immobility, even catalepsy and of an intense desire to understand what the author so gravely and so earnestly is saying to them that their attention is sooner or later captured completely. [1964]

(In Erickson, 1980, Vol. I, chap. 10, p. 285)

Defined simply, a "confusion technique" is one based upon the presentation to the subjects of a series of seemingly but only loosely related ideas actually based upon a significant thread of continuity not readily recognized, leading to an increasing divergence of associations, interspersed with an emphasis on the obvious, *all of which preclude subjects from developing any one train of association, yet stirs them increasingly to need to do something until they are ready to accept the first clear-cut definitive suggestion offered.* [circa 1940's]

(In Erickson, 1980, Vol. I, chap. 11 pp. 293–294)

Unable to do anything, interrupted so suddenly in the initiation of what he was going to do, too astonished by the author's completely nonpertinent behavior, utterly at a loss for something to do, and hence, completely susceptible to any clearly comprehensible suggestion of what to do fitting to the total situation that he responded relievedly to the simple quiet instruction the author offered. [1964]

(In Erickson, 1980, Vol. I, chap. 10, p. 288)

They begin to wonder but they don't know what they are wondering about. That is very confusing!

(Erickson, Rossi & Rossi, 1976, p. 106)

This goal is an urgent pressing need on the part of the subject to have the confusion of the situation clarified. Hence, the suggestion of a trance state as a definitive idea is readily accepted and acted upon. [1959]

(In Erickson, 1980, Vol. I, chap. 8, p. 204)

To summarize this example, a train of physical activity was initiated in this subject. As she followed along in the development, first one and then another nonverbal suggestion of a motor type was offered just long enough to permit her to become aware of it, but before she could respond another had taken its place. Each suggestion in itself was acceptable, but each time she was precluded from a response although a need to respond was being increasingly developed. [circa 1940's]

(In Erickson, 1980, Vol. I, chap. 11, pp. 295–6)

A basic consideration is a seemingly incidental or unintentional interference with the subjects' spontaneous responses to the reality situation. This leads to a state of uncertainty, frustration and confusion in the subjects, which in turn effects ready acceptance of hypnosis as a means of resolving the situation. [1959]

(In Erickson, 1980, Vol. I, chap. 8, p. 203)

As the subjects try, conditioned by their early cooperative response to the hypnotist's apparent misspeaking, to accommodate themselves to the welter of confused, contradictory responses apparently sought, they find themselves at such a loss that they welcome any positive suggestion that will permit a retreat from so unsatisfying and confusing a stiuation. [1952]

(In Erickson, 1980, Vol. I, chap. 6, p. 159)

They don't know what to do. So then the therapist can tell them what to do.

(Erickson, Rossi & Rossi, 1976, p. 107)

And the subject's own state of mental uncertainty and eagerness to comprehend would effect the same sort of readiness to accept any comprehensible communication by pantomime as is effected by clear-cut definite communications in the Confusion Technique. [1964]

(In Erickson, 1980, Vol. I, chap. 14, p. 331)

The rapidity, insistence, and confidence with which the suggestions are given serve to prevent the subjects from making any effort to bring about a semblance of order. [1952]

(In Erickson, 1980, Vol. I, chap. 6, p. 159)

You're keeping them off balance by asking and not answering questions. You are keeping them reaching out hopefully.

(Erickson & Rossi, 1981, p. 101)

To make her awfully uncertain as to her state of awareness. And if she's uncertain about her state of awareness, then she can rely upon me to clarify it. [1959]

(In Erickson, 1980, Vol. I, chap. 9, p. 224)

The calculated vagueness of some of the instructions forced their unconscious minds to assume responsibility for their behavior. Consciously they could only wonder about their inexplicable situations, while they responded to it with corrective, unconscious reactions.

(Erickson, 1954a, p. 173)

Repeated efforts to devise and deliver a Confusion Technique for the sake of practice only will soon teach the user of more conventionalized, ritualistic, traditional, verbalized techniques a greater fluency in speech, a freedom from rote suggestions, a better understanding of the meaning of suggestions, and a greater ease in shifting one's own patterns of behavior in response to observed changes in the patients, and in shifting from one set of ideas to another. [1964]

(In Erickson, 1980, Vol. I, chap. 10, p. 291)

It [confusion technique] serves excellently to teach experimenters a facility in the use of words, a mental agility in shifting their habitual patterns of thought, and allows them to make adequate allowances for the problems invoked in keeping the subjects attentive and responsive. Also it allows experimenters to recognize and to understand the minimal uses of behavioral changes with the subject. [1964]

(In Erickson, 1980, Vol. I, chap. 10, p. 284)

It became possible to utilize his acceptance of stimulation of his behavior by a procedure of pausing and hesitating in the completion of an interjection. This served to effect in him an *expectant dependency* upon the writer for further and more complete stimulation. [1959]

(In Erickson, 1980, Vol. I, chap. 8, p. 179)

As she developed an attitude of expectation for the writer's silent interruptions, his movements were deliberately slowed and made with slight, hesitant pauses, which compelled her to slow down her own behavior and to await the writer's utilization of her conduct. [1959]

(In Erickson, 1980, Vol. I, chap. 8, p. 180)

Nobody likes hesitation.

(Erickson & Rossi, 1981, p. 66)

You ought always to use hesitation and emphasis. On that particular occasion I just threw in some, not for any particular purpose except to demonstrate that I can use variations whenever I please. And I don't ever want to get stuck by a subject learning a rigid pattern. [1959]

(In Erickson, 1980, Vol. I, chap. 9, pp. 241–242)

You use a direct authoritative suggestion in this situation where you see a patient in an uncertain state. When she is uncertain, you help her by taking over firmly. Just as when a child is uncertain about something, you say, "I'll tell you when to go...Now!" That's the same sort of thing. That is acceptable as help since patients have a long history of having accepted help in such circumstances.

(Erickson, Rossi & Rossi, 1976, p. 169)

In understanding this technique, it may be well to keep in mind the patter of the magician which is not intended to inform but to distract so that his purposes may be accomplished.

(Erickson, 1954 d, p. 112)

A magician makes his living out of that. He utilizes your ability not to see what he is doing.

(Erickson, Rossi & Rossi, 1976, p. 217)

Nor is there any reason for the patient to be led to understand the techniques and levels of communication, any more than does the surgical patient need to have a full comprehension of the surgical techniques to be employed. [1964]

(In Erickson, 1980, Vol. I, chap. 13, p. 301)

It ruins a magician's act if he explains to you how he did it. You've taken it out of the alien frame of reference and put it into the ordinary frame of reference.

(Erickson & Rossi, 1981, p. 247)

Create a Conscious-Unconscious Dissociation

As described earlier, the goal of focusing attention inward is the eventual focusing of all awareness and response through the unconscious mind. When this occurs, there is effected a dissociation between conscious and unconscious functioning, with the functions of the conscious mind receding into the background of awareness or disappearing altogether and the functions of the unconscious mind absorbing attention entirely. This dissociation may occur automatically in response to the progressively increased internal focus of awareness or it may be initiated and facilitated by the presentation of particular stimuli or tasks. The assignment of one task to the conscious mind and another to the unconscious can result in a dissociative experience. The use of two different tones of voice or two different levels of meaning can accomplish the same end. Simply reassuring subjects that there is no longer any reason for them to listen consciously to what is being said and that they can just relax and drift off while their unconscious takes over the responsibility of doing so is often quite sufficient. A gradual shift into a simpler, more literal manner of speaking may also enable a dissociation to occur because the subjects are thereby forced to focus upon the hypnotist's words through their unconscious minds in order to comprehend them effectively.

In some respects, any of the situations discussed previously as possible stimuli to initiate an internal focus of attention can also be considered to be dissociative stimuli. Any inward focusing of awareness is a minor or embryonic form of dissociation which the hypnotist can then amplify and deepen to establish the complete dissociation desired for a deep trance.

Thus it [hypnosis] may be defined as an artificially enhanced state of suggestibility resembling sleep wherein

there appears to be a normal, time-limited and stimulus-limited dissociation of "conscious" from the "subconscious" elements of the psyche. This dissociation is manifested by a quiescence of the "consciousness" simulating normal sleep and a delegation of the subjective control of the individual functions, ordinarily conscious, to the "subconsciousness."

(Erickson, 1934, p. 611)

In appearance and nature this somnambulistic state is an experimental equivalent to the states of dissociation in dual personalities.

(Erickson, 1934, p. 612)

In other words, dissociation phenomena, whether spontaneous or induced, can be used in a repetitious manner to establish a psychological momentum to which subjects easily and readily yield. [1952]

(In Erickson, 1980, Vol. I, chap. 6, p. 166)

The author would like to have him retell his story slowly, carefully, with his eyes closed, and to give it in good detail, letting his unconscious mind (he was a college graduate) take over all dominance, and that, as he related his story, he was to specify in full and comprehensive detail exactly what it was he wished in relation to cigarettes, but that during his narrative he would find himself going unaccountably into a deep and deeper trance without any interruption of his story. [1964]

(In Erickson, 1980, Vol. IV, chap. 19, p. 210)

And when a patient says, "I don't want to do this," I say, "okay, then I'll take care of it while you do this other." So they can dissociate.

(Erickson, Rossi & Rossi, 1976, pp. 246–247)

Also, by suggesting a sleeping of the body and wakefulness of the mind, a state of dissociation was induced. [1952]

(In Erickson, 1980, Vol. IV, chap. 27, p. 259)

It [telling subjects they do not need to listen] depotentiates consciousness and thereby potentiates the unconscious functioning.

(Erickson & Rossi, 1981, p. 183)

Allow Plenty of Time

Different subjects move through different phases of the induction process at different rates. Some take a much longer time than others to learn to allow their attention to remain focused, to direct their attention internally or to experience dissociation. The effective hypnotist is the patient hypnotist who is willing to allow subjects to progress at their own speed. If anything, subjects should be encouraged to slow down and to explore their experiences at each step along the way.

The need for the allotment of sufficient time becomes even more crucial when it comes time for subjects to begin using the hypnotist's suggestions to create their own internal realities. As subjects drop their typical reality orientations or normal mental sets and begin replacing them at an unconscious level with the mental sets suggested to them by the hypnotist, the construction and adoption of those new mental sets takes time. It takes time to become comfortable and familiar with the "hypnotized" mental set. It takes time to create and become comfortable with the mental sets necessary to experience hallucinations or dissociative movements. Subjects should be given plenty of time to respond to suggestions and should not be expected to experience the suggested event immediately.

Similarly, subjects should be given plenty of opportunities to experience the process of becoming hypnotized. Providing subjects with several induction, deepening, and waking experiences in succession before any hypnotic work is attempted will considerably increase their comfort and ability to respond to the process and will probably prove to be much more productive for everyone involved than an immediate attempt to utilize the first trance secured.

How long does it take to develop a trance? How long does it take to develop physiological sleep? ... When you are sufficiently prepared psychologically, you can develop a trance just as quickly. [1964]
(In Erickson, 1980, Vol. I, chap. 15, p. 346)

You can go as deeply in the trance as you wish, the only thing is that you don't know when.
(Erickson & Rossi, 1977, p. 43)

Unfortunately even among those endeavoring to do scientific work, the attitude that hypnosis is miraculous and minimizes time requirements is still prevalent. [1967]
(In Erickson, 1980, Vol. I, chap. 2, p. 19)

Unfortunately, much published work has been based upon an unrecognized belief in the immediate omnipotence of hypnotic suggestions and a failure to appreciate that responsive behavior in the hypnotic subjects, as in unhypnotized persons, depends upon a time factor. Hypnotic subjects are often expected, in a few moments, to reorient themselves completely psychologically and physiologically, and to perform complex tasks ordinarily impossible in the non-hypnotic state. [1952]
(In Erickson, 1980, Vol. I, chap. 6, p. 142)

The oversight and actual neglect of time as an important factor in hypnosis, and the disregard of the individual needs of subjects account for much contradiction in hypnotic studies. Published estimates of the hypnotizability of the general population range from 5 - 70 percent and higher. The lower estimates are often due to a disregard of time as an important factor in the development of hypnotic behavior. [1952]

(In Erickson, 1980, Vol. I, chap. 6, p. 143)

The essential consideration seems to be the provision of a sufficient period of time to permit the development of a mental set conducive to the behavior. Unless this period of time is allowed, the subject's response, while in accord with the suggestions given, will be marked to the critical observer by inhibitions, denials, avoidances, and blockings not in keeping with a valid experiential response. [circa 1960's]

(In Erickson, 1980, Vol. II, chap. 29, p. 306)

I also want to emphasize the absolute importance of the element of time itself in securing hypnotic phenomena. This consideration has been sadly neglected despite the general recognition of the fact that time itself constitutes an absolute function of all forms of behavior and that the more complicated the form of behavior, the more significant is the time element. [circa 1960]

(In Erickson, 1980, Vol. II, chap. 29, p. 304)

The expectation of practically instantaneous results from the spoken word indicates an uncritical approach which militates against scientifically valid results. [1952]

(In Erickson, 1980, Vol. I, chap. 6, p. 142)

Of great importance in inducing trance states and trance behavior is the allotment of sufficient time for the

subject to make those neuro- and psychophysiological changes necessary for certain types of behavior. To rush or force a subject often defeats the purpose. [1944]
(In Erickson, 1980, Vol. IV, chap. 2, p. 18)

The necessity of a time-taking procedure of suggestion as a measure of permitting the subject, who is receiving such suggestions, to acquire the "mental set" by means of which there can be reestablished at the levels of mentation characteristic of any suggested age without interference from subsequently acquired experience. [1939]
(In Erickson, 1980, Vol. III, chap. 20, p. 204)

The ordinary deep trance, rapidly induced, with the subject given direct and emphatic suggestions, does not permit the gradual and effective development of what may be called the "mental set" which is requisite for the execution of complicated behavior free from the influence of waking patterns of behavior. [1939]
(In Erickson, 1980, Vol. II, chap. 3, pp. 25–26)

Easy hypnotizability may indicate a need to allow adequate time for a reorientation of the subject's total behavior to permit full and sustained responses. [1952]
(In Erickson, 1980, Vol. I, chap. 6, p. 142)

After he had been given about 20 minutes to develop the "mental set" essential to their performance, he was told to proceed with his task. [1944]
(In Erickson, 1980, Vol. II, chap. 4, p. 41)

It is hardly reasonable to expect a hypnotized subject, upon the snap of the fingers or the utterance of a simple command, to develop at once significant, complex, and persistent changes in behavioral functioning. Rather, it is to be expected that time and effort are required to permit a development of any profound alterations in behavior. Such alteration must presumably arise from neuro- and psychophysiological changes and processes within the subject, which are basic to behavioral manifestations, and not from the simple experience of hearing a command spoken by a hypnotist. [1944]

(In Erickson, 1980, Vol. II, chap. 4, p. 50)

Apparently, the element of time is an important factor in securing a neuropsychological state which will permit the subject to accept and act upon a suggestion freely and completely and without inhibitions and limitations deriving from customary waking habits and patterns of behavior. [1939)

(In Erickson, 1980, Vol. II, chap. 3, p. 26)

The employment of hypnosis as a therapeutic agent or as a laboratory method of experimentation requires, for valid results, a training process extending over several hours. [1970]

(In Erickson, 1980, Vol. IV, chap. 1, p. 6)

And it takes time to get out of one pattern and into another.

(Zeig, 1980, p. 316)

Some subjects require extensive instruction in a number of regards; others can themselves transfer learnings in one field to a problem of another sort. [1952]

(In Erickson, 1980, Vol. I, chap. 6, p. 145)

The more extensive and varied a subject's hypnotic experience is, the more effectively a subject can function in complicated problems. [1952]

(In Erickson, 1980, Vol. I, chap. 6, p. 143)

She was given extensive training to teach her to respond in accord with her own unconscious pattern of behavior. [1952]

(In Erickson, 1980, Vol. I, chap. 6, p. 152)

In this training procedure subjects may be hypnotized, awakened, rehypnotized, and reawakened repeatedly, with each of the trance and waking states employed to teach them by slow degrees a facility of control over mental faculties and an organization of responses that increases the degree of dissociation between consciousness and subconsciousness, thus establishing in effect but not in actuality a dissociated hypnotic personality. [1939]

(In Erickson, 1980, Vol. IV, chap. 1, p. 6)

Awakening and putting a patient back into trance repeatedly is a way of deepening trance.

(Erickson & Rossi, 1979, p. 253)

I didn't want it to be a one time thing because that closes it off. When you have a second trance you can have a third, a fourth, a fifth, and that knowledge allows a continuation of the thought, "I can have a trance ten years from now."

(Zeig, 1980, p. 353)

The time required to induce the first deaf state ranged from twenty to forty minutes, an interval indicated by previous experience with other subjects as requisite to achieve the "mental set" permitting a consistent, reliable state of deafness to develop.

(In Erickson, 1980, Vol. II, chap. 10, p. 84)

Ordinarily, a total of four to eight hours of initial induction training is sufficient. Then, since trance induction is one process and trance utilization is another — to permit the subjects to reorganize behavioral processes in accord with projected hypnotic work, time must necessarily be allotted with full regard for their capacities to learn and to respond. [1952]

(In Erickson, 1980, Vol. I, chap. 6, p. 143)

I've seen patients for as long as 16 consecutive hours ...I've seen patients for 12 hours, for eight hours, preferably for four hours, and often for two or three hours depending upon the patient's problems and the degree of urgency. Usually I like to see a patient for only one hour.

(Erickson & Rossi, 1981, p. 18)

A special technique of suggestion was devised by which subjects in the stuporous trance could slowly and gradually adjust themselves to the demands of the somnambulistic trance. Usually an hour or more was spent in systematic suggestion, building up the somnambulistic state so that all behavior manifested was in response to the immediate hypnotic situation, with no need on the part of the subjects to bring into the situation their usual responses to a normal waking situation. Essentially this training was directed to a complete inhibition of all spontaneous activity while giving complete freedom for all responsive activity. [1938]

(In Erickson, 1980, Vol. II, chap. 10, p. 82)

The author has so often emphasized the need for spending four to eight or more hours in inducing trances and training subjects to function adequately before attempting hypnotic experimentation or therapy. [1952]

(In Erickson, 1980, Vol. I, chap. 6, p. 145)

I can afford the time.

(Zeig, 1980, p. 334)

Maintain the Trance

Trance induction, trance utilization, and trance maintenance are three different components of the hypnotic session. The effective hypnotist must help the subject with all three. In a sense, they must all be accomplished almost simultaneously. To accomplish this, suggestions designed to induce or deepen the trance, suggestions to maintain the depth already achieved, and suggestions to elicit additional alterations in mental set and response must be interspersed throughout the hypnotic process. It does no good to induce a deep trance if that depth is lost as soon as the first hypnotic suggestion is offered.

Although this may appear to be a difficult, confusing task for the hypnotist, the necessary shifting of attention from one purpose to another actually encourages the hypnotist to present guidance and instructions in such a manner that it is increasingly difficult for the subject's conscious mind to follow the shifts or to take issue with any particular suggestion. Working with more than one purpose in mind seems to be something of a confusion technique in and of itself, one that eventuates in a further withdrawal of the conscious mind, an increased dissociation, and a more satisfactory hypnotic response.

Experience with many subjects discloses a frequent tendency to return to a lighter trance state when given complicated hypnotic tasks. Such subjects for various reasons are thereby endeavoring to ensure adequate functioning by enlisting the aid of conscious mental processes. [1952]

(In Erickson, 1980, Vol. I, chap. 6, p. 142)

Trance induction is one thing, and trance utilization is another. [1952]

(In Erickson, 1980, Vol. I, chap. 6, p. 147)

And to use it [hypnosis] for therapeutic purposes, it must be maintained.

(Erickson & Rossi, 1981, p. 188)

During a technique of suggestions for trance induction and trance maintenance, hypnotherapeutic suggestions can be interspersed for a specific goal. [1966]

(In Erickson, 1980, Vol. IV, chap. 28, p. 266)

Combining psychotherapeutic, amnestic, and posthypnotic suggestions with those suggestions used first to induce a trance, and then to maintain that trance, constitutes an effective measure in securing desired results. [1966]

(In Erickson, 1980, Vol. IV, chap. 28, p. 267)

Such an interspersing of therapeutic suggestions among the suggestions for trance maintenance may often render the therapeutic suggestions much more effective. The patients hear them, understand them, but before they can take issue with them or question them in any way, their attention is captured by the trance maintenance suggestions. [1966]

(In Erickson, 1980, Vol. IV, chap. 28, p. 266)

Once the hypnotic trance has been induced, there is need to keep a subject in the trance until the necessary work has been completed. This is best done by instructing the subjects to sleep continuously, to let nothing disturb them, to enjoy their trance state, and above all to enjoy their feeling of comfort, satisfaction, and full confidence in themselves, their situation, and their ability to meet adequately and well any problem or task that may be presented to them. [1944]

(In Erickson, 1980, Vol. IV, chap. 2, p. 18)

Maintain a Belief in Success

Ideally, both the hypnotist and the subject should believe firmly from beginning to end that the hypnotic process is going to succeed. At minimum, the hypnotist should demonstrate this conviction of success openly and obviously all the way through and lead the subject to share in this conviction during the hypnotic experience itself. Nothing should be done that could possibly undermine the subject's belief in the success of the hypnotic process.

Accordingly, the hypnotist should endeavor to create or elicit behaviors or internal events that ratify or validate trance responsiveness for the subject and that justify an expectation of future responsivity. Suggestions should be given in such a manner that failure is impossible, that they will lead at least to the appearance of success or complicance. If the hypnotist has any uncertainty about the subject's ability or willingness to accept and act upon a particular suggestion, that suggestion should not be presented in a direct manner. Instead, a suggestion that calls for an otherwise inevitable response, an all-encompassing suggestion or inescapable double-bind suggestion should be used.

Furthermore, whenever a compliant hypnotic response is received, it should be acknowledged, praised and used later as the basis for additional suggestions. In this way the hypnotic process becomes a naturally evolving coherent structure which builds upon its own successes.

> **You're emphasizing the fact that she's going to respond, that she's all set to respond. [1959]**
> *(In Erickson, 1980, Vol. I, chap. 9, p. 209)*

Failure in attempts at hypnotic therapy always increases the difficulty of further efforts at therapy. Hence, for the benefit of the individual patient, extensive care and effort is always warranted.[1944]

(In Erickson, 1980, Vol. IV, chap. 2, p. 23)

Every effort should be made to make the subjects feel comfortable, satisfied, and confident about their ability to go into a trance, and the hypnotist should maintain an attitude of unshaken and contagious confidence in the subject's ability. A simple, earnest, unpretentious, confident manner is of paramount importance. [1944]

(In Erickson, 1980, Vol. IV, chap. 2, p. 18)

You keep validating your suggestions as you go along.

(Erickson & Rossi, 1979, p. 375)

All suggestions are used to reinforce, substantiate, and validate others.

(Erickson & Rossi, 1981, p. 218)

Validate the suggestion by commenting on it. [1959]

(In Erickson, 1980, Vol. I, chap. 9, p. 240)

Not knowing what will develop, better have plenty of set-ups that you can use. A multitude of preliminary suggestions offers an opportunity for subsequent selection and use. [1959]

(In Erickson, 1980, Vol. I, chap. 9, p. 217)

You have to lay the foundation. [1959]

(In Erickson, 1980, Vol. I, chap. 9, p. 255)

All your suggestions in therapy should be a connected whole.

(Erickson & Rossi, 1979, p. 252)

A good technique keeps referring back. [1959]
(In Erickson, 1980, Vol. I, chap. 9, p. 232)

Get Subjects To Do It

It is best not to accept total responsibility for controlling or directing everything that happens during the hypnosis session. Teachers do not expect themselves to teach their students everything. Students need to be given homework and free time to explore and use the things they are learning. The concepts they discover on their own and the abilities they master through unsupervised practice will be more significant, interesting, and long-lasting than anything told them by the teacher.

Hypnotherapists need to adopt this "teacher" perspective. Subjects must be given free time to explore and to master their hypnotic abilities. They must be encouraged to become familiar with the potentials of the state of mind in which they now find themselves. They must be given the freedom to learn what they can do and the motivation to apply that learning effectively. Finally, and most importantly, they must be provided with the opportunity to give themselves suggestions, especially suggestions having a therapeutic orientation. The use of indirect implications, metaphors, analogies, multiple options, puns, or deliberate mispronunciations can be invaluable in stimulating these internally-originated self-suggestions. Frequently, however, the hypnotist should just get out of the picture entirely, leaving subjects to their own devices with only the simple expectation of interesting and beneficial results of some unknown, and perhaps unknowable, type. Both brief and lengthy pauses of this sort may allow the induction and utilization processes to progress smoothly.

Then situations were devised in which the subjects had ample time and opportunity to discover and to develop their abilities to respond to the demands made of them with as little interference from the hypnotist as possible. [1944]

(In Erickson, 1980, Vol. 2, chap. 4, p. 36)

The crucial step of bridging the gap between light hypnosis and a deep trance can often be accomplished easily by letting the subject assume the entire responsibility for this further progress instead of resorting to the use of overwhelming, compelling suggestions by the hypnotist. [1945]

(In Erickson, 1980, Vol. IV, chap. 3. p. 32)

In therapy this is often the way you get patients to become aware of their capabilities. You are essentially giving them the freedom to use themselves. Patients come to you because they don't feel free to use themselves.

(Erickson, Rossi & Rossi, 1976, p. 292)

This is the Experiential Mode of Hypnotic Induction. You let the subject experience his own behavior and toy with it. It is an experiential phenomenon by which the self teaches the self by studying dissociated frames of reference, frames of reference that are unfamiliar.

(Erickson & Rossi, 1981, p. 242)

You let them have an opportunity to experience their trance state without necessarily giving them anything to do. You leave them to their own devices. It deepens the trance. They become more aware of what they can do. They become more facile in their capacities.

Erickson, Rossi & Rossi, 1976, p. 141)

Here I am excluding myself so the patient must initiate his own inner exploration. [1976–78]

(In Erickson, 1980, Vol. I, chap. 23, p. 481)

I'm giving Dr. S an opportunity for inner experiential learning in this trance, which she won't know about until the time is right to use it.

(Erickson, Rossi & Rossi, 1976, p. 291)

He was allowed to continue in the trance for an additional thirty minutes while the author left the room. [1964]

(In Erickson, 1980, Vol. I, chap. 13, p. 313)

And so I continue and let subjects deepen their own trances because what they are doing is more important, and they can continue. I continue my hand levitation suggestions, knowing that they are useless and serving no purpose except to give the subjects opportunity to deepen their own trance experiences. [1976–78]

(In Erickson, 1980, Vol. I, chap. 23, p. 490)

She did not accept the suggestions offered her by the author; she accepted only the opportunity offered to reach understandings in her own way, taking advantage of the author's suggestions as a means but nothing more. [1964]

(In Erickson, 1980, Vol. I, chap. 15, p. 348)

And the subject takes credit for it. You're not telling the subject to "do this, do that." So many therapists tell their patients how to think and how to feel. That is awfully wrong.

(Erickson, Rossi & Rossi, 1976, p. 101)

So you don't have to depend upon verbal constructions because you want your patient to do a lot of things. You don't want to have to tell the patients everything they are to do... Therefore you build up a situation so they are free to respond on their own initiative.

(Erickson & Rossi, 1981, p. 214)

Thus, suggestions are given to the subject, but the execution of them, the rapidity and time of response, and their effectiveness are made the responsibility of the subject, and they are contingent upon processes taking place within him and related to his own needs. [1945]

(In Erickson, 1980, Vol. IV, chap. 3, p. 32)

Because it is his own creative effort he is less likely to reject it than if it was simply thrust upon him as a direct statement.

(Erickson & Rossi, 1979, p. 259)

Now I have stressed this because I want to impress upon you the tremendous importance in *offering your suggestions not as the thing the patient is to do but as the stimulus to elicit patient behavior in accordance with individual body learnings, individual psychological experiences.*

(Erickson & Rossi, 1979, p. 137)

The more participation you can get from them, the better. [1959]

(In Erickson, 1980, Vol. I, chap. 9, p. 212)

R: You facilitate the patient's saying the suggestions to themselves.
E: Yes, cause them to say it to themselves!

(Erickson & Rossi, 1981, p. 28)

It's always much better to have patients make important suggestions to themselves.

(Erickson & Rossi, 1979, p. 285)

Acceptance of such help is neither an expression of ignorance nor of incompetence: rather, it is an honest recognition that deep hypnosis is a joint endeavor in which the subject does the work and the hypnotist tries to stimulate the subject to make the necesary effort.

(Erickson & Rossi, 1979, p. 61)

"Direct suggestion...does not evoke the re-association and reorganization of ideas, understandings, and memories so essential for an actual cure. ...Effective results in hypnotic psychotherapy...derive only from the patient's activities. The therapist merely stimulates the patient into activity, often not knowing what that activity may be. And then he guides the patient and exercises clinical judgment in determining the amount of work to be done to achieve the desired results."

(Erickson & Rossi, 1979, p. 9)

Summary

The hypnotic induction process consists of fixating a subject's attention so intensely upon internal events and away from external reality that there is created a dissociation whereby the ordinary conscious frame of mind disappears from awareness and is replaced by the perspectives of the unconscious mind. The hypnotist accomplishes this focused redirection of attention by direct or indirect verbal and non verbal techniques designed to elicit ideomotor responses, to create boredom, confusion, or surprise, and to initiate a dissociation between the operations of the conscious and the unconscious minds.

Subjects should be allowed to use whatever length of time is necessary for them to progress into a deep trance state. Trance maintenance instructions should be intermingled with whatever additional induction or deepening techniques are provided along the way. Circumstances should be arranged so that subjects experience successful hypnotic responsivity and all successes should be used to validate the trance state to the subject. Eventually, the responsibility for a successful induction and utilization of hypnosis should be turned almost completely over to the subjects. Long pauses should be included to allow and encourage the subjects to explore their own unconscious potentials and to give themselves appropriate therapeutic suggestions. In this way, hypnosis can be used to help subjects learn more effective methods for assessing and utilizing their own potentials and experientially acquired learnings.

CHAPTER ELEVEN

UTILIZING HYPNOSIS THERAPEUTICALLY: GENERAL CONSIDERATIONS

Within an Ericksonian framework, the behaviors and goals of the psychotherapist and of the hypnotherapist are almost identical. The primary difference is the presence or absence of a special state of mind (hypnosis) in the patient. This state of mind can enhance the effectiveness of what the therapist says or does and can enable patients to be more receptive to their own experiences and unconscious perceptions, abilities, and knowledge. The same goals, roles, attitudes, and techniques of interaction are applicable in both situations. Hypnosis itself is merely a circumstance offering increased leverage to the therapist and increased freedom to the patient. It is a tool for making therapy easier and not a form of therapy in and of itself. The obvious parallels between the following general comments by Erickson about hypnosis and the general comments made by him about psychotherapy should demonstrate this point quite clearly.

Hypnosis is Only a Tool

Any therapeutic situation is an appropriate situation for the use of hypnosis. Although hypnosis is not always necessary to accomplish therapeutic goals, it can usually make it easier to do so. In fact, Erickson evidently believed that hypnosis could facilitate the development of almost all the ingredients of successful psychotherapy. He maintained that hypnosis could be used to establish a positive relationship with patients, to secure their attention, to enhance their cooperation, to increase their acceptance of responsibility for change, and to develop more conceptual flexibility and responsivity to their own potentials for objectively based perception, understanding, and response.

In spite of the advantages that hypnosis offers, Erickson emphasized on numerous occasions that it is not a miracle worker. Hypnosis should not be used to demand or to suggest directly the desired changes in personality, emotion, or behavior. Such an approach will usually be futile or will only produce short-lived alterations at best. Rather, hypnosis should be used to facilitate the learning and therapeutic reorganization necessary to allow the desired changes to occur in a natural and permanent manner. Changes in personality, cognition, emotion, or behavior should be an outgrowth of the learning allowed by hypnosis and not a direct expression of specific hypnotic suggestions.

> **As for the type of case warranting the use of hypnosis, the answer is simply any case in which you wish full, free, and easy cooperation to the patient's fullest capacity. [circa 1950's]**
>
> *(In Erickson, 1980, Vol. IV, chap. 21, p. 227)*

> **To repeat: all patients who come to you seeking the help, the inspiration, and the motivation they need to**

recover and maintain recovery can benefit from hypnosis. [1957]

(In Erickson, 1980, Vol. IV, chap. 5, p. 49)

What are some of the uses of hypnosis in psychiatry? The first, and I think the primary, use of it should be in establishing a good personal relationship with the patient. [1957]

(In Erickson, 1980, Vol. IV, chap. 5, p. 49)

Indeed, hypnosis offers the patient a sense of comfort and an attitude of interest in his own active participation in his therapy. [1945]

(In Erickson, 1980, Vol. IV, chap. 3, p. 34)

Hypnosis was used solely as a modality by means of which to secure their co-operation in accepting the therapy they wanted. [1964]

(In Erickson, 1980, Vol. IV, chap. 19, p. 207)

In other words, they were induced by hypnosis to acknowledge and act upon their own personal responsibility for successfully accepting the previously sought and offered but actually rejected therapy. [1964]

(In Erickson, 1980, Vol. IV, chap. 19, p. 207)

Usually, however, hypnotic questioning serves to elicit the information more readily than can be done in the waking state, but the entire process of overcoming the resistance and reluctance depends on the development of a good patient-physician relationship rather than upon hypnotic measures, and the hypnosis is essentially, in such situations, no more than a means by which the patient can give the information in a relatively comfortable fashion.

(Erickson, 1939a, pp. 401-02)

I regard hypnotic techniques as essentially no more than a means of asking your subjects (or patients) to pay attention to you so that you can offer them some ideas which can initiate them into an activation of their own capacities to behave. [1960]

(In Erickson, 1980, Vol. II, chap. 31, p. 315)

It is possible to use hypnosis as a method by which you can secure patients' complete attention. It is then possible to focus their attention and to create a state of receptivity by such stimulation so that they function in accordance with those relevant past learnings. [1960]

(In Erickson, 1980, Vol. II, chap. 31, p. 375)

Also of paramount importance is the fact that the hypnotized patient is in a receptive state for psychotherapy. The difficulty involved in getting patients to accept therapeutic suggestions directly constitutes the greatest obstacle in psychotherapy. Hypnosis renders the person receptive.

(Erickson, 1934, p. 61)

In hypnosis, however, individuals are more open to ideas, and they more readily consent to examine them. [1960]

(In Erickson, 1980, Vol. II, chap. 31, p. 321)

Hypnosis, facilitating as it does a receptiveness and a responsiveness to ideas, is of value in every aspect wherein instruction, advice, counsel, guidance, direction, reassurance, comfort, and all those manifold values of interpersonal relationships are so significant. [circa 1950's]

(In Erickson, 1980, Vol. IV, chap. 21, p. 228)

Hypnosis is a modality by which can be elicited with greater than ordinary ease those patterns of behavior, thinking and feeling more conducive to the welfare of the individual and his society than to the promotion of some school of interpretative and speculative theoretical concepts and formulations. [1965]

(In Erickson, 1980, Vol. I, chap. 29, p. 542)

It [hypnosis] is not a miracle worker, even though its results sometimes seems to be miraculous. Rather, it is an effective measure by which one can slowly, carefully, and thoroughly elicit, as a result of careful suggestions, forms of behavior, emotional reactions, insights and understandings which would be impossible or nearly so in the ordinary waking state in which the subject's attention to a chosen field cannot be so completely secured and rigidly fixed as it can be in hypnosis.

(Erickson, 1941b, p. 17)

Hypnosis is not an absolute answer...Rather it is no more than one of the adjuvants or synergistic measures that can be employed to meet the patient's needs. [1959]

(In Erickson, 1980, Vol. IV, chap. 27, p. 255)

Hypnosis, like every other psychotherapeutic procedure, should be looked upon as a means of approach to the problem and not as the royal road to the achievement of miracles. [1932]

(In Erickson, 1980, Vol. I, chap. 24, p. 493)

Hypnosis is not a cure. [1970]

(In Erickson, 1980, Vol. IV, chap. 6, p. 74)

There is really no such thing as hypnotherapy. There is *therapy* wherein you use hypnotic modalities, hypnotic understandings, hypnotic approaches, and that sort of thing. But hypnosis in itself is not a therapy.

(ASCH, 1980, Taped Lecture, 7/18/65)

In this author's understanding of psychotherapy, if a patient wants to believe in a "hypnotic miracle" so strongly that he will undertake the responsibility of making a recovery by virtue of his own actual behavior and continue that recovery, he is at liberty to do so under whatever guise he chooses, but neither the author nor the reader is obliged to regard the success of the therapy as a hypnotic miracle. [1964]

(In Erickson, 1980, Vol. IV, chap. 19, p. 207)

It's true that direct suggestion can effect an alteration in the patient's behavior and result in a symptomatic cure, at least temporarily. However, such a "cure" is simply a response to suggestion and does not entail that reassociation and reorganization of ideas, understandings and memories so essential for actual cure. *It is this experience of reassociating and reorganizing his own experiential life that eventuates in a cure, not the manifestation of responsive behavior which can, at best, satisfy only the observer.* [1948]

(In Rossi, 1973, p. 19)

In my own hypnotic work I have, as an experimental approach to personality problems, attempted over a period of years to build up new personalities in hypnotic subjects, only to realize the futility of such attempts. [circa 1940's]

(In Erickson, 1980, Vol. III, chap. 24, p. 264)

It is possible to build up in the hypnotic subject pseudo-personalities, but these are extremely limited in character and extent of development, and they obviously are temporary, superimposed manifestations. [circa 1940's]

(In Erickson, 1980, Vol. III, chap. 24, p. 264)

> **The stimuli emanating from reality and those from memory trances within the brain are fundamentally different in their components, and it smacks of the miraculous to assume that a time limited procedure could establish a fundamental alteration of the psychological habits established in a lifetime. [1932]**
>
> *(In Erickson, 1980, Vol. I, chap. 24, p. 497)*

Hypnosis Increases Access to Potentials

Hypnosis is just another means toward the goal of enabling patients to use their own potentials. It gives them the opportunity to reorganize their learnings and to take responsibility for their own therapeutic gains. The hypnotic state serves the same purpose as the therapeutic climate discussed previously. The induction of an hypnotic condition is simply the creation of a comfortable setting wherein the patient can follow the leads or implications of the therapist and can cooperate in the therapeutic process more easily and more completely. Hypnosis does not provide patients with new capacities, but allows them easier access to and more effective utilization of their experiences and pre-existing abilities, knowledge, and potentials. Hypnosis merely makes it easier for both the patient and the therapist to conduct therapy and to focus effectively upon the problems under consideration; it does not alter the basic goals of therapy nor does it alter significantly the procedures and principles relevant to the accomplishment of those goals.

> **I'm like all other doctors. I can't help you either. But there is something that you know, but you don't know that you know it. As soon as you find out what it is that you already know, but don't know you know, you can begin having dry beds.**
>
> *(Zeig, 1980, p. 81)*

There is a strong normal tendency for the personality to adjust if given an opportunity. [1955]

(In Erickson, 1980, Vol. IV, chap. 56, p. 505)

Properly oriented, hypnotic therapy can give the patient that necessary understanding of his own role in effecting his recovery and thus enlist his own effort and participation in his own cure without giving him a sense of dependence upon drugs and medical care. [1954]

(In Erickson, 1980, Vol. IV, chap. 3, p. 34)

Hypnotic psychotherapy is a learning process for the patient, a procedure of reeducation. [1948]

(In Erickson, 1980, Vol. IV, chap. 4, p. 39)

Hypnosis facilitates exceedingly effective learnings that would be impossible otherwise except by prolonged effort and therapy. [1960]

(In Erickson, 1980, Vol. II, chap. 31, p. 316)

Go into a deep trance because you have got billions of brain cells that will function and you will learn all that there is to learn.

(Zeig, 1980, p. 49)

It [hypnosis] serves to permit them to learn more about themselves and to express themselves more adequately. [1948]

(In Erickson, 1980, Vol. IV, chap. 4, p. 38)

It [hypnosis] is gaining acceptance because of its valuable ability to enlist as fully as possible the patient's own capabilities and potentialities at both psychological and physiological levels of functioning. [circa 1950's]

(In Erickson, 1980, Vol. IV, chap. 21, p. 225)

Hypnosis is in fact the induction of a peculiar psychological state which permits subjects to reassociate and reorganize inner psychological complexities in a way suitable to the unique items of their own psychological experiences. [1944]

(In Erickson, 1980, Vol. III, chap. 21, p. 207)

Successful hypnotic psychotherapy should be systematically directed to a reeducation of patients, a development of insight into the nature of their problems, and the promotion of their earnest desires to readjust themselves to the realities of life and the problems confronting them. [1944]

(In Erickson, 1980, Vol. IV, chap. 2, p. 22)

This is essentially a physician-patient relationship that permits the physician to enable the patient to capitalize upon every positive thing he has to reach a satisfactory adjustment in life rather than become psychologically invalided. [1944]

(In Erickson, 1980, Vol. IV, chap. 2, p. 22)

In other words, the hypnotic state derives from, or results in, an attentiveness and a receptiveness to ideas and understandings as well as a readiness to function responsively to the ideas themselves without a need to establish them as stimuli emerging from or constituting a part of the existing objective reality external to the self! As a result, the reality or validity of ideas and suggestions in hypnosis which act as stimuli to elicit responses based upon experiential learnings transcends in importance and significance the irrelevant, coincidental, or concomitant aspects of objective reality. [1958]

(In Erickson, 1980, Vol. II, chap. 19, p. 195)

Hypnosis was used for the specific purpose of placing the burden of responsibility for therapeutic results upon the patient himself after he himself had reached a definite conclusion that therapy would not help and that a last resort would be a hypnotic "miracle." [1964]

(In Erickson, 1980, Vol. IV, chap. 19, p. 207)

The use of hypnosis as a technique of deliberately shifting from the therapist to the patient the entire burden of both defining the psychotherapy desired and the responsibility for accepting it. [1964]

(In Erickson, 1980, Vol. IV, chap. 19, p. 211)

Again she was assured that her own behavior would be employed to produce effective results. [1960]

(In Erickson, 1980, Vol. IV, chap. 16, p. 186)

The subject cannot be forced to do things against his will, but rather he can be aided in achieving desired goals.

(Erickson, 1954b, pp. 22–23)

Indeed, in medical hypnosis the result obtained should derive primarily from the subject's activity and participation since it is his needs and problems that must be met. [1945]

(In Erickson, 1980, Vol. IV, chap. 3, p. 33)

Effective results in hypnotic psychotherapy, or hypnotherapy, derive only from the patient's activities. [1948]

(In Erickson, 1980, Vol. IV, chap. 4, p. 39)

The hypnotic subject can participate actively in his own hypnotic trance in an indefinite but nonetheless significant manner, and in direct relation to his own needs; and

that hypnotic technique oriented to this understanding can reasonably offer the hypnotic patient an opportunity to deal with his own needs and problems in accord with his own psychological structure and experiences. [1945]
(In Erickson, 1980, Vol. IV, chap. 3, p. 33)

Requisite to effective hypnotherapy — and the same holds true for experimental hypnosis — is the adequate communication of ideas and understandings to the hypnotized person. Since the object of hypnotherapy is not the intellectual clarification of understandings but the attainment by the patient of personal goals, this cannot be achieved by a simple reliance upon the inherent values of the ideas and understandings to be presented. Rather, communications need to be presented in terms of the patient's personal and subjective needs, learnings, and experiences, whether reasonable or unreasonable, recognized or unrecognized, so that there can be an acceptance and a response and a feeling of personal fulfillment. [1960]
(In Erickson, 1980, Vol. IV, chap. 16, p. 181)

And you use hypnosis for the patient to discover, he can do things.
(Zeig, 1980, p. 93)

Hypnosis cannot create new abilities within a person, but it can assist in a greater and better utilization of abilities already possessed, even if these abilities were not previously recognized. [1970]
(In Erickson, 1980, Vol. IV, chap. 6, p. 54)

Thus, a favorable setting is evolved for the elicitation of needful and helpful behavioral potentialities not previously used, or not fully used or perhaps misused by the patient. [1966]
(In Erickson, 1980, Vol. IV, chap. 28, p. 263)

It [hypnosis] serves to elicit and to release the actual patterns of behavior and response existing within the patient and available for adequate and useful expression of the personality. [1965]

(In Erickson, 1980, Vol. I, chap. 29, p. 542)

Hypnosis could help him only by making more available to him his own potentials for self-help. [1966]

(In Erickson, 1980, Vol. IV, chap. 18, p. 193)

I'd like to have you be aware of the fact that you yourself possess a lot of potentials of which you are unaware, just as your patients possess potentials of which they are unaware. And you use hypnosis as a means of communicating ideas and understandings to your patients, but also use it as a means of becoming aware that you too possess unrealized potentialities and capabilities and interests that you ought to develop.

(ASCH, 1980, Taped Lecture, 7/16/65)

Hypnosis can allow you to divide up your patient's problems.

(Erickson & Rossi, 1981, p. 6)

In other words, I use hypnosis to govern the way in which things are presented to the patient.

(Erickson & Rossi, 1981, p. 19)

There can be achieved no transcendence of abilities, no implantation of new abilities, but only the potentiation of the expression of abilities that may have gone unrecognized or not fully recognized. [1970]

(In Erickson, 1980, Vol. IV, chap. 6, p. 54)

Hypnosis is essentially that sort of concept, i.e., a way to offer stimuli of various kinds that will enable patients in response to those stimuli to utilize their own experiential learnings. **[1960]**

(In Erickson, 1980, Vol. II, chap. 31, p. 316)

In this type of phenomenon [post-hypnotic behavior] lies probably the greatest medical and experimental value of hypnosis, since it permits a direction and a guidance of behavior, but only in terms of the patterns of response belonging to the individual.

(Erickson, 1954b, p. 23)

Hypnosis offers an opportunity to control and direct thinking, to select and exclude memories and ideas, and thus to give the patient the opportunity to deal individually and adequately with any selected item of experience. **[1945]**

(In Erickson, 1980, Vol. IV, chap. 3, p. 34)

In other words, the hypnotic technique serves only to induce a favorable setting in which to instruct patients in a more advantageous use of their own potentials of behavior. **[1966]**

(In Erickson, 1980, Vol. IV, chap. 28, p. 262)

Hypnotherapeutic benefits, especially in such cases as reported here, are markedly contingent upon a varied and repetitious presentation of ideas and understandings to insure an adequate acceptance and responsiveness by the patient. **[1959]**

(In Erickson, 1980, Vol. IV, chap. 27, p. 261)

I teach my patients to listen carefully to my words and to follow my train of suggestions closely. **[1960]**

(In Erickson, 1980, Vol. II, chap. 31, p. 318)

Actually, the sole purpose of these purported and repetitious explanations is merely to offer or to repeat various suggestions and instructions without seemingly doing so. [1964]

(In Erickson, 1980, Vol. I, chap. 13, p. 306)

Hypnosis is a state of awareness in which you offer communications with understandings and ideas to a patient and then you let them use those ideas and understandings in accord with their own unique body learnings, their physiological learnings. Once you get them started, they can then proceed to utilize a wealth of other experiences. [1960]

(In Erickson, 1980, Vol. II, chap. 31, p. 323)

Throughout life there are various conditions of learning for individuals that involve their total functioning as organic creatures, where blood circulation, neural and muscle behavior, and other organ systems participate most actively. Whenever you set up the right kind of stimuli, you can elicit some of these experientially conditioned behaviors. [1960]

(In Erickson, 1980, Vol. II, chap. 31, p. 315)

But this experiential learning is unconsciously acquired and is elicited by stimuli not even intended to do so but which set into action mental processes within the listener at an involuntary level, often uncontrollable. [1964]

(In Erickson, 1980, Vol. I, chap. 13, p. 327)

Stimuli can then be given to take advantage of existing, but unrealized, body learnings. [1970]

(In Erickson, 1980, Vol. IV, chap. 6, p. 75)

Hypnosis can be used to elicit the learnings acquired by the human body, but unrealized by the person. [1970]

(In Erickson, 1980, Vol. IV, chap. 6, p. 75)

Hypnosis Helps Overcome Conscious Barriers

Most of the barriers to therapeutic progress are attributable to the functions of the conscious mind. Psychopathology and inadequate or inappropriate use of experiential learnings and underlying potentials are usually produced in the first place by the irrational biases, conditionings, and limiting concepts of the conscious mind. In these instances, therapeutic change requires an alteration of the erroneous or unproductive conscious patterns of thought, perception, or response. But, as noted previously, the conscious mind will defend itself against such changes and protect itself from all internal or external assaults upon its organization. Furthermore, the conscious mind tends to be distracted by irrelevancies and is also unable to allow the potentials of the unconscious mind to be accessed or employed effectively. Therefore, even when problems stem from unconscious beliefs or understandings, correction of them is made difficult or impossible by the mere presence of conscious activities.

Luckily, hypnosis offers a pathway around or through these conscious barriers. Attention is captured and focused upon the pertinent issues and experiences more easily in a hypnotic state and the conscious defenses and biases become less and less operative as contact with externalities diminishes. The patterns of thought that normally cause misunderstandings, distortions, and limitations are replaced by an increased openness to new ideas and a refreshing clarity of perception. The comfort and quiet awareness of even a mild hypnotic condition enables patients to participate more freely, to discuss themselves more openly, to examine issues more calmly and to profit from their experiences more directly. Even if these were the only beneficial consequences of hypnosis, they certainly would warrant its widespread application.

It [hypnosis] gives the patient an opportunity to reassociate and reorganize the psychological complexities and disturbances of his psychic life under special conditions that permit him to deal with his problems constructively; free from overwhelming distress. [1945]

(In Erickson, 1980, Vol. IV, chap. 3, p. 33)

You must realize that hypnosis allows you to come back to a particular idea, or fear, or anxiety so that it is never necessary to ask a patient to experience too much distress or emotional discomfort at any one time.

(Erickson & Rossi, 1981, p. 5)

The rationale for the use of hypnosis in the healing arts is the beneficial effect of restriction of the patient's attention to those items of behavior and function pertinent to his well-being. [1970]

(In Erickson, 1980, Vol. IV, chap. 6, p. 54)

Hypnosis allows freedom and ease in structuring the therapeutic situation and renders the patient much more accessible. [1965]

(In Erickson, 1980, Vol. IV, chap. 58, p. 523)

But in a state of hypnosis the field of conscious awareness is limited and tends to be restricted to exactly pertinent matters, other considerations being irrelevant. [1970]

(In Erickson, 1980, Vol. IV, chap. 6, p. 55)

The less disturbed they are by such outer distractions, the more focused is their energy on therapy.

(Erickson, Rossi & Rossi, 1976, p. 6)

R: A major function of psychotherapy is to let unimportant things fade into the background and only the relevant things come into the foreground. That's what hypnotherapy does *par excellence.*

E: That's right and R didn't take hold of these background things.

I let her render them into the background.

(Erickson & Rossi, 1979, p. 310)

In a hypnotic state the patient gains a more acute awareness of his needs and capabilities. He is freed from mistaken beliefs, false assumptions, self-doubts and fears which might otherwise stand in the way. [1957]

(In Erickson, 1980, Vol. IV, chap. 5, p. 49)

Thereby the patients are prevented from intruding unhelpfully into a situation which they cannot understand and for which they are seeking help. At the same time, a readiness to understand and to respond is created within the patient. Thus, a favorable setting is evolved for the elicitation of needful and helpful behavioral potentialities not previously used, or not fully used or perhaps misused by the patient. [1966]

(In Erickson, 1980, Vol. IV, chap. 28, pp. 262-263)

When a person goes into a trance, you bounce him around and keep him whirling and then you tell him to work quietly on that problem. You have first detached him from his conscious mental sets. You have broken the connections that have been stopping him from working on his problem. That is a very important thing.

(Erickson, Rossi & Rossi, 1976, p. 196)

You use the trance state so that you can get around the self-protection which the neurosis provides on an unrecognized level. The neurotic is self-protective of the neurosis. [1973]

(In Erickson, 1980, Vol. III, chap. 11, p. 100)

I'm not going to let her conscious mind grab onto anything that she can dispute! You move away from dispute.

(Erickson & Rossi, 1981, p. 105)

E: These shifts from negative (won't) to the positive (will) and sometimes the shift from positive to negative are keeping the patient in a constant state of movement. You change the mind this way and back...

E: You don't let the patients get a set. A mental set they can stay with...

E: You don't want them with *their* mental set.

R: You keep them in movement so they will have to grasp onto your mental set?

E: Yes, the mental set you want to work with. You keep them in flux so you can constantly orient them. But you aren't telling them, "I want you to pay attention to this one thing."

(Erickson, Rossi & Rossi, 1976, p. 175)

I asked her, "How do you *feel?*" because I did not want her *thinking*.

(Erickson & Rossi, 1979, p. 291)

Constant alertness must be exercised to prevent any undue thinking that might break down the established psychological orientation.

(Erickson, 1954c, p. 264)

I don't want her conscious programs to depotentiate it!

(Erickson, Rossi & Rossi, 1976, p. 291)

By this general measure new trance states can be secured free from the limitations deriving from various factors such as the subject's mental set, deliberate conscious intentions regarding trance behavior, misconcep-

tions, and the continuance of waking patterns of behavior. [1941]

(In Erickson, 1980, Vol. 1, chap. 19, p. 403)

Hypnosis Facilitates Learning

Hypnosis enables patients to learn from experienced events which they would otherwise tend to recoil from, overlook, or distort. Hypnosis thereby allows the business of therapy (i.e. experientially based learning) to progress more efficiently toward the final goal of objective perception, acceptance and competence within a reality which previously had caused problems or symptoms. Hypnosis helps remove the conscious barriers to this process and facilitates a more meaningful use of the patient's resources.

Hypnosis enables patients to confront their problems or difficulties head-on instead of downplaying or denying them. They can meet their enemies directly and somewhat comfortably in the trance state and can be encouraged to discover new or more competent ways to cope with them. Experiences can be created which encourage or demand a therapeutic response and communications can be offered which achieve an alteration in understanding. Past learnings can be marshalled and applied in new ways to the problem via direct or indirect suggestions for that outcome.

As in a non-hypnotic psychotherapeutic situation, questions may be asked to focus the individual's attention on pertinent issues or to initiate an application of previous learnings to the present problem. Vague instructions or implied directives may be employed to force patients to generate their own internally based solutions. Metaphorical, analogical, or symbolic descriptions of the presenting problems may transform them sufficiently to allow patients to develop metaphoric or symbolic modes of response which can then be applied directly to their own circumstances. Hypnosis can be used to teach the person apparently new skills (e.g. anesthesia, dissociation, etc.) which can then be applied to their real life problems. Finally, hypnosis can be used to break down mental sets, to provide untried alternative sets or to bypass conscious mental sets altogether.

What all of this means when translated into specifics is that a large part of the hypnotherapeutic process is conducted in exactly the same manner, using exactly the same strategies and verbalizations as ordinary Ericksonian psychotherapy in the conscious state. The only significant difference is that the patient is hypnotized while the therapeutic learning process is conducted. This change in the patient's state of mind does not necessarily have a dramatic effect on what the therapist does; it only makes the patient more responsive by diminishing conscious barriers. Even when the patient moves into a deep trance state and begins functioning at an unconscious level of awareness, what the therapist attempts to do remains similar to what is attempted in waking therapy. The therapist's options increase at that point — as does the patient's responsiveness — but it is important to note once more that hypnosis, even deep hypnosis, merely facilitates the therapeutic process. It does not really change the fundamental goals or procedures employed; it just expands their applicability and enhances the capacity of the patient to learn from them.

> **And you need to learn to look at things that are unpleasant — without fear, with a willingness to understand, and with a willingness to learn how well you can adjust. And you do it without a sense of discouragement or fear.**
>
> *(Erickson & Lustig, 1975, Vol. 2, p. 3)*

Yes, and I made her give a commitment, a total commitment. The thing is, you wouldn't do therapy with her except with the actual problem present. You can't remove a wart unless the patient brings the wart into the therapy room.

(Erickson & Rossi, 1979, p. 315)

That's right, made her fears a reality I could work on, a reality I could then put in that chair si.e was sitting in and leave there.

(Erickson & Rossi, 1979, p. 315)

That's right, there was a body threat in both. I had to make it so that it might all turn out terrible. I could not get a commitment by just asking her to imagine herself in a locked room. It had to be *this room*, something that would be truly horrible.

(Erickson & Rossi, 1979, p. 315)

She had to have her psychological problem with her at the time that I treated her. She then went into trance quite easily. She was actually committed to do anything. She had no freedom of any kind. She was in a state of total commitment. Once in a trance state I had her board a plane and ride through a storm in her imagination. It was sickening to see; she actually went through a kind of convulsion. It was horrible to watch.

(Erickson & Rossi, 1979, pp. 315-316)

But you did live through that spanking...and you can live through other troubles.

(Erickson & Lustig, 1975, Vol. I, p. 8)

What one does in hypnosis is primarily to get a patient interested in ideas, memories, understanding, or a concept of any kind. As the patients deal with these they can develop understanding. [1959]

(In Erickson, 1980, Vol. III, chap. 4, p. 28)

And you need to learn the things, and discover later how you can use those learnings.

(Erickson & Lustig, 1975, Vol. I, pp. 5–6)

In brief the Hypnotic Corrective Emotional Experience, however simple it may appear, is a highly complex restructuring of subjective experiences that can be initiated very simply and then gently guided toward a therapeutic goal. Essential is good clinical attentiveness to the patient's behavior, a confident awareness that one can delay, even halt, and nullify hypnotically whatever is taking place, and postpone, modify, or reinforce the structured situation leading to a therapeutic goal. [1965]

(In Erickson, 1980, Vol. IV, chap. 58, p. 524)

The Corrective Emotional Experiences vary in relation to the individual and in relation to his problem. The essential task is to structure the therapeutic situation in such fashion that emotions are greatly intensified, all behavior inhibited, and the need for behavior intensified. Then, and not until then, an opportunity for directed behavior with a special significance is given. [1965]

(In Erickson, 1980, Vol. IV, chap. 58, p. 523)

Then, as a result of some concrete or tangible performance, the patient develops a profound feeling that the repressive barriers have been broken, that the resistance has been overcome, that the communication is actually understandable and that its meaning can no longer be kept at a symbolic level.

(Erickson, 1954d, p. 128)

The experimental therapy consisted of using simple hypnotic trances and hypnotic regression to permit a reeducation of the two patients in a progressively greater control of their condition and with a progressive alteration of symptomatology to render it less severe. [1965]

(In Erickson, 1980, Vol. IV, chap. 10, p. 133)

The process of inducing a trance should be regarded as a method of teaching patients a new manner of learning something, and thereby enabling them to discover unrealized capacities to learn, and to act in new ways which may be applied to other and different things. [1948]

(In Erickson, 1980, Vol. IV, chap. 4, p. 36)

By employing hypnosis a communication of special ideas and understandings ordinarily not possible of presentation was achieved in relation to personality needs and subjective attitudes toward weight reduction. Each was enabled to undertake the problem of weight loss in accord with long-established patterns of behavior but utilized in a new fashion. [1960]

(In Erickson, 1980, Vol. IV, chap. 16, p. 187)

You never forget the problem at hand, but you translate it into many other avenues of the patient's experience. You utilize their other experiential learnings to deal with their current problem.

(Erickson & Rossi, 1979, p. 248)

And each person can put past experiences and learnings together in a way that is satisfying.

(Erickson & Lustig, 1975, Vol. II, p. 5)

The patient needs help, and he does not know where to look, so I'd better focus his looking with a question.

(Erickson, Rossi & Rossi, 1976, p. 165)

They are questions; they fixate attention and call upon thoughts and associations that are inevitable in her future.

(Erickson & Rossi, 1979, p. 194)

That's the way you change a subject quickly: Ask a question.

(Erickson & Rossi, 1981, p. 101)

I don't answer her question directly but ask her a question that would evoke her own experiential learning.

(Erickson & Rossi, 1979, p. 293)

By such indirect suggestion the patient is enabled to go through those difficult inner processes of disorganizing, reorganizing, reassociating, and projecting of inner real experience to meet the requirements of the suggestion. [1948]

(In Erickson, 1980, Vol. IV, chap. 4, p. 39)

The calculated vagueness of some of the instructions forced their unconscious minds to assume responsibility for their behavior. Consciously they could only wonder about their inexplicable situations, while they responded to it with corrective, unconscious reactions.

(Erickson, 1954a, p. 173)

In working at a problem of difficulty, you try to make an interesting design in the handling of it. That way you have an answer to the difficult problem. Become interested in the design and don't notice the backbreaking labor. In therapy that is often a very delightful thing to do.

(Erickson, Rossi & Rossi, 1976, p. 258)

You are transforming one task into another. You alter the tension.

(Erickson & Rossi, 1979, p. 157)

Yes, I'm now transforming the phobia problem by placing it into a frame of reference of dealing with intellectual tasks, where she is really an expert.
(Erickson & Rossi, 1979, p. 333)

Therefore it was reasoned that it would be well to create a learning situation that would bypass the possible psychogenic elements. This could be done with a newly created learning situation which could then be associated with childhood learning situations. [1965]
(In Erickson, 1980, Vol. IV, chap. 33, p. 319)

This is a two-level communication dealing with his problem in a metaphorical way.
(Erickson & Rossi, 1979, p. 257)

Yes, these two-level communications are like the secret language of childhood.
(Erickson & Rossi, 1979, p. 265)

We don't know which meanings her unconscious will act upon.
(Erickson & Rossi, 1976, p. 159)

***R:* What are you trying to convince with these validating analogies from everyday life? The conscious or the unconscious?**
***E:* The unconscious knows all about these things!**
***R:* You're telling the unconscious what mental mechanisms to use by analogy.**
***E:* Yes.**
(Erickson, Rossi & Rossi, 1976, p. 218)

Always impressing upon her the need for an unconscious retention of the ideas. [1965]
(In Erickson, 1980, Vol. IV, chap. 20, p. 221)

Hypnosis Allows Unconscious Psychotherapy

Perhaps the most intriguing consequence of the hypnotic state, especially the deep hypnotic state, is the complete removal of the conscious mind from the situation. Normally psychotherapy is brought about by motivating the person to experience an internal or external event in a manner that will stimulate a conscious reorganization. But there are instances where the conscious mind is so distorted, closed, rigid, or defensive that no approach can break through and trigger any change at all. Even the comfort of a mild hypnotic episode may be inadequate to lower the conscious barriers to new learning and response. What is needed in these situations is a complete removal of the patient's inhibiting conscious mind so that it cannot intrude unhelpfully and interfere with the normal healing process. Appropriate experiential learning simply will not occur with some patients as long as the conscious mind is present at all. Deep hypnosis can eliminate the conscious mind in these cases and enable the patient to progress without conscious participation or awareness. Tremendous strides in self-evaluation, self-exploration, and re-learning can be made in such a condition without conscious distortions or distress.

There is no particular reason to limit such an application of deep hypnotic dissociation solely to the most difficult or intransigent patients. Except in those few cases where the time and energy necessary to teach patients how to rely exclusively upon their unconscious minds exceeds the time it would take to approach their problems on a more conscious level, deep hypnosis can be a valuable and efficient aid.

Hypnosis enables the hypnotherapist to exchange ideas and information directly with the patient's unconscious. It frees the unconscious to apply its capacities fully to the problem at hand. Most importantly, however, it can enable patients to learn to trust, to communicate with, and to use that vast range of hidden resources stored within their own unconscious minds. Perhaps the single most important thing a hypnotherapist must teach patients during the pre-induction, induction, and suggestion process is that they can and should trust their unconscious minds completely and rely upon them faithfully. Once patients have learned this, then the psychotherapeutic process, and their lives in general, can proceed more smoothly and efficiently. The unconscious can then be given free rein to do what it can do; and what it can do, with or without the aid of a therapist, is to acquire the understandings, undergo the reorganizational experiences, and develop the motivations necessary to accomplish the therapeutic purposes.

About six hours were spent determining the fact that there was no approach to him to be made at the conscious level. [circa 1936]
(In Erickson, 1980, Vol. IV, chap. 53, p. 476)

In a similar manner many emotional problems can be solved more easily without conscious thinking.
(Erickson & Rossi, 1979, p. 173)

An unconscious conflict may be resolved unconsciously. [1944]
(In Erickson, 1980, Vol. III, chap. 21, p. 216)

It [hypnosis] allows the physician to approach directly the subconscious of the person with its disturbing conflicts. It often serves as a gateway past his resistances and allows approaches to many difficulties which otherwise could not be attacked.
(Erickson, 1934, p. 612)

Hypnosis offers both to the patient and the therapist a ready access to the patient's unconscious mind. It permits a direct dealing with those unconscious forces which underlie personality disturbances, and it allows a recognition of those items of individual life experiences significant to the personality and to which full consideration must be given if psychotherapeutic results are to be achieved. [1945]

(In Erickson, 1980, Vol. IV, chap. 3, p. 34)

Hypnosis alone can give the ready, prompt, and extensive access to the unconscious, which the history of psychotherapy has shown to be so important in the therapy of acute personality disturbances. [1945]

(In Erickson, 1980, Vol. IV, chap. 3, p. 34)

I made up my mind that you should have free access to what your conscious mind knows about your body but does not know that it knows, and what your body knows freely but that neither your conscious nor your unconscious mind openly knows. *You might as well use well all knowledge that you have,* body or mind knowledge, and use all of it well.

(Erickson & Rossi, 1979, p. 436)

The role in hypnotic psychotherapy of this special state of awareness ["unconscious"] is that of permitting and enabling patients to react, uninfluenced by their conscious mind, to their past experiential life and to a new order of experience which is about to occur as they participate in the therapeutic procedure. This participation in therapy by the patients constitutes the primary requisite for effective results. [1948]

(In Erickson, 1980, Vol. IV, chap. 4, p. 37)

One of the greatest advantages of hypnotherapy lies in the opportunity to work independently with the unconscious without being hampered by the reluctance, or sometimes actual inability, of the conscious mind to accept therapeutic gains. [1948]

(In Erickson, 1980, Vol. IV, chap. 4, p. 40)

I break up her conscious set. Her questions are on the conscious level but the answers require that she make a search at the unconscious level.

(Erickson & Rossi, 1976, p. 156)

We both want to know the cause of your behavior. *We both know that that knowledge is in your unconscious mind.*

(Erickson, 1954d, p. 122)

I would like you to learn that no matter what any person believes, your belief, your unconscious knowledge is all that counts.

(Erickson, Rossi & Rossi, 1976, p. 198)

It's his conscious mind that's perplexed. I verify that by adding that his unconscious understands a lot more than he does. I keep out of the situation; don't say, "I know what's going on." I say, "*Your* unconscious knows."

(Erickson & Rossi, 1979, p. 256)

I set her up to place unconscious understandings on whatever I say. *They will be her unconscious understandings.* She is not limited or biased by my ideas.

(Erickson & Rossi, 1979, p. 172)

And it is very important for a person to know their unconscious is smarter than they are. There is a greater wealth of stored material in the unconscious. We know the unconscious can do things, and it's important to assure your patient that it can. They have to be willing to let their unconscious do things and not depend so much on their conscious mind. This is a great aid to their functioning.

(Erickson, Rossi & Rossi, 1976, p. 9)

Your unconscious will know what to do and how to do it. You will yield absolutely to that need and give full expression to me.

(Erickson & Rossi, 1979, p. 240)

Your unconscious will carry out the thing that needs to be done.

(Erickson & Rossi, 1977, p. 50)

He knew unconsciously how to respond.

(Erickson & Rossi, 1981, p. 211)

"You've said that your conscious mind is uncertain and confused. And that's because the conscious mind does forget. And yet we know the unconscious does have access to so many memories and images and experiences that it can make available to the conscious mind so you can solve that problem."

(Erickson, Rossi & Rossi, 1976, p. 67)

Yes, because whenever your conscious mind does not understand, it says, "Wait a minute, that will come to me." What are you saying? In effect you are saying, "My unconscious will help me."

(Erickson & Rossi, 1981, p. 208)

R: That is a very important learning because it enables her to recognize the value of exploring her unconscious and its capacities, which are greater than her conscious mind believes.
E: That's right.

(Erickson, Rossi & Rossi, 1976, p. 173)

The patient had better believe in his own unconscious.
(Erickson & Rossi, 1979, p. 257)

Her resistance isn't toward me or toward learning. *She just doesn't quite trust her unconscious mind to do all the learning necessary.*
(Erickson, Rossi & Rossi, 1979, p. 162)

"Shut up with your conscious mind and its foolish requests for medicine, and let your unconscious mind attend to its task!" ·
(Erickson & Rossi, 1979, p. 240)

He doesn't need to move, he doesn't need to talk, he doesn't need to do anything except let his unconscious mind take over and do everything. And the conscious doesn't have to do anything — it's usually not even interested.
(Erickson & Lustig, 1975, Vol. 2, p. 2)

It is sufficient that only your unconscious mind becomes aware.
(Erickson & Rossi, 1981, p. 72)

And your willingness to rely upon your unconscious mind to do anything that can be of interest or value to you is most important.
(Erickson, Rossi & Rossi, 1976, p. 68)

You have to rely on the unconscious.
(Erickson, Rossi & Rossi, 1976, p. 207)

You can trust your unconscious mind.
(Erickson & Rossi, 1979, p. 366)

She was to allow her unconscious to deal with her problem, instead of her conscious mind. [1938]
(In Erickson, 1980, Vol. III, chap. 17, p. 175)

Subjects often need to be taught to realize their capabilities to function adequately, whether at a conscious or an unconscious level of awareness. [1952]
(In Erickson, 1980, Vol. I, chap. 6, p. 145)

I wanted her to learn to use her unconscious. I did not know where or how, and I did not try to tell her where or how.
(Erickson & Rossi, 1981, p. 108)

She was instructed that her unconscious could and would so govern her conscious mind that she could learn about hypnosis and her hypnotic experience in any way that was satisfying and informative to her as a total personality. [1952]
(In Erickson, 1980, Vol. I, chap. 6, p. 157)

One of the first considerations in undertaking hypnotic psychotherapy centers around the differentiation of the patient's experience of having a trance induced from the experience of being in a trance state....Both the therapist and the patient need to make this differentiation, the former in order to guide the patient's behavior more effectively, the latter in order to learn to distinguish between conscious and unconscious behavior patterns. [1948]
(In Erickson, 1980, Vol. IV, chap. 4, pp. 36–37)

To ensure such differentiation, the trance induction should be emphasized as a preparation of the patient for another type of experience in which new learnings will be utilized for other purposes in a different way. [1948]
(In Erickson, 1980, Vol. IV, chap. 4, p. 37)

Thus the patient accepts hypnotic suggestions, and acts upon them without conscious awareness and without building defense reactions. In so doing he allows them to become a valid part of his mental patterns, all the more so since fundamentally, if not immediately, he does desire aid against his conflicts. By this means he can be given new mental equipment wihich does not have to pass the protective scrutiny of his "consciousness."

(Erickson, 1934, p. 613)

How many more mentally ill patients, hopelessly sick, might be economically rehabilitated if physicians understood hypnosis as a modality of communication of ideas, understandings and useful unrealized self-knowledge contained in what is popularly called the unconscious? [1957]

(In Erickson, 1980, Vol. IV, chap. 6, p. 74)

No way you can consciously instruct the unconscious!
(Erickson & Rossi, 1977, p. 43)

You have to do things in your own way and you don't know what your way is.

(Erickson & Rossi, 1977, p. 43)

In a very delightful way of doing it, in a careful unconscious thinking it out, you can devise a mastery of your own functions so that you can work out patterns of function.

(Erickson & Rossi, 1979, p. 338)

Your unconscious mind has learned a lot — it knows it can function by itself. Your conscious mind can learn from it, can use the learning that the unconscious mind has, as well as the learning your unconscious mind can reach back into the past and single out.

(Erickson & Lustig, 1975, Vol. I, p. 9)

Conscious activity was relatively unimportant in the therapeutic situation, that *the only thing of paramount*

importance was the reorganization of unconscious think-
ing taking place without conscious awareness. [1956]
(In Erickson, 1980, Vol. IV, chap. 49, p. 441)

But utilizing hypnosis as a technique of deliberately and intentionally shifting to the patients their own burden of responsibility for therapeutic results and having them emphatically and repetitiously affirm and confirm in their own expressed verbalizations of their own desires, needs and intentions at the level of their own unconscious mentation, forces the therapeutic goals to become the patient's own goals. [1964]
(In Erickson, 1980, Vol. IV, chap. 19, p. 211)

The man really wanted to do things. I carefully told his unconscious that his conscious mind did not yet have the new brain patterns that he needed. So I'm going to keep his conscious mind angry and resentful so he will work while you [his unconscious] help him build more and more brain patterns. [circa 1965]
(In Erickson, 1980, Vol. IV, chap. 34, p. 326)

Allow Unconscious Psychotherapy to Remain Unconscious

In an hypnotic state of mind the patient's unconscious can be allowed to develop the desired therapeutic understandings. The therapist can assist in and facilitate this process by providing general instructions, guidance, or helpful experiences to the unconscious, but must allow the unconscious to acquire therapeutic understandings and abilities in its own time and in its own way. While patients have their attention highly focused on internal events and are responding purely through the filter of their unconscious mind, the hypnotherapist can direct their attention to particular memories, thoughts, abilities, or other experiences that they would be unable to access or use in their normal state of awareness. Furthermore, patients can examine their problem areas objectively and report what they find to the hypnotherapist who can then use that information to guide further re-learnings and reorganizations or to elicit additional hypnotic responses that will demonstrate useful alternative modes of solution or reaction.

Hypnotherapists must be very careful not to intrude in an unwarranted fashion or to attempt to impose their own relatively uninformed solutions upon patients. Patients must have their privacy and unique personality needs protected at all times. They should be helped to resolve their problems in their own ways, even at an unconscious level, and should be encouraged to share no more of their unconscious understandings with the therapist than they believe to be useful or safe at the time.

Similarly, patients should be allowed to transfer the results of their unconscious therapeutic endeavors to their conscious minds in their own time and in their own way. Sometimes the therapy that occurs at an unconscious level will remain unconscious permanently, with neither the therapist nor the patient ever knowing exactly what happened or what issues were involved. All that is known by either is that the unconscious was given the opportunity to deal with the matter and that the desired alterations in emotion, thought, or behavior occurred. On other occasions, the patient may be aware of the unconscious activities and the therapist not or vice versa. Usually, however, both the therapist and the patient eventually will be provided with some conception of the therapeutic occurrences and reorganizations, but only when it is appropriate and useful for the patient.

The role of the hypnotherapist in this process is neither to pry for details nor to confront the patient's conscious mind with them. The therapist merely provides the opportunity for a transfer of the unconscious therapeutic understandings to the conscious mind by stimulating pockets of renewed conscious awareness throughout the hypnotic procedure and by offering suggestions to the unconscious mind regarding the various methods it might wish to use to transfer those understandings (e.g. dreams, sudden insights, or slips of the tongue).

Usually such a transfer or integration of unconscious and conscious awareness will not occur unless the conscious mind acquiesces. It may even be necessary actually to ask for conscious permission from the person before suggesting such a transfer. Erickson also recommended that the unconscious be allowed to make up its own mind how and when to accomplish any breakthroughs. Forcing too much awareness too soon can generate resistance or confusion, whereas not encouraging or allowing enough awareness when the time is ripe can retard progress unnecessarily.

> **The assumption that the unconscious must be made conscious as rapidly as possible often leads merely to the disorderly mingling of confused, unconscious understandings with conscious confusions and, therefore, a retardation of therapeutic progress. [1948]**
> *(In Erickson, 1980, Vol. IV, chap. 4, p.48)*

> **For example, many psychotherapists regard as almost axiomatic that therapy is contingent upon making the unconscious conscious. When thought is given to the unmeasurable role that the unconscious plays in the total experiential life of a person from infancy on, whether asleep or awake, there will be little expectation of doing more than making some small parts of it conscious. Furthermore, the unconscious as such, not as transformed**

into the conscious, constitutes an essential part of psychological functioning

(Erickson, 1953, p. 2)

You protect the patient. You're protecting the conscious mind by keeping that self-understanding unconscious.

(Erickson, Rossi & Rossi, 1976, p. 256)

The suggestion was offered that her needs could be met in a remarkably adequate fashion and in a manner that would please and intrigue her without emotional repercussions of any sort. She was urged to accept this idea of this possibility, even though she did not know exactly what was meant. [circa 1950's]

(In Erickson, 1980, Vol. IV, Chapter 44, p. 389)

Whatever the strength and nature of the hypnotic relationship, it does not alter the sanctity of one's personal privacy. This belongs, apparently, to the waking state upon which it depends for protection.

(Erickson, 1939a, p. 401)

People have a lifetime of learning that talking in your sleep is socially unacceptable. It's surprising how many people fear they will betray themselves by speaking in their sleep or trance.

(Erickson, Rossi & Rossi, 1976, p. 131)

I don't need to know what your problem is for you to correct it.

(Erickson & Rossi, 1979, p. 172)

So, the patient doesn't have to know that psychotherapy is being done....the therapist doesn't have to know why the patient needs psychotherapy.

(Zeig, 1980, p. 153)

And in doing psychotherapy, don't try to dig up everything all at once. Dig up the safe thing when it's a deep repression.

(Zeig, 1980, p. 57)

She protested that they had been forgotten events. Therefore, they ought to remain forgotten, and she declared emphatically that she would not remember them when she awakened.

(Erickson, 1954c, p. 276)

She also declared that she did not want to remember consciously any of the memories previously recovered in hypnosis, since they had "once been forgotten and might as well stay that way."

(Erickson, 1954c, p. 277)

Now in the back of our mind, which is a common phrase, we know a lot of things; and sometimes we have trouble getting those things into the front of our mind.

(Erickson & Lustig, 1975, Vol. 2, p. 3)

An experimental procedure was employed which in some manner permitted the patient's unconscious, distorted and disorganized in its functioning, to achieve a satisfactory role in her total experiential life, and to do so without becoming a part of the conscious.

(Erickson, 1953, p. 6)

The subject's unconscious was provided with special learning and then, later, an opportunity was created in which that special learning could become manifest in response to inner personal needs.

(Erickson, 1954c, p. 282)

There should be a careful search of her unconscious mind of all possible ways and means of controlling, alter-

ing, changing, modifying, re-interpreting, lessening, or in any other way doing whatever was possible to meet her needs. [1964]
(In Erickson, 1980, Vol. I, chap. 13, p. 322)

Now there are many different ways in which the mind can function in which the unconscious can join with the conscious. Many different ways in which the unconscious can avoid the conscious mind without the conscious mind knowing that it has just received a gift.
(Erickson, Rossi & Rossi, 1976, p. 68)

The only important thing is for your unconscious to see to it that you really feel comfortable with all the memories you do have.
(Erickson & Rossi, 1979, p. 305)

It [unconscious] also learned that we could learn a lot without intruding upon the personality.
(Erickson, Rossi & Rossi, 1976, p. 207)

Insuring that the patient learns both to share unconscious activity and to withhold it from conscious awareness greatly speeds psychotherapy. [1964]
(In Erickson, 1980, Vol. I, chap. 13, p. 305)

Too many hypnotherapists try to recover the total experience all at once.
(ASCH, 1980, Taped Lecture, 8/8/64)

Now there are discoveries you make. Some are personal and belong only to you, and some can be shared with certain others, and some can be shared with others in general.
(Erickson & Rossi, 1979, p. 388)

And sometimes we can have a secret between your unconscious and me.

(ASCH, 1980, Taped Lecture, 8/8/64)

The little item of having a "secret understanding" between the subjects' unconscious minds and the hypnotist has many times proved to be remarkably effective as a means of securing deep trances in otherwise aggressively resistant subjects. [1952]

(In Erickson, 1980, Vol. I, chap. 6, p. 158)

There is no more reason why hypnotic therapy should consist of an explanation of the patient's symptoms to the patient without regard to the the patient than that this should be the process of analysis. [1939]

(In Erickson, 1980, Vol. III, chap. 23, p. 253)

Because you are dealing with a person who has both a conscious mind and an unconscious mind, achieving good results with a patient in a deep trance does not mean that the patient will benefit from it in the ordinary waking state. There has to be an integration of unconscious learnings with conscious learnings....And therefore it is essential to integrate the unconscious learnings with the conscious learnings....Therefore, in dealing with patients it is always necessary to decide how rapidly and how thoroughly they will need to integrate what they learn unconsciously with what they learn consciously.

(Erickson & Rossi, 1981, p. 6)

Often the entire process of communication is unconscious, and a sudden irruption into the conscious mind may complete a long process of unrecognized communication. [1966]

(In Erickson, 1980, Vol. II, chap. 34, p. 353)

In hypnotic psychotherapy too often suitable therapy may be given to the unconscious, but with the failure by the therapist to appreciate the tremendous need of either enabling the patient to integrate the unconscious with the conscious or of making the new understandings of the unconscious fully accessible, upon need, to the conscious mind. [1948]

(In Erickson, 1980, Vol. IV, chap. 4, p. 40)

Hypnosis also offers the opportunity of dealing with the patient at two levels of awareness, so that the patient can safely approach a complete understanding of a traumatic experience that was previously repressed as intolerably painful — that is, at an unconscious level of mentation and then at a level of conscious awareness.

(Erickson & Rossi, 1979, pp. 358-359)

Thus in hypnotherapy, one tries to do hypnotherapy at an unconscious level but to give the patient an opportunity to transfer that understanding and insight to the conscious mind as far as it is needed.

(Erickson, 1977b, p. 21)

At the same time that the psychiatrist gave the patient permission to face the facts unconsciously, he gave her conscious mind the right to be free from its obsessive preoccupation with the problem. [1938]

(In Erickson, 1980, Vol. III, chap. 17, p. 175)

Thus, bit by bit, he could integrate his unconscious learnings with his conscious behavior in a corrective fashion which would lead to good adjustment. [1948]

(In Erickson, 1980, Vol. IV, chap. 4, p. 45)

When the answer is "shared," especially if the conscious opinion is opposite in character, the patient shows amazement, and sometimes unwillingly admits to the self an awareness or strong feeling that the unconscious answer is unquestionably correct. [1964]

(In Erickson, 1980, Vol. I, chap. 13, p. 305)

A direct link was established between conscious and unconscious systems of thought and feeling which surrounded the parental figures,...There was almost immediate relief from seriously disturbing neurotic and emotional symptoms. [1938]

(In Erickson, 1980, Vol. III, chap. 17, p. 176)

Properly, hypnotherapy should be oriented equally about the conscious and unconscious, since the integration of the total personality is the desired goal in psychotherapy. [1948]

(In Erickson, 1980, Vol. IV, chap. 4, p. 40)

And then the results of that unconscious functioning can become conscious. But first they have to get beyond their conscious understanding of what is possible.

(Erickson, Rossi & Rossi, 1976, p. 10)

The importance of the recovery of lost memories in psychotherapy is fully established, and hypnosis often proves a royal road to those memories, although it still leaves the task of integrating that memory into the waking life of the patient a painstaking task for the therapist. [1944]

(In Erickson, 1980, Vol. IV, chap. 2, p.20)

In some aspects of the patient's problem direct reintegration under the guidance of the therapist is desirable; in other aspects the unconscious should merely be made available to the conscious mind, thereby permitting a spontaneous reintegration free from any immediate influence by the therapist. [1948]

(In Erickson, 1980, Vol. IV, chap. 4, p. 40)

You want to deal with the unconscious mind, bring about therapy at that level, and then to translate it to the conscious mind.

(Erickson, 1977b, p. 21)

Nor is there any necessary reason why analytically informed investigators or therapists who in these days are using hypnotism should forcibly thrust upon their patients the material which has been gained from the unconscious under hypnosis, merely because in a more naive period before anything was understood about the forces of resistance, the traditional hypnotist proceeded in that ruthless fashion. [1939]

(In Erickson, 1980, Vol. III, chap. 23, p. 253)

It is possible in the hypnotic as in the waking state to secure information from the unconscious and then to so motivate the total personality that there will be an increasing interplay of conscious and unconscious aspects of the personality, so that the former gradually overcomes the resisting forces and acquires an understanding of the latter. [1939]

(In Erickson, 1980, Vol. III, chap. 23, p. 253)

R: In deep trance it is possible to place suggestions so deeply that there is no bridge to consciousness where they can be expressed. Those suggestions cannot be therapeutically effective.

E: That is why I build bridges.

(Erickson & Rossi, 1979, p. 177)

By working separately with the unconscious there is then the opportunity to temper and to control the patient's rate of progress and thus to effect a reintegration in the manner acceptable to the conscious mind. [1948]

(In Erickson, 1980, Vol. IV, chap. 4, p. 41)

Each patient's unconscious was provided with a wealth of formulated ideas unknown to the conscious mind. Then, in response to the innate needs and desires of the total personality, the unconscious could utilize those ideas in translating them into realities of daily life as spontaneous responsive behavior in opportune situations.

(Erickson, 1954c, p. 282)

Now, all of the things I've said to you will come back translated into your own language, into your own ways of understanding. And, in the future, you will discover sudden insights, sudden understanding, a sudden thought that you hadn't thought of before. It will only be your unconscious mind, feeding to your conscious mind things that you already knew, but you didn't know that you knew. Because we all do our own learning in our own way.

(Zeig, 1980, p. 224)

R: Allow the unconscious to take over: let the unconscious be dominant to permit latent and therapeutic response potentials to become manifest. That is the essence of your approach, isn't it?
E: Yes.

(Erickson & Rossi, 1981, p. 74)

Special understandings for the future were developed in their unconscious minds, and their actual life situations presented the reality opportunities to utilize those ideas in responsive behavior in accord with their inner

needs and desires.

The fashion in which the patients made their fantasies a part of their reality life was in keeping with the ordinary natural evolution ˙of spontaneous behavior responses to reality.

(Erickson, 1954c, pp. 282–283)

Then, once she had achieved her goals, at the level of unconscious motivation she felt compelled to verbalize her original presenting complaint but with a totally different meaning and perspective. [1965]

(In Erickson, 1980, Vol. IV, chap. 20, p. 222)

Summary

Hypnosis is a therapeutic tool which increases access to hidden potentials, helps overcome conscious barriers, and allows therapeutic learnings to be gained by the unconscious first and later shared with the conscious on an "as-acceptable" basis. Hypnosis merely facilitates the normal psychotherapeutic process and is not in itself a form of therapy.

CHAPTER TWELVE

UTILIZING HYPNOSIS THERAPEUTICALLY: SPECIFIC TECHNIQUES

Although hypnosis does not significantly alter the goals and procedures of psychotherapy, it does enable the patient to do, to experience, and to learn many things that ordinarily would be difficult or impossible. This is especially true as the patient learns to function more fully at an unconscious level during the trance process. In some cases, patients may be able to progress very nicely on their own if simply placed in a deep trance and instructed to use their new found skills to do whatever is necessary. Other patients will learn what they need to learn with a minimal amount of indirect or general guidance during their trance experience.

The majority of patients, however, seem to require special training and direction if they are to learn how to apply their hypnotic capacities constructively. In such circumstances the hypnotherapist must be prepared to take a more active role in the teaching and self-exploration process. Where necessary, the hypnotherapist should be familiar with the specific techniques used by Erickson to elicit information, to stimulate effective plans for future progress, to initiate an objective evaluation of internal and external realities, to resurrect repressed memories, and to secure a reevaluation of them. Techniques to accomplish such ends and general considerations regarding their application are the subjects of the material presented in this chapter.

Ideomotor Responses

There are numerous occasions when a patient simply cannot consciously produce the information necessary for successful therapy. Either conscious concerns and inhibitions prohibit it or the information is located exclusively within the unconscious and is not consciously available to the person. In either case, it may be advantageous to solicit information directly from the unconscious without conscious awareness or participation.

Simply asking a deeply hypnotized individual to report verbally the desired information probably will not work. Most subjects use their *conscious* minds to speak to the hypnotist, returning to conscious awareness to report on what they observed while their awareness was directed toward unconscious functioning. Talking to hypnotized subjects is rather like asking dreamers to report on their dreams; what is obtained is movement in and out of the sleep state with intermittent verbal reports on the progress of the dream as it has unfolded thus far. Although this type of reporting may be quite sufficient for maintaining an ongoing awareness of what the subject is experiencing, it is hardly adequate for accessing deeply repressed, highly emotionally charged material. The likelihood is that either the unconscious will continue to protect the conscious mind and provide no information or that the conscious mind will deny or distort whatever is provided to it.

It is possible to initiate a verbal interaction directly with a hypnotized subject's unconscious, but most subjects find it difficult to learn how to allow themselves to engage in automatic or unintentional speaking. It is much easier for most people to learn to allow automatic or unconscious motor responses such as finger movements. Hypnotized subjects can be trained to allow these unconscious responses to occur without conscious intention or awareness. Next, they can be instructed that movement of a finger on one hand will mean "Yes" and movement of a finger on the other "No". The unconscious answers to a variety of questions can be secured in this manner and much unconscious information gained.

Some hypnotists establish an elaborate code for finger signaling, with each finger representing a slightly different meaning such as "Maybe" or "Never". Others rely upon unconscious movements of the head or feet. Apparently it makes no real difference which ideomotor systems of communication are used. When a small weight on the end of a string, called a Chevreal pendulum, is held between the thumb and first finger and allowed to swing freely it can move in different directions in response to barely noticeable ideomotor movements. These movements can be used to provide valuable unconscious information just as finger movements can. The Ouija Board is a classic example of this principle of ideomotor movement. The major advantage to the use of finger signaling seems to be that it is relatively easily transformed into automatic drawing or automatic writing.

None of the ideomotor signaling systems requires a deep trance in order to be used successfully. In fact, normally alert people can provide very satisfactory unconscious responses if they are provided with an ideomotor outlet for unconscious responses and then given a competing task to occupy or divert their conscious awareness. People often doodle while occupied with other tasks and the productions secured in this manner may be as full of unconscious symbolic signals as the automatic drawing of a deeply hypnotized subject. It should be remembered that the solicitation of a simple ideomotor response such as finger movement or arm levitation was often used by Erickson as an induction device because people evidently have to enter at least a mild dissociative state in order to allow the ideomotor signal to occur. This dissociative response can therefore be used to signal the onset of a brief trance state, to validate the trance process for the subject, and to enhance the dissociative internal focus of attention so necessary for hypnosis and for unconscious communications.

By teaching a patient to expand upon minor ideomotor movements, automatic writing or automatic drawing eventually can be elicited. Such responses open up a direct door into the understandings of the unconscious. Unfortunately, the products obtained via automatic movements often contain a variety of puns, metaphors, or symbolic communications which may be difficult or impossible to decipher. The use of such coded communications by the unconscious may be diminished if the hypnotist assures the unconscious that what is communicated will be kept secret from the patient's conscious mind and used protectively. Sometimes, however, these coded messages serve the same purpose as dreams, their message presented in a symbolic fashion which the patient's conscious mind cannot or will not comprehend until it is thoroughly prepared to do so. Then, in a flash of insight, the meaning becomes clear and the transfer of therapeutic learning from the unconscious to the conscious is experienced.

You cannot force them [patients], but you can get them to disclose more completely when you provide an ideomotor outlet for responses that are not available to consciousness.

(Erickson & Rossi, 1981, p. 145)

By...widening the conscious gap between the conscious and unconscious parts of the psyche, it might be possible to secure communications from the unconscious more simply than can be done when both parts of the personality are using the single vehicle of speech. [1939]

(In Erickson, 1980, Vol. III, chap. 17, p. 174)

If, however, by some method, one could allow the various aspects of the psyche to express themselves simultaneously with different simple and direct methods of communication, it would be conceivable at least that each part could express itself more clearly and with less internal confusion and resistance. [1939]

(In Erickson, 1980, Vol. III, chap. 17, p. 174)

Automatic drawing and automatic writing may offer an accessory method of approach to the unconscious. [1939]

(In Erickson, 1980, Vol. III, chap. 23, p. 252)

The essential technical consideration in the simultaneous performance of two separate and distinct tasks, each at a different level of awareness, which is not ordinarily possible at a single level of awareness, consists in the provision of some form of motivation sufficient to set into action a train of learned activity which will then continue indefinitely at one level of awareness, despite the initiation or continuation of a different train of activity at another level. [1941]

(In Erickson, 1980, Vol. I, chap. 19, p. 410)

I'm telling her she can have her conscious *false* beliefs about not being able to do automatic writing but I believe she can. Again, I'm speaking to her unconscious.
(Erickson & Rossi, 1976, p. 159)

Some people, a lot of people, think that they must go through the same learning process in automatic writing by which they learned ordinary writing. So they show their belief.
(Zeig, 1980, p. 222)

The vertical or horizontal lines thus secured were later found to be an excellent approach to the teaching of automatic writing to difficult subjects. [1961]
(In Erickson, 1980, Vol. I, chap. 5, p. 135)

Yes, usually [in automatic writing] there is an economy of effort.
(Erickson & Rossi, 1979, p. 405)

Additionally, one never tells the patient that an unconscious reply is almost always characterized by a strong element of perseveration. [1964]
(In Erickson, 1980, Vol. I, chap. 13, p. 305)

This perseveration of ideomotor activity, however, is much briefer in duration if the unconscious mind wishes the conscious mind to know; the time lag and the dissociated character are greatly reduced, although the unconscious answer may be considerably delayed as the unconscious mind goes through the process of formulating its reply and the decision to share or not to share. [1964]
(In Erickson, 1980, Vol. I, chap. 13, p. 305)

There seemed to be no interference by the automatic writing with the conscious waking performance. [1941]
> *(In Erickson, 1980, Vol. I, chap. 19, pp. 409–410)*

It suggests that when only one form of communication is used, the struggle between the expressive and repressive forces may be intensified. [1938]
> *(In Erickson, 1980, Vol. III, chap. 17, p. 174)*

It is possible that the presence of such a well organized dual personality may be an essential precondition for the successful use of such devices as automatic drawing or writing, mirror gazing, and the like, since they would seem to depend upon a rather high degree of hysterical dissociation. [1939]
> *(In Erickson, 1980, Vol. III, chap. 23, pp. 251–252)*

In the translation of automatic writing, as in the interpretation of dreams, each element may be made to do double and triple duty. [1940]
> *(In Erickson, 1980, Vol. III, chap. 18, p. 186)*

When she said this was "strange" writing, that means it is foreign to her consciousness. You have to be aware of the possible double meaning words like "sun" that could be "son". You always look for those possibilities. I may have my ideas about what it means but I'm not going to ask her to betray it.
> *(Erickson & Rossi, 1979, p. 410)*

When a person in a trance says something you know is a lie, you better look it over because it has another meaning....

Yes. In some way the person is telling the truth. A

truth seen from a totally different point of view. And bear in mind that you as the therapist also have your own set and rigid points of view to deal with.

(Erickson, Rossi & Rossi, 1976, p. 256)

You can make the unconscious known without making it known. You make it known by automatic writing. You make it unknown by folding the paper and putting it away til consciousness is ready for it.

(Erickson & Rossi, 1976, p. 166)

You cover it up so she will feel safer: You are not trying to pry...I don't pry, I don't read it at that point myself.

(Erickson & Rossi, 1979, p. 397)

Projection Into the Future

Erickson's primary focus of attention was on the future adjustments of his patients rather than upon their past failures. Thus, the primary question confronting the hypnotherapist, at least from Erickson's perspective, should be, "What can I or my patient do *now* that will lead to enhanced adjustment in the future?" This is an intriguing and important question. Unfortunately, most psychotherapists take it upon themselves to answer it themselves and to prescribe what *they* have determined will eventuate in the changes *they* believe are desirable.

Erickson, on the other hand, recognized that the patient is the only person in a position to answer this question realistically, because the patient is the only person who is privy to the unique patterns of attitudes, needs and events governing his or her life. Although objective information and judgements regarding realistic possibilities for the future are impossible for the conscious mind to access, the unconscious mind is capable of such determinations.

This argument forms the basis for what I believe is the most fascinating, unique, and potentially beneficial therapeutic approach ever developed by Erickson: the hypnotic projection of the person into an imagined successful future with a subsequent review of the responses and experiences that have led to that outcome followed by a posthypnotic suggestion directed to the individual's unconscious which will lead the person to do those specific things that the unconscious has thus indicated will result in success. *This process is the essence of Erickson's therapeutic approach.* Almost all of his therapeutic interventions can be best described as variations on this basic theme. First, there is an objective determination by the therapist and/or the patient of the way things will be once the problems or difficulties have been resolved. Next there is an objective determination of a feasible sequence of events leading from the present situation to that goal state. Finally, the therapist does something which will ensure that the patient will actually do those things that are required to move out of the present situation and into the goal state.

In a standard psychotherapeutic setting the therapist typically must rely upon a skillful utilization of existing needs, attitudes, and motivations in order to propel the patient into the desired responses. In a hypnotherapeutic setting, however, the hypnotist can use post-hypnotic suggestions to enable the patient to respond almost automatically in the ways needed. Thus, successful therapeutic outcomes can virtually be guaranteed using this post-hypnotic predetermination process. (For a more extensive discussion of this strategy see Erickson, M.H., Pseudo-orientation in time as a hypnotherapeutic procedure, *Journal of Clinical and Experimental Hypnosis*, 1954, *2*, 261–283 and Havens, R.A., Posthypnotic predetermination of therapeutic progress, *American Journal of Clinical Hypnosis,* in press.)

The feasibility and utility of this approach obviously is dependent upon several factors. First of all, it is dependent upon the ability of the unconscious mind to fantasize about the future in ways that are realistic projections of present circumstances. The unconscious evidently is quite adept at this feat and can construct a remarkably accurate image of future possibilities because it is uninfluenced by normal conscious fantasies, needs, and restrictions. This therapeutic strategy also is dependent upon eventual compliance with the projected sequence of "curative" responses, and the capacity of hypnotic subjects to absorb and comply with post-hypnotic suggestions seems to enhance the likelihood of this happening. In fact, Erickson's discussions of cases where future projection and post-hypnotic predetermination procedures were employed suggest the possibility of almost miraculous outcomes.

It is not necessary or always desirable for patients to be consciously aware of their projected curative activities. When aware of what needs to be done, many patients will intrude along the way and change the course of events unhelpfully by imposing their conscious preferences or defenses. In most cases it is probably preferable to allow an amnesia for the unconscious projections to develop and to initiate cooperation from the unconscious via post-hypnotic suggestions. Subsequently, patients will tend to respond in the required manner with no conscious awareness that they are doing so. From their perspective, one thing will just lead to another and their problems will seem to resolve themselves.

Future projection can also be used to gain access to deeply repressed information. By projecting patients into the future beyond that point where the repressed material would finally have surfaced, patients can be allowed to look back upon their imagined breakthroughs and to describe what occurred on these occasions rather dispassionately. The repressive barriers have already been broken and the emotional turmoil has already been dealt with, at least from their imaginary future perspective. They are being asked simply to remember and describe what has already happened. It is normally desirable to suggest or construct an amnesia for such remembrances in order to protect the conscious mind and to allow repressed material to stay repressed until the conscious personality is ready to become aware of it. The hypnotherapist, however, will have gained a helpful understanding of the directions in which the patient's attention needs to be guided.

> **This technique was formulated by a utilization of those common experiences and understandings embraced in the general appreciation that practice leads to perfection, that action once initiated tends to continue and that deeds are the offspring of hope and expectancy. These ideas were utilized to create a therapy situation in which the patient could respond effectively psychologically to desired therapeutic goals as actualities already achieved.**
> *(Erickson, 1954c, p. 261)*

> **Thus, the patient was enabled to achieve a detached, dissociated, objective, and yet subjective view of what he believed at the moment he had already accomplished.**
> *(Erickson, 1954c, p. 261)*

> **It [orienting S's to the future] permits elaboration of hypnotic work in fuller accord with the subject's total personalities and unconscious needs and capabilites. It often permits the correction of errors and oversights before they can be made, and it furnishes a better understanding of how to develop suitable techniques. Subjects employed in this manner can often render in-**

valuable service in mapping out procedures and techniques to be employed in experimentation and therapy. **[1952]**

(In Erickson, 1980, Vol. I, chap. 6, p. 165)

Subjects oriented from the present to the actual future, instructed to look back upon proposed hypnotic work as actually accomplished, can often, by their "reminiscence," provide the hypnotist with understandings that can readily lead to much sounder work in deep trance. **[1952]**

(In Erickson, 1980, Vol. I, chap. 6, p. 165)

Then she was reoriented to a time actually three months in the future and thereby was enabled to offer a "reminiscent" account of her therapy and recovery. **[1952]**

(In Erickson, 1980, Vol. I, chap. 6, p. 164)

Thus, they [conscious fantasies] represent accomplishments apart from reality, complete in themselves, and expressive, recognizedly so to the person, of no more than conscious, hopeful, wishful thinking.

Unconscious fantasies, however, belong to another category of psychological functioning. They are not accomplishments complete in themselves, nor are they apart from reality. Rather, they are psychological constructs in various degrees of formulation for which the unconscious stands ready, or is actually awaiting an opportunity, to make a part of reality. They are not significant merely of *wishful desire* but rather of *actual intention* at the opportune time.

(Erickson, 1954c, pp. 281-282)

There was no running away of the imagination, but a serious appraisal in fantasy form of reality possibilities in keeping with their understandings of themselves.

(Erickson, 1954c, p. 283)

They were fantasies in keeping with their understandings of actually attainable goals.

(Erickson, 1954c, p. 283)

For these patients, apparently, the establishment of a dissociated state, in which they could feel and believe that they had achieved certain things of benefit to them, gave to them the profound feeling of accomplished realities which, in turn, resulted in the desired therapeutic reorientation.

(Erickson, 1954c, p. 283)

When I first began the study of hypnosis, I wondered greatly about verbal technique. You take a subject in the present time, and you're offering him ideas that are to affect his future. You're also to distract his mind from the present. And you're to take his mind away from surrounding reality and direct it to his inner world of experience...and I build up an acceptance of all those statements of the future because I deprive him of the privilege, of the right, of the possibility of disputing the future. I bring the remote future closer and closer to the present.

(Erickson & Rossi, 1981, p. 254)

Such future dates are best selected by the subject, since the hypnotist might choose one inauspicious for the situation.

(Erickson, 1954c, p. 263)

You present new ideas and new understandings and you relate them in some indisputable way to the remote future. It is important to present therapeutic ideas and posthypnotic suggestions in a way that makes them contingent on something that will happen in the future.

(Erickson & Rossi, 1975, p. 148)

When I associate her current hypnotic learning with *inevitable* things that will happen to her child, I'm extending these learnings into her future as an unrecognized posthypnotic suggestion.

(Erickson & Rossi, 1979, p.298)

Special understandings for the future were developed in their unconscious minds, and their actual life situations presented the reality opportunities to utilize those ideas in responsive behavior in accord with their inner needs and desires.

(Erickson, 1954c, p. 282)

The subject's unconscious was provided with special learning, and then, later, an opportunity was created in which that special learning could become manifest in response to inner personal needs.

(Erickson, 1954c, p. 282)

Hypnotic and post-hypnotic suggestions can be given in the form of a manifestation of interest in the patient's comfort, in explanations and in reassurances, all of which are worded to extend indefinitely into the future with the implied time limit of *goals satisfactorily reached.* [1964]

(In Erickson, 1980, Vol. I, chap. 13, p. 309)

By this measure [posthypnotic suggestion] subjects can be given instructions in the trance to govern their future

behavior, but only to a reasonable and acceptable degree. [1944]

(In Erickson, 1980, Vol. IV, chap. 2, p. 21)

Such use of posthypnotic phenomena offers extensive opportunities for direction and guidance of behavior in terms of the individual's needs and patterns of response without dependency upon immediate guidance and relationships.

(Erickson, 1970, p. 996)

In this phenomenon [post-hypnotic suggestion] lies the greatest therapeutic advantage of hypnosis, since thereby the subject can be given suggestions to guide his later conduct.

(Erickson, 1934, p. 612)

Revivification

Revivification is the recollection of an event with such clarity, intensity, and detail that it becomes an experience of seemingly reliving the original event. This intense reorientation into the past is quite possible with hypnosis and can be remarkably useful therapeutically. Total displacement in time and space and re-immersion into the past can provide an opportunity for the person to discover things long forgotten, both strengths and weaknesses. It can allow patients to relive an event and to respond more constructively to the experience than they did originally. It can be used to resurrect old, more effective patterns of response or to remind patients of positive aspects of their past. It can focus their awareness upon events that were misunderstood initially, especially when that misunderstanding has led to problems in the present. Stimulating an awareness of the genesis of existing attitudes or reactions can enable the person to gain a more reasonable perspective on the present. Within hypnosis it is even possible to alter the subjective experience of time in such a manner that patients can re-experience practically their entire lives in the span of several minutes. Such an all-encompassing review may provide immeasurable leaps in objective self-understanding and self-appraisal.

Revivification requires more than a simple instruction to return to the past. With most patients it is first necessary to remove their conscious orientation to the present and then gradually to move their focus of awareness further and further back in time. Once a dissociation from the present and a reorientation into the past have been obtained by direct or indirect suggestion, then the vivid and detailed memories of the unconscious can be released and experienced as actualities. It must be kept in mind, however, that repressed memories were repressed for a reason and subjects should not be plunged back into those experiences without some form of protection such as the dissociative perspective or amnesias discussed later in this chapter.

> **Rather than hypnotically treating a patient suffering from a phobia for doorknobs by telling him in the trance to forget his phobia, to overcome it, to realize its foolishness, one tries instead by hypnosis to elicit indirectly and adequately the story of the genesis of that phobia and to build up in him anew his own forgotten and repressed patterns of normal behavior toward doorknobs.**
>
> *(Erickson 1941b, p. 17)*

The procedure of hypnotic reorientation to a past event makes possible the reliving of that experience as if in the

course of the actual original development, thus excluding the modifying effects of the perspective and the secondary emotional reactions which obtain in the normal waking state and permitting revival of the experience in a more sequential order and in greater detail than is possible in the normal state. [1937]

(In Erickson, 1980, Vol. III, chap. 6, p. 52)

In brief, there are three highly important considerations in hypnotic psychotherapy that lend themselves to effective therapeutic results. One is the ease and readiness with which the dynamics and forms of the patient's maladjustments can be utilized effectively to achieve the desired therapy.

Second is the unique opportunity that hypnosis offers to work either separately and independently, or, jointly with different aspects of the personality, and thus to establish various nuclei of integration.

Equally important is the value of hypnosis in enabling the patient to recreate and to vivify past experiences free from present conscious influences, and undistorted by his maladjustment, thereby permitting the development of good understandings which lead to therapeutic results. [1948]

(In Erickson, 1980, Vol. IV, chap. 4, p. 48)

It was assumed that by means of this procedure a "removal" of the complex could be effected, since the patient could thus relive it at a conscious level and thereby might gain an insight into his reactions. [1935]

(In Erickson, 1980, Vol. III, chap. 28, p. 327)

Hypnosis offers a means of reaching an eventual understanding of the processes entering into the development of various behavioral phenomena. [1962]

(In Erickson, 1980, Vol. II, chap. 33, p. 348)

So can hypnosis be applied to the calling forth of even long-forgotten patterns of response. [1939]
(In Erickson, 1980, Vol. IV, chap. 1, p. 11)

But we all grow up, having lost some things that we forgot about — and if we ever do remember them, we will see them differently than when it happened.
(Erickson & Lustig, 1975, Vol. 2, p. 7)

You'll just remember, "Yes, when I was a little kid I was scared." That's the way you'll remember it. You will be able to laugh about it and take an adult person's view.
(Erickson & Rossi, 1979, p. 322)

You have those learnings in adult life, you can correct them, but there is no real need to correct them. They should be appreciated...
Psychotherapy using hypnosis, taking note of past memories in their purity without any need to correct them. As you should want to know what they are. We learn to recognize those individual memories without correcting them. You then have the opportunity to assess, evaluate, the components of a total understanding.
(Erickson, Rossi & Rossi, 1976, p. 214)

As the subject became sufficiently reassured, she was able to face the sources of her terror and finally could recover the lost memories while gazing into a mirror under hypnosis. [1939]
(In Erickson, 1980, Vol. III, chap. 23, p. 252)

I like to initially regress my psychiatric patients to something pleasant, something agreeable...I impress upon them that it is tremendously important to realize that there are some good things in their past, and those good things form the background by which to judge the severity of the present.

(Erickson & Rossi, 1981, p. 13)

Furthermore, recent experimental work by Platonov and Prikhodivny (1930), among others, has indicated that regression in a hypnotic state to an earlier period of life is possible, with the reestablishment of its corresponding patterns of behavior uninfluenced by subsequently acquired skills. [1937]

(In Erickson, 1980, Vol. III, chap. 6, p. 49)

And she can remember at any level that she wishes. I know that I can remember what happened at three weeks old. If I can so can others.

(Erickson & Rossi, 1979, p. 391)

I admit to her that there is a way of losing memories by a loss of brain cells, but I affirm that is not the case with her.

(Erickson & Rossi, 1979, p. 287)

I'm emphasizing her own natural memory patterns, rather than having her rely on some way of remembering she was artificially taught.

(Erickson & Rossi, 1979, p. 283)

Normal adults may be "regressed" by hypnotic suggestion literally to a state of infancy, with this regression including not only intellectual and emotional patterns of response but even muscular reflex responses. [1939]

(In Erickson, 1980, Vol. IV, chap. 1, p. 11)

The first confusion technique I worked out was for the purpose of inducing regression.

(ASCH, 1980, Taped Lecture, 8/8/64)

Suggestions are offered to effect a dissociation from the immediate environment and then to emphasize the unimportance of the identity of the day of the week and then of the month, culminating in an amnesia for time, place, and situation, but with an awareness of the general identity of the self. [circa 1940's]

(In Erickson, 1980, Vol. IV, chap. 46, p. 425)

Thus there has been a rapid and easy mention of realities of today gradually slipping into the future with the past becoming the present and thereby placing the mentioned realities, actually of the past, increasingly from the implied present into the more and more seemingly remote future. [1964]

(In Erickson, 1980, Vol. I, chap. 10, p. 263)

I removed reality and got her back in time.

(Zeig, 1980, p. 305)

Now go deeply into trance, so that your unconscious can deal with that vast store of memories that you have.

(Erickson & Lustig, 1975, Vol. 1, p. 3)

Some external thing has no real value to them, but the images they have within are of value. Furthermore, you're only talking about what did occur in their past. It is their past and I'm not forcing anything upon them.... They did learn many, many images. They can be pleased and select any image they want.

(Erickson, Rossi & Rossi, 1976, p. 8)

So you have a whole bank full of memories and understandings, and all I do is say something that touches upon those memories. Yesterday when I said, "Try to stand up," I tapped into your memory bank to a time when you couldn't stand up. And there was a time

**when you couldn't sit down because you didn't know
what "sit down" meant.**

(Erickson & Rossi, 1979, p. 231)

**Thus the role of the hypnotist was limited strictly to
the initiation of the process of reliving, and once started
it continued in accord with the *actual experiential patterns of response individual to the subject*. [circa 1960]**

(In Erickson, 1980, Vol. II, chap. 29, p. 303)

**So she has a tremendous amount of freedom to explore
all these possibilities in her past — and all this by implication.**

(Erickson & Rossi, 1979, p. 413)

Dissociation

Although the hypnotic state increases comfort, diminishes
defenses, and increases the flexibility of the conscious mind, it
does not do so completely or permanently. The conscious
mind remains unable to deal with many internal events such as
memories, thoughts or different perspectives. Frequently,
however, patients can consciously review various internal
events more objectively if they are trained to assume a
dissociative, objective perspective upon them. This dissociative
condition is similar to the conscious/unconscious dissociation
developed in deep trance, except that the conscious mind remains relatively more alert and active and thus develops
understandings from those things which pass through
awareness. Awareness, learning, and understanding are not
relegated totally to the unconscious mind but to a dissociated,
more objective, or detached conscious mind. The unconscious
is employed to help the conscious mind learn how to experience this dissociative phenomenon and the contents of the

unconscious usually form the bulk of the material reviewed from this objective perspective. The activity of the conscious mind, however, is not suppressed and the unconscious mind is not the only mode of awareness used. Instead, hypnotized subjects are allowed to view memories, thoughts, and ongoing experiences as if they belonged to someone else. They can review the life events of a child with no immediate awareness that that child is themself. They can review the thought patterns or response tendencies of an individual, with no awareness that they are that individual. They are thereby given the opportunity to review and assess a great variety of events from a detached, objective perspective and to develop a more appropriate analysis of their internal and external realities.

Subjects also can be dissociated along lines of demarcation other than the subjective-objective dimension. For example, they can be separated from their emotional life, their intellectual life, or their physical life. They can be allowed to experience a present or past event on one or another of these levels only. By limiting the input to one channel and dissociating patients from the other elements of the event, they can be allowed to experience tolerable chunks of it at a time and to integrate these various aspects into a totality as their understanding develops. Use of this jig-saw reconstruction frequently enables subjects to remember aspects of events that were repressed because of their intense emotional impact, because of the intolerable cognitive meaning derived from them, e.g. "Mommy hate me," or because of the physical discomfort involved. Understanding is allowed to develop as the subject remembers and comprehends detached elements of the original situation and slowly reintegrates these elements into a new, more objective comprehension of it. Painful or difficult material can be approached more easily when it is presented piecemeal or in any fashion that buffers its impact.

Probably of even greater significance is the opportunity hypnosis gives the patient to dissociate himself from his problems, to take an objective view of himself, to make an inventory of his assets and abilities, and then, one by one, to deal with his problems instead of being overwhelmed with all of them without being able to think clearly in any direction. [1945]

(In Erickson, 1980, Vol. IV, chap. 3, p. 34)

In contrast to the functioning of the ordinary state of conscious awareness, hypnosis permits a dissociation of ideas and attitudes in one relationship and a vivification and intensification of others in another relationship, thereby facilitating a much more effective examination, identification, and evaluation of wishes, fears, beliefs, and understandings. In this way clear comparison of intrinsic values, a recognition of conflicts, and an integration of understandings can be more readily effectuated. [circa 1940's]

(In Erickson, 1980, Vol. IV, chap. 46, p. 425)

You have such a total freedom for exploring and solving problems when you put the patient in the observer modality.

(Erickson, 1980, Vol. IV, p. 396)

You remove the subjective and let the objective work.

(Erickson, 1980, Vol. IV, p. 394)

The detached, objective observer can recover childhood perceptions with an adult's understanding. This is a valid characteristic of trance. The detached observer is a center pole and fixed reality about which the patient can explore many childhood experiences in adult words. Memory is not all of one piece; it's always fragments of adult and child interacting.

(Erickson & Rossi, 1979, p.420)

She was not allowed to interpose her resistances between herself and therapy, but put into a situation of objectively examining them. [1964]

(In Erickson, 1980, Vol. I, chap. 10, pp. 289–290)

Thus the patient, as an observant, objective, judicious third person, through the mechanisms of repression and projection, viewed freely, but without recognition, a panorama of his own experiential life, a panorama which permitted the recognition of faults and distortions without the blinding effects of emotional bias. [1948]

(In Erickson, 1980, Vol. IV, chap. 4, p. 44)

You can see things better in such a dissociative state. Dissociation helps you realize different experiential states. If these different experiential states do not know each other, the observation of them can be all the more objective.

(Erickson & Rossi, 1979, p. 417)

The objective observer that sees and describes current realities can also alter and change earlier childhood realities.

(Erickson & Rossi, 1979, p. 418)

What you're doing is taking something which is a personal experience and rendering it into an objective matter.

(Erickson, 1980, Vol. IV, p.394)

It [putting the patient into the observer modality] removes the questionable aspects of the experience from the patient's awareness. It allows him to objectify that thing, and then he can be curious about it as an objective phenomenon.

(Erickson, 1980, Vol. IV, p. 394)

Hypnotically, of course, it is very easy to induce a deep trance and reorient patients completely, even to depersonalize them.

(Erickson & Rossi, 1981, p. 9)

Notice how I accept and reinforce the depersonalization by using "it" and contrasting it with the part of her that I address as "you." She can *see* what she is writing, but this in itself implies she will not *know* what she is writing. You can see without knowing. I can just see those books, for example. Her questions and the strange feeling are all characteristic of the dissociative process.

(Erickson & Rossi, 1979, p. 400)

Dissociation, a detachment or separation of subjective from objective values, another highly complicated phenomenon, is of particular significance in effecting specialized learnings (for example anesthesia or emotional objectivity) without arousing impeding or obstructing subjective reactions.

(Erickson, 1970, p. 996)

He could see himself depicted in various situations and at different times in his life. Thereby he could observe his behavior and reactions, make comparisons and contrasts, and note the thread of continuity in his reaction patterns from one age level to the next.

(Erickson, 1954c, p. 262)

Further, induced states of dissocation can be established, exploratory measures developed, and vital information obtained which otherwise would be inaccessible both to the patient and to the therapist.

(Erickson, 1934, pp. 612-613)

The suggestion was offered, to which he readily assented, that he might like to begin with a brief but comprehensive review of the past as depicted in crystal ball scenes.

(Erickson, 1954c, p. 264)

Then by means of dream activity, a situation was created whereby the subject, without assuming the responsibility, could circumvent the repression. [1933]

(In Erickson, 1980, Vol. III, chap. 5, p. 44)

It [dreaming something unreported] gives the subjects a sense of liberty which is entirely safe and yet can be in accord with any unconscious ideas of license and freedom in hypnosis. It utilizes familiar experiences in forgetting and repression. It gives a sense of security and confidence in the self, and it also constitutes a posthypnotic suggestion to be executed only at the subject's desire. [1952]

(In Erickson, 1980, Vol. I, chap. 6, pp. 150–151)

Dreams give us the opportunity to relive past events and appraise them critically from an adult perspective.

(Erickson & Rossi, 1979, p. 473)

To uncover that memory and return it to you is not likely to occur all at once. What is likely to happen is that you'll remember a little bit here and next week a little bit there.

(Erickson & Rossi, 1979, p. 282)

Various bits of the incident recovered in that jigsaw fashion allow you to eventually recover an entire, forgotten traumatic experience of childhood...that had been governing this person's behavior...and handicapping his life very seriously.

(Erickson & Rossi, 1981, p. 7)

Now I think that in hypnotherapy that you had better recognize the tremendous importance of indifference, of detachment and this possibility of extracting only one fragment here and another fragment there.

(ASCH, 1980, Taped Lecture, 8/8/64)

The dissociation of intellectual content from emotional significances often facilitates an understanding of the meaningfulness of both. Hypnosis permits such dissociation when needed, as well as a correction of it. [1948]

(In Erickson, 1980, Vol. IV, chap. 4, p. 48)

You then point out to a patient that it is perfectly possible to remember the intellectual facts of something but not the emotional content, and vice versa.

(Erickson & Rossi, 1979, p. 348)

All right, and now can you understand you have two responses; intellectual and emotional?

(Erickson & Rossi, 1979, p. 342)

He was immediately interrupted and extensive hypnotic instructions were given that he report only on what he himself saw and did and that he was not to try to understand the situation.

(Erickson, 1954c, p. 265)

I always distinguish between thinking and feeling: Thinking can be valid but it's limited; a feeling can be anything even though it's an illusion from a rational point of view.

(Erickson & Rossi, 1979, p. 291)

This is specious reasoning, but it is the "emotional reasoning" that is common in daily life, and daily living is not an exercise in logic. [1966]

(In Erickson, 1980, Vol. IV, chap. 28, p. 267)

Now we move in three different ways. It may be intellectually, it may be emotionally and we move motorically by moving around. Some move more than others.

(Zeig, 1980, p. 52)

We have our affective, or our emotional life, and we have our cognitive, or intellectual life. And we are taught from the very beginning to emphasize our intelligence as if that were really the important thing. But, the important thing is the person on all those levels.

(Zeig, 1980, p. 52)

Now, when patients have deeply repressed memories, that doesn't mean they haven't got them. And sometimes the best way to dig out those repressions, those horrible memories, is to have them bring out the emotion, or the intellectual part, or the motoric part. Because emotions alone don't tell the story. The intellectual part alone is like reading something in a storybook, and the memory reactions don't mean anything at all.

(Zeig, 1980, p. 56)

You separate the emotional and intellectual content because so often people cannot face the meaningfulness of an experience. People cry and do not know why they cry, they feel suddenly elated and know not why. In using regression therapeutically you first recover the emotions in trance to help the patient recognize them. Then put the patient back in a trance; this time leave the emotions buried and let the intellectual content be recognized. Then put them back in a trance a third time and put the cognitive and emotional aspects together and then have them come out of trance with a complete memory.

(Erickson & Rossi, 1979, pp. 317–318)

In other words, one can split off the intellectual aspects of a problem for a patient and leave only the emotional aspects to be dealt with. One can have a patient cry out very thoroughly over the emotional aspects of a traumatic experience. Or, one can do it in a jigsaw fashion — that is, let him recover a little bit of the intellectual content of the traumatic experience of the past, then a little bit of the emotional content — and these different aspects need not necessarily be connected.

(Erickson & Rossi, 1981, p. 7)

We are giving the patient new possibilities and we are taking away the undesirable qualities. Usually it's best to have patients experience the emotion first and later the intellectual, because after they have experienced the emotions so strongly, they have a need to get the intellectual side of it.

(Erickson & Rossi, 1979, p. 330)

Then she sought circumscribed therapy, only circumscribed therapy. This was presented to her in such a fashion that, even as she had circumscribed everything, she was in a position to enlarge properly her whole problem. Her thinking about her problem had been emotionally repressed, largely at an unconscious level. Her therapy permitted her to do the same type of thinking but to include in it not only the events leading to her problem but the emotional values dating all the way back to her childhood. [1965]

(In Erickson, 1980, Vol. IV, chap. 20, p. 222)

You can also have a patient hallucinate a protective shield or an opaque cloth, and you can have that shield or cloth get thinner and thinner and more and more transparent in order to view the area of anxiety, you can stop the transparency at any stage you choose.

(Erickson, 1980, Vol. IV, p. 396)

Amnesias

Amnesia, or the absence of a memory for the experiences of a particular segment of time, it a common, everyday phenomenon. Everyone is amnesic for a vast number of the experiences and learnings of early childhood and everyone develops new amnesias from one day to the next. Some are relatively brief, as when you momentarily forget what it was you were saying or were about to do, and others are more permanent as when you experience and then forget a dream. Some amnesias even develop as a direct result of waking suggestions given to us by ourselves or others. A casual "Oh, forget it!" can produce remarkably effective results. Whatever "it" was often becomes totally obliterated from awareness.

Erickson was interested in the everyday occurrences of amnesia because amnesia can be a very useful ability for a hypnotherapeutic patient to have and the study of the circumstances which initiate amnesias in everyday life can provide an arsenal of techniques for developing amnesias in patients. Amnesia is a simple, straightforward method of protecting patients. After patients have recognized their ability to forget any event that happens to them during hypnosis, they can allow themselves to experience many previously avoided things with the full assurance that if any event is too unpleasant or calls for too much change they can and will simply forget it.

One interesting feature of this capacity for amnesia is the fact that even forgotten events represent acquired experiential learning which can be applied usefully later on, although the person may have no idea when or where that learning was acquired. Many pathological conditions seem to be expressions of inappropriate experiential learning which has not or cannot be corrected because patients do not even know that it is there. They may have forgotten the original learning situation altogether because of a trauma leading to repression or simply because of an innocuous amnesia. In any event, even though the precipitating situation may have been forgotten, the faulty learning obtained from it can live on and continue to influence the person's adjustment. A creative hypnotherapist, such as Erickson, can utilize these consequences of amnesia to generate new, productive learnings with no conscious memory of the trance experiences which led to that learning. As a consequence, the conscious mind is prevented from intruding unhelpfully upon or changing the unconscious learning or understandings gained from those experiences.

In fact, Erickson usually initiated an amnesia in his subjects for the entire trance experience, thereby relegating the learnings acquired during it to the unconscious and enabling the person to develop an awareness of them only as circumstances permitted. He typically accomplished this by the simple expedient of making a few remarks as the subject emerged from the trance which related to or continued a conversation begun prior to the induction. The reorientation thus required takes subjects back to the beginning of trance and sets the trance experience off as a separate, encapsulated, dissociative phenomenon which they then have difficulty remembering.

Erickson evidently preferred such indirect approaches over the more direct suggestions of forgetting which often have the paradoxical effect of enhancing the subject's memory. A rough rule of thumb of Erickson's seems to have been: Never try to get subjects to do something by asking them directly to do it if, instead, you can create a stimulus condition or experience which will elicit the desired response in a natural, normal, and unrecognized fashion.

Specific amnesias are everyday occurrences. Their study and analysis offer a wide field of therapeutic and theoretical interest through the understanding they afford of the mechanisms of repression and the means of removing, overcoming, or circumventing repressive forces. [1933]

(In Erickson, Vol. III, chap. 5, p. 38)

We tend spontaneously to forget the parts or details of a situation when we are fixated or motivated by the total Gestalt or major goal of that situation. [circa 1960's]

(In Erickson, 1980, Vol. III, chap. 8, p. 59)

Something well learned can be meaningless when encountered out of context, thus giving an effect comparable to a failure of recognition and such as may occur in amnesia. [circa 1950's]

(In Erickson, 1980, Vol. III, chap. 7, p. 56)

The primary differences between hypnotically induced amnesias and those of everyday life are that the former can be intentionally controlled or directed by others, while those of daily life are not easily amenable to external direction but are dependent upon processes within the person for their manifestation. [circa 1960's]

(In Erickson, 1980, Vol. III, chap. 8, p. 58)

Amnesia resulting from direct suggestion is a phenomenon that occurs in everyday life most commonly in relation to children, though it also occurs in relation to adults. [circa 1960's]

(In Erickson, 1980, Vol. III, chap. 8, p. 62)

Here the amnesia is evidently due to the loss of an important associative connection caused by an outer inter-

ruption that momentarily distracts the person and "breaks his train of thought." [circa 1960's]

(In Erickson, 1980, Vol. III, chap. 8, p. 60)

You can forget anything. You forget that you had to learn to lift your head as an infant. You had to learn how to move your hand. And one time you didn't even know it was your hand.

(Erickson & Rossi, 1981, p. 47)

You can be sitting with a newly-made friend whose name you know when suddenly another train of thought comes along, and you find that you have forgotten his name, an easy thing to do unintentionally in the waking state, but also easy to do upon simple request in the hypnotic state. [1962]

(In Erickson, 1980, Vol. II, chap. 33, p. 347)

In the ordinary state of awareness, then, direct suggestions can be given to elicit amnesias. In this author's experience, however, such suggestions are most effective if given in a casual, nonrepetitive fashion and under circumstances involving some form of increased emotion.... Repetition of the instruction to forget produced a better recollection of it than of the other "neutral" items. [circa 1960's]

(In Erickson, 1980, Vol. III, chap. 8, p. 64)

There can be separate states of awareness that develop spontaneously in ordinary life: they are independent of each other, and can give rise to a total amnesia. If this can occur spontaneously, why then should there be any doubt that similar situations can be set up psychologically in order deliberately and intentionally to evoke hypnotic amnesias? [circa 1960's]

(In Erickson, 1980, Vol. III, chap. 8, p. 62)

One can secure all of that information from the patient via regression which gives you complete understanding of many aspects about your patient, and then awaken the patient with a total amnesia of what he has told you. The patient doesn't know what he is talking about, but you know what he is talking about. And therefore, you can guide the patient's thinking and speaking closer and closer to the actual problem. You can detect the significant words that refer to the traumatic experience of which he is consciously unaware and thus understand the deeper implications of what he is talking about.

(Erickson & Rossi, 1981, p. 7-8)

You don't have to remember. The important thing is to have certain experiences recorded in your mind. Some day their presence will be of service to you. It is necessary for you to be aware that you know they are there.

(Erickson, Rossi & Rossi, 1976, p. 260)

Also, hypnosis allows ready retreat if the patient is not yet ready, without there being any loss of therapeutic gains already made. [1965]

(In Erickson, 1980, Vol. IV, chap. 58, p. 523)

You can be free to inquire into yourself instead of dropping dead when you discover something you don't want to know about yourself. Just *forget* it. You don't know how much your unconscious wants you to know.

(Erickson & Rossi, 1977, p. 50)

Thus, in the trance state, the subject can remember vividly long-forgotten, even deeply repressed experiences, recount them fully and still have a complete amnesia for them when aroused from the trance state. This ability is remarkably useful in experimental work, since it permits the recovery of memories otherwise unavailable, and hence the exploration of the experiential past of the subject.

(Erickson, 1954b, p. 23)

In other words, the amnesia enables patients to be confronted with material belonging to their own experiential lives but which, because of the induced repression, is not recognized by them as such. Then it becomes possible for those patients to reach a critical objective understanding of unrecognized material from their own life experience, to reorganize and reassociate it in accord with its reality significances and their own personality needs. [1948]

(In Erickson, 1980, Vol. IV, chap. 4, p. 42)

In undertaking hypnotherapy it is important in the early stages to have the patient develop an amnesia for some innocuous memory, then to restore that memory along with some other unimportant but forgotten memory. [1948]

(In Erickson, 1980, Vol. IV, chap. 4, p. 42)

I facilitate a certain flexibility in mental functioning when I remind her ,how easily her pleasure and fear can be "removed and reassumed."

(Erickson & Rossi, 1979, p. 347)

You ask a question, and then before an answer can be given, you say a lot of meaningful things, and then you go back to the original question. You've thereby drawn a blanket over the meaningful material; you've put a parenthesis around it. This is a very important principle of producing hypnotic amnesia in order to prevent the patient's consciousness from negating meaningful questions.

(Erickson & Rossi, 1981, p. 101)

We develop an "I don't know" set to facilitate hypnotic amnesia.

(Erickson & Rossi, 1981, p. 103)

This measure of reorientation in time by reawakening trains of thought and associations preceding trance inductions, in this author's experience, is far more effective in inducing post-hypnotic amnesia than direct, forceful suggestions for its development. One merely makes dominant the previous thought patterns and idea associations. [1964]

(In Erickson, 1980, Vol. I, chap. 15, p. 348)

You thus emphasize that the patient undoubtedly covered up many things that didn't need to be covered up. So why not uncover every one of those things that are safe to uncover and be sure to keep covered up the things that are not safe to uncover?

(Erickson & Rossi, 1979, p. 348)

Amnesic barriers may be overcome by an item of experience serving to arouse associations related to the forgotten data. [circa 1950's]

(In Erickson, 1980, Vol. III, chap. 7, p. 55)

Pain Control

Perhaps because he was subjected to intense, chronic pain stemming from his various physical ailments, Erickson was very interested in the use of hypnosis to control the experience of pain. He used it on himself and he used it for the benefit of numerous patients. His reports of the rapid and effective alleviation of pain, even in the most debilitating cases of cancer, with none of the incapacitating effects of drugs have been substantiated by similar reports from many other authors. Actually, no other beneficial use of hypnosis has received such widespread acknowledgement, application, and research support. The hypnotic control of pain has become an established fact which has led to its widespread use for this purpose.

Erickson developed numerous techniques for teaching patients how to control or eliminate their experiences of pain. Readers are referred to Erickson & Rossi's *Hypnotherapy: An exploratory casebook*, Irvington Publishers, 1979, pp. 94–142 for an extended discussion of this topic. In many respects, however, Erickson's approaches to the problem of using hypnosis to alleviate pain were not substantially different from his applications of hypnosis in other problem situations. The same dynamics were utilized and hypnosis played essentially the same role that it did in all other therapeutic applications. Evidently, the alleviation of physical pain, emotional pain and psychological pain all call for similar procedures.

Erickson recognized that all people have an existing ability to minimize, ignore or even forget physical discomfort, an ability they display every day in one way or another. His goal, therefore, was to teach people how to apply these naturally occurring phenomena or previously learned capacities to their present pain. Hypnosis was used simply to facilitate that learning process.

Some people can learn to develop an anesthesia for a specific pain by learning how to use the same mechanisms that they have used previously to ignore the glasses on their noses or the pressure of their feet on the floor. Some can learn to focus their attention so intensely upon things other than their pain that the pain recedes from awareness, or they can be helped to re-experience a previous anesthesia and to bring that anesthesia into the present. They can be asked to imagine and describe a state of complete comfort in such detail that their imagined condition becomes their experienced reality. They can be allowed to develop whatever degree of anesthesia they can personally accept and tolerate. They can even move the discomfort to another area of their body and can change the intensity or quality of it to suit their needs.

In some instances, simply placing the person in a trance and instructing the unconscious to produce comfort will suffice, whereas in others a more elaborate training program must be developed using regressions, revivifications, dissociations, amnesias, metaphors, and indirect forms of communication. Some of Erickson's most creative, complex and indirect forms of intervention were developed in an effort to assist pain sufferers. For example, he talked to one man about tomatoes and interspersed his comments with suggestions for relaxation and comfort. This man had refused hypnosis, but Erickson utilized his interest in gardening and his desire for relief to provide him with comfort nonetheless. The man learned how to experience comfort without ever realizing that he was doing so.

Pain in any area of our physical, emotional, or intellectual lives is debilitating and calls for professional intervention. No matter where the pain is located, hypnosis can and should be used to help the person learn how to respond most comfortably and effectively to it and to eliminate its source if possible.

Nobody likes pain.
(ASCH, 1980, Taped Lecture, 7/18/65)

Pain is a threatening thing. It threatens the integrity and the continuance of the self.
(ASCH, 1980, Taped Lecture, 7/18/65)

Pain is a complex, a construct, composed of past remembered pain, of present pain experience, and of anticipated pain of the future. Thus, immediate pain is augmented by past pain and is enhanced by the future possibilities of pain. [1967]

(In Erickson, 1980, Vol. IV, chap. 24, p. 238)

Because pain is a complex, a construct, it is more readily vulnerable to hypnosis as a modality of dealing successfully with it than it would be were it simply an experience of the present. [1967]

(In Erickson, 1980, Vol. IV, chap. 24, p. 238)

And what does pain mean to a person? It means disability. Disability of a very large extent.

(ASCH, 1980, Taped Lecture, 7/18/65)

Cultural and individual psychological patterns are of as much and perhaps greater importance than the physiological experience of pain. [1959]

(In Erickson, 1980, Vol. IV, chap. 27, p. 256)

Apparently, the patient's fixed, psychological understanding was that dental work must absolutely be associated with hypersensitivity. When this rigid understanding was met, dental anesthesia could be achieved, in a fashion analogous to the relaxation of one muscle permitting the contraction of another. [1958]

(In Erickson, 1980, Vol. I, chap. 7, p. 169)

Acceptance of his neurotic belief and employing it to create hypnotically an area of extreme hypersensitivity met his need to be able to experience pain without having to do so. [1965]

(In Erickson, 1980, Vol. IV, chap. 20, p. 218)

So you must not make the mistake of trying to take too much away.

(Erickson & Rossi, 1979, p. 277)

And so for the rest of the hour, I continued offering her suggestions about her pain, rejection of pain, without telling her to reject the pain.

(ASCH, 1980, Taped Lecture, 2/2/66)

If you can get your patients' attention in some way so that they can be induced to use their learnings, you can abolish the pain. It doesn't matter whether you keep them awake, or keep them asleep, or keep them in a state of dual awareness. [1960]

(In Erickson, 1980, Vol. II, chap. 31, p. 317)

You have anesthesia of various parts of your body, and you use it every day. You have forgotten the shoes on your feet, the glasses on your face, the collar on your neck. You recognize them very promptly when you pay attention to them. By inducing sensory changes in the patient you bring about these changes by utilizing the experiential learning of their everyday life. [1959]

(In Erickson, 1980, Vol. III, chap. 4, p. 31)

People can learn so simply to turn pain, catalepsy, or any other subjective experience on and off. [1973]

(In Erickson, 1980, Vol. IV, chap. 29, p. 280)

One of the best measures for teaching extended pain relief is to teach the patient to let catalepsy persist. [1973]

(In Erickson, 1980, Vol. IV, chap. 29, p. 279)

Once the patients begin to develop a light trance, I speed the process more rapidly by jumping steps, yet retaining my right to mention pain so that patients know that I do not fear to name it and that I am utterly confident that he will lose it because of my ease and freedom in naming it, usually in a context negating pain in favor of absence or diminution or transformation of pain. [1964]

(In Erickson, 1980, Vol. I, chap. 10, p. 286)

Now this is a challenge to her. When I told her that she would not be able to describe the relief, the comfort, the kind of feelings she would *like* to have, I was literally putting her in a bind to describe them. And as surely as she started to describe them she would want to sense them, because how better can you describe a thing? How well can you describe a visual scene except by closing your eyes and visualizing it and looking at the various parts of your visualization? She literally had to sense the various feelings of comfort that she wanted to have.

(ASCH, 1980, Taped Lecture, 2/2/66)

The unconscious has many foci of attention, and when you withdraw that from any part of your body, you don't destroy your intellectual, conscious comprehension of that part, but it becomes an object because the unconscious foci of attention are withdrawn.

(Erickson & Rossi, 1981, p. 251)

Now the next thing you should bear in mind is that when you take away the sense of feeling, anesthesia or analgesia, you've asked your patient to make a different kind of reality orientation.

(Erickson & Rossi, 1979, p. 132)

R: The unconscious can take a general instruction like "relieve the pain." But the unconscious does not follow a

specific instruction about how to do it exactly.
E: **That's right. I have the thought "I'd like to get rid of this pain." That's enough!**

(Erickson & Rossi, 1977, p. 44)

Then you leave it to your unconscious....you can't know how it's achieved without keeping it [pain] with you.

(Erickson & Rossi, 1977, p. 45)

Terminating A Trance

All good trances must come to an end and, within an Ericksonian framework, they should all come to a good end. Poor termination of a trance can erase many of the potential benefits from it and may generate confusion or even hostility. Proper termination procedures, on the other hand, can enhance the benefits of the hypnotic episode, can ratify its reality, and can leave the subject feeling remarkably relaxed, comfortable, and optimistic.

Emergence from a hypnotic state of mind involves a general reorientation of awareness away from internal events outward toward external realities. It also requires a massive shift in mental set from those systems of perception, understanding and response typical of the unconscious back into the patterns of the ordinary conscious mind. This transition must be handled carefully.

The transition into normal wakefulness should be a natural, comfortable awakening process which proceeds in accordance with the needs and desires of the patient. Rather than a sudden demand for immediate wakefulness upon the hypnotist's signal, subjects usually should be given the time and opportunity to drift back into a normal state in their own way. The hypnotist can provide indirect cues that facilitate this reorientation process, such as a shift into a more normal tone of voice, breathing rate, and speaking rate, but subjects, like babies, should emerge when they are ready.

On the other hand, according to Erickson, subjects should not be allowed to linger for very long in the twilight state between waking and hypnotic orientation. In this state the new unconscious learning may become prematurely available to conscious awareness. Furthermore, Erickson indicated that it was desirable to establish a clear line of demarcation for the trance state in order to set it off as a unique and valid experience in its own right. Hence, he used the previously mentioned initiation of amnesia for the entire trance process by immediately reintroducing a pre-trance topic of conversation when subjects open their eyes or begin moving about physically to re-orient themselves. Their resultant amnesia makes the hypnotic episode seem real. Erickson also asked subjects if they were fully awake or if they could describe what had happened to them. Such questions were asked to further ratify the trance experience to subjects, i.e. to demonstrate that something different and potentially useful actually did happen to them.

Erickson always praised his subjects and thanked them for their helpful participation. He did this before, during, and after a trance episode. Such comments relax potential subjects, provide support to hypnotized subjects, and ratify the value of the hypnotic experience to subjects emerging from trance. Even if nothing of particular significance had happened during the trance, Erickson wanted to avoid discouragement. If something important had been learned, he did not want conscious skepticism to undo it.

You have them close their eyes because there is a whole lifetime of experience of having their eyes closed before they awaken.

(Erickson, Rossi & Rossi, 1976, p. 105)

I didn't ask you to wake up. (Laughter) I let your conscious mind take over.

(Zeig, 1980, p. 45)

Yes. It was a distraction. You don't want too much self analysis immediately. A person fresh out of trance is still lingering close to it, and unconscious knowledge is easily available. You don't know if that should be used yet. So you distract them.

(Erickson, Rossi & Rossi, 1976, p. 53)

Now what I had to do was to awaken her and distract her so whatever she has done can remain at the unconscious level. I don't want it shoved into a conscious frame of reference.

(Erickson, Rossi & Rossi, 1976, p. 294)

All this rather slow and elaborate awakening procedure is to get her away from any traumatic unconscious material that her conscious mind is not yet ready to handle.

(Erickson & Rossi, 1979, p. 309)

The implication of my question, "What happened to you?" is that something did happen. In his answer he is validating verbally that his first experience was a trance.

(Erickson & Rossi, 1981, p. 220)

I'm using them [questions] to ratify the trance, and I'm directing his attention to various things. And I'm not telling him! I'm just asking for information. You ask for in-

formation about all of the things you want him to be
aware of unconsciously.

(Erickson & Rossi, 1981, p. 206)

Her recognition that "the breathing was sort of more
like sleep breathing" is another ratification of trance.

(Erickson & Rossi, 1981, p. 95)

Yes, that is the purpose in having them describe the
sensations. It ratifies trance.

(Erickson & Rossi, 1981, p. 93)

Yes, it [the question "Are you fully awake?"] really
ratifies trance to his unconscious mind, and his conscious
mind can think anything it pleases.

(Erickson & Rossi, 1981, p. 202)

Even with a light trance you ask them to explain how
light the trance was. But they are ratifying that there was
a trance. [1959]

(In Erickson, 1980, Vol. I, chap. 9, p. 228)

If there is evidence of trance, their unconscious knows
it. I don't have to prove it!....That is a sheer waste of
time, and it arouses a patient's hostility.

(Erickson & Rossi, 1981, p. 105)

When she awakened, I thanked her again, because it is
very important to thank the patient's unconscious mind
as well as the conscious mind.

(Zeig, 1980, p. 182)

You always give praise to the unconscious.

(Erickson & Rossi, 1979, p. 183)

Give credit wherever you can.

(Zeig, 1980, p. 347)

We can reinforce the value of that experience by speaking well of it to the patient even though we do not know exactly what it is referring to. You don't know how long the patient will need to digest the new material. It could be a day or a week or whatever. So you need not see patients on a rigid schedule. It is best to let them call when they need to. A therapist should have flexibility in his schedule to accommodate the patient's needs.

(Erickson & Rossi, 1979, p. 382)

Yes, and giving her permission for failures. *All the failures will prove an improvement.*

(Erickson & Rossi, 1979, p. 205)

The author is well aware of the deadliness of skeptical disparaging remarks and of the engendering of iatrogenic disease. [1964]

(In Erickson, 1980, Vol. I, chap. 13, p. 326)

The final interview was simply one of a deep trance, a systematic, comprehensive review by her within her own mind of all of her accomplishments and the gentle request to believe with utter intensity in the goodness of her own body's potentials in meeting her needs and to be *"highly amused* when the skeptics suggest that you have had remissions before followed by relapses." [1964]

(In Erickson, 1980, Vol. I, chap. 13, p. 326)

You now know that you can, you are confident. In fact, you have succeeded, and there is nothing that you can do to keep from succeeding again and again. [1958]

(In Erickson, 1980, Vol. I, chap. 7, p. 172)

Summary

Ideomotor responses of various sorts can be used as communication systems for the unconscious in addition to their use as induction enhancing devices. Ideomotor signal systems, which allow unconscious communications to be conveyed without conscious awareness, can be developed into the more complex and informative process of automatic writing. Information which might otherwise be unavailable can be secured in this manner from the unconscious.

The unconscious also has the capacity to project awareness into an imaginary but plausible future, thus creating an awareness of the potential paths to therapeutic success. It can equally well project awareness into the past, allowing a revivification of previous life events. The hypnotized subject can experience these and other alterations in awareness from the dissociative perspective of an objective observer or the subject can be led to develop an amnesia for all such occurrences.

No matter what hypnotized subjects learn during the hypnotic episode, be it how to control pain or how to view themselves, their pasts, or their present situations more objectively, the trance termination process plays an important role in determining how well such learning is absorbed and transferred into ordinary living. Proper termination procedures must be employed to ensure that the trance experience will be viewed as a valid phenomenon and to allow the learning and abilities developed during trance to be utilized effectively when needed.

Throughout his work Erickson was ever mindful of the old maxim, "As a man thinketh in his heart, so he is." He was highly dependent upon the ephemeral realm of beliefs and attitudes to work his so-called miracles. As a result, he did whatever he could to prevent unproductive, self-defeating beliefs and to instill useful and productive ones. Furthermore, he himself knew that he could use hypnosis and therapy to provide enormous benefits to others and this knowledge motivated and enabled him to do so. As the material in the final chapter of this book indicates, anyone who would do psychotherapy or use hypnosis probably should have an equally intense belief about hypnosis and the unconscious, a belief that can probably be gained only through personal experience.

CHAPTER THIRTEEN

BECOMING A HYPNOTHERAPIST

Anyone who sets off to become an effective and dynamic hypnotherapist in the tradition of Milton H. Erickson is undertaking an incredibly difficult and complex journey. Gaining the perspective and skill necessary to engage in effective psychotherapy is, in and of itself, a monumental endeavor. Adding the task of becoming a proficient hypnotist who can use the hypnotic process in a therapeutic setting probably magnifies several times the effort and dedication required.

Luckily, Erickson mapped the way for the rest of us. He observed and explored the terrain and furnished us with the general description of people provided in Section I of this book. He located and defined our objective when he described the goals, perspectives, and processes of therapy and hypnosis presented in the second and third sections of this book. Finally, as indicated by the quotations presented in this chapter, he charted the obstacles and described the best routes for us to take if we would follow in his footsteps.

Overcoming Skeptics

Like Erickson, prospective hypnotherapists must resist the numerous cultural and professional prejudices against the practice of hypnotherapy and must accept the very real possibility of rejection or misunderstanding from colleagues. Although the situation may not be as bad as it was when Erickson began his work, it is far from ideal. There are many attitudes and misunderstandings, even within the field of hypnosis, which can lead the prospective hypnotherapist astray. These may turn out to be difficult to resist and have the potential for redirecting thoughts and energies away from the perpectives and actions Erickson recommended and used. Of course, all hypnotherapists must decide for themselves which approach is most productive and useful for them, but they should take care not to adopt a particular attitude just because it is easier or more popular.

He had sought hypnotherapy by the author, who at that time was working under the joint supervision of the departments of psychology, psychiatry, and pharmacology and a psychiatrist-lawyer, all of whom acted as his sponsors to prevent the Dean of the College of Liberal Arts from expelling him for daring to deal with the black art of hypnosis. [circa 1960's]

(In Erickson, 1980, Vol. III, chap. 8, p. 67)

Hypnosis was a topic which the author had been most emphatically forbidden by the authorities of the Colorado General Hospital even to mention under threat of

dismissal from his internship and refusal of his application for examination for a state license to practice
medicine.

(Erickson, 1973, p. 92, Footnote 3)

Hypnosis was a forbidden subject because it required
understanding.

(Erickson & Rossi, 1981, p. 247)

The whole field of hypnotic research is still so
undeveloped that there is very little general understanding
either of how to hypnotize a subject satisfactorily for experimental purposes, or of how to elicit the hypnotic
phenomena which are to be studied after the subject has
been satisfactorily hypnotized. [1964]

(In Erickson, 1980, Vol. II, chap. 24, p. 301)

There are any number of attitudes taken to disprove
the legitimacy of hypnotic experiments and the concepts
one deals with in hypnosis despite their occurrence in the
ordinary course of human events. [1962]

(In Erickson, 1980, Vol. II, chap. 33, p. 342)

The simple fact that analogous conditions can develop
both in everyday life and in hypnotic states should be
ample warrant to accept those of the hypnotic state as
sufficiently valid to justify scientific examination. [1962]

(In Erickson, 1980, Vol. II, chap. 33, p. 347)

The readiness to accept, not to discard, to examine,
not to disparage, each item of behavior that seems related
to hypnosis is most important. We need to take the attitude that there are things we do not know or understand, and because we do not understand them, we ought
not attempt to offer comprehensive formulations of hypnosis as a total phenomenon, but rather endeavor to

identify manifestations as such and examine their relation to each other. [1962]

(In Erickson, 1980, Vol. II, Chapter 33, p. 349)

The validity of hypnotic phenomena lies within the phenomena themselves, and is not to be measured by standards applicable to another category of phenomena. [1967]

(In Erickson, 1980, Vol. I, chap. 2, p. 71)

I think that hypnosis can best be investigated by a careful searching of the great varieties of human behavior which can be modified or changed or influenced by the hypnotic state. [1960]

(In Erickson, 1980, Vol. II, chap. 31, p. 325)

The job of laboratory research is to discover what does happen rather than to discount the validity of the patient's experience. [1962]

(In Erickson, 1980, Vol. II, chap. 33, p. 348)

The easiest way is to *not* understand and call it a fake. That's an avoidance of understanding.

(Erickson & Rossi, 1981, p. 246)

The unfamiliar is unacceptable unless you can make it very mystical.

(Erickson & Rossi, 1981, p. 248)

Unfortunately both the American Medical Association and the American Psychiatric Association have done much to discourage the use of scientific hypnosis by medically competent men who have already demonstrated their ability to deal well and successfully with patients of all kinds under conditions of all manner of stress and strain. [1964]

(In Erickson, 1980, Vol. I, chap. 28, p. 539)

Increasing Awareness

Anyone can become an effective hypnotherapist if they are willing and able to become aware of and to learn the variety of things Erickson indicated were necessary. Careful observation of normal and abnormal behavior, the understanding of conscious and unconscious modes of functioning, and the effort necessary to recognize and adopt multiple frames of reference are the primary prerequisites.

> **Any person willing to learn the psychological principles involved can perform hypnosis. It is purely a matter of technic, a technic of convincing and persuasive suggestion similar to that utilized every day in ordinary commercial life for quite other purposes.**
>
> *(Erickson, 1934, p. 611)*

> **The field of hypnosis is open to any person willing to qualify by interest, study, and experience, and the intelligent use of hypnosis depends essentially upon a background and foundation of personal interest and training. [1945]**
>
> *(In Erickson, 1980, Vol. IV, chap. 3, p. 28)*

> **Clinically, and through our own daily experience, we know many varieties of behaviors can occur. In the use of hypnosis clinically it is our obligation to be aware of these possibilities and to utilize them. [1962]**
>
> *(In Erickson, 1980, Vol. II, chap. 33, p. 348)*

> **Only an awareness of what constitutes behavior deriving from the unconscious mind of the subjects enables the hypnotist to induce and to maintain deep trances. [1952]**
>
> *(In Erickson, 1980, Vol. I, chap. 6, p. 146)*

> **Yes, it [hypnosis] is difficult. You have to learn to recognize different frames of reference.**
>
> *(Erickson & Rossi, 1981, p. 249)*

> **As they [hypnotists] understand the way they are thinking, they have to entertain the idea of how the other fellow thinks in relation to these words. In that way you can learn to respect the *frame of reference* of the other person.**
>
> *(Erickson & Rossi, 1981, p. 255)*

Increasing Flexibility

Learning to be an effective hypnotherapist does not mean learning *the* technique to use with everyone. It should be apparent by now that Erickson believed that every patient requires a unique approach. Imitation of anyone, even Erickson, or the recitation of a memorized patter is not the road to success. Every hypnotherapist must develop a personal style that is comfortable and flexible enough to be modified by each patient's unique constellation of needs and learnings.

> **An awareness of the variability of human behavior and the need to meet it should be the basis of all hypnotic techniques. [1952]**
>
> *(In Erickson, 1980, Vol. I, chap. 6, p. 140)*

> **The able hypnotist is the one who is able to adapt technique to the personality needs of each subject. Thus, some subjects want to be dominated, others coaxed, still others to be persuaded. [1944]**
>
> *(In Erickson, 1980, Vol. IV, chap. 2, p. 17)*

Hypnotic techniques and procedures should vary according to the subject, circumstances, and the purposes to be served. [1945]

(In Erickson, 1980, Vol. IV, chap. 3, p. 28)

A good operator varies the details of his technique from subject to subject, fitting it to the peculiarities of each personality.

(Erickson, 1977b, p. 22)

Therefore, the more fluidity in the hypnotherapist, the more easily you can actually approach the patient.

(Erickson, 1977b, p. 22)

Moods, attitudes, and understandings often change in the subjects even as they are undergoing a trance induction, and that there should be a fluidity of change in technique by the operator from one type of approach to another as indicated. [1964]

(In Erickson, 1980, Vol. I, chap. 1, pp. 15–16)

It should never be assumed that the subject's understanding of instructions is identical with that of the hypnotist. [1941]

(In Erickson, Vol. I, chap. 19, p. 399)

You must attune your vocabulary to the individuality of each listener.

(Erickson & Rossi, 1981, p. 28)

You always use the patient's own words and experience as much as possible for trance induction and suggestion.

(Erickson, Rossi & Rossi, 1976, p. 29)

The hypnotist must implant his suggestions in the vast aggregate of mental reactions and patterns accumulated throughout the subject's lifetime.

(Erickson, 1934, p. 611)

The hypnotists, not the subjects, should be made to fit themselves into the hypnotic situation. [1952]

(In Erickson, 1980, Vol. I, chap. 6, p. 161)

Properly, hypnotists should have a good appreciation of their own personality and capabilities so that they may adapt themselves to the specific personality needs of each subject. [1944]

(In Erickson, 1980, Vol. IV, chap. 2, p. 17)

There is an equally important need for the hypnotist to use that technique which permits him to express himself most satisfactorily and effectively in the special interpersonal relationship which constitutes hypnosis. [1945]

(In Erickson, 1980, Vol. IV, chap. 3, p. 30)

Now the next thing I want to stress is *the tremendous need for each doctor to work out a method of suggestion for himself.*

(Erickson & Rossi, 1981, p. 3)

Remember that whatever way you choose to work must be your own way, because you cannot really imitate someone else. In dealing with the crucial situations of therapy, you must express yourself adequately, not as an imitation.

(Haley, 1967, p. 535)

To initiate this type of therapy you have to be yourself as a person. You cannot imitate somebody else, but you have to do it in your own way.

(Erickson & Rossi, 1979, p. 276)

**You need to extract from the various techniques the
particular elements that allow you to express yourself as a
person.**

(Haley, 1967, p. 534)

**Express your own personality only to the extent that it
is requisite to meet the patient and get that patient to
respond to you.**

(Haley, 1967, p. 535)

Experiencing Hypnosis

When Erickson sought to train hypnotherapists he did not
just lecture to them, *he hypnotized them.* There are several
possible explanations for this. First, because experience is the
best teacher, it makes sense to experience what it is you wish
to learn about. Secondly, because the hypnotist is basically attempting to teach the subject how to experience a particular
set of internal events, it is reasonable to believe that the
teacher should have learned to experience those events also. It
is often difficult for someone who has never participated in a
particular endeavor to teach others how to do it. Furthermore,
Erickson discovered that almost anyone who had been hypnotized could hypnotize someone else, an observation that was
partially responsible for his frequent use of relatively unsophisticated but very hypnotizable subjects to hypnotize some
of his most resistant subjects.

Finally, and perhaps most significantly, Erickson suggested
that hypnotherapists themselves should be able to participate
directly in the hypnosis process before and during their hypnotherapeutic sessions. Being hypnotized themselves evidently
allows hypnotherapists to stay with their psychotherapy patients and hypnotic subjects more effectively, to develop a

feeling for their subjects' potential responses to particular suggestions and thus, to present suggestions in a more meaningful manner. It also allows hypnotherapists to respond from within the perspective of their own unconscious and thus to understand the experiences and communications of the deeply hypnotized subject more effectively. This, in turn, enables them to communicate in terms that are appropriate to the unconscious understandings of each subject.

An even more facinating, and perhaps more controversial, component of Erickson's attitudes regarding the desirability of the hypnotherapist being able to enter a hypnotic state at will is his proposition that hypnotherapists can enter an autohypnotic state prior to a therapeutic session and allow their unconscious to plan the approaches and interventions that *it* will use with that patient. Then during the session itself, by virtue of the autohypnotic state, the hypnotherapists' unconscious mind is allowed to carry out its plans without conscious interference or distractions. The success of this approach is predicated upon the assumption that the therapist's unconscious has been provided with a wide background of careful observations and a reasonable understanding of the goals of therapy, but it is no less intriguing for that. Erickson's use of autohypnosis before and during therapy sessions was at least partially responsible for his remarkable successes and for his ability to generate creative and insightful interventions on the spot. If we were to speculate on the source of his reputation for mystical and magical abilities, we might conclude that his unfettered use of his unconscious mind was responsible. Obviously there was much more to it than that, as indicated by the large quantity of material presented previously in this book, but the ability to utilize one's own unconscious mind in the creation of metaphors, in the deciphering of a patient's unconscious productions and in the presentation of hypnotic suggestions certainly would be advantageous to anyone.

The one thing in the use of hypnosis is this: you really ought to know more about it than your patients do. You ought to know it so thoroughly that no matter what develops in the situation you can think of something, you can devise something, that will meet your patient's needs.

(Erickson & Rossi, 1981, p. 21)

Now S has been trying to get some rational understanding of hypnosis. She doesn't realize that to learn to swim you have to get in the water to actually experience it. Intellectual book knowledge about swimming won't do it. She has been trying to get in the trance and understand. But she should just get in the water first.

(Erickson, Rossi & Rossi, 1976, p. 237)

S offers me the handicap of intellectual desire to keep her knowledge available for use with her own patients.

(Erickson, Rossi & Rossi, 1976, p. 100)

Experience is the only teacher, and careful study of behavior manifestations is necessary. [1952]

(In Erickson, 1980, Vol. I, chap. 6, p. 148)

The hypnotic experience of learning to differentiate waking behavior from trance behavior in the same subject provides a general background of understanding by means of which one learns to recognize integration. [circa 1940's]

(In Erickson, 1980, Vol. III, chap. 24, p. 263)

The reality to the self of the subject's hypnotic behavior and its recognition by the hypnotist is essential to induce and to permit adequate functioning in the trance state. [1952]

(In Erickson, 1980, Vol. I, chap. 6, p. 148)

Indeed, long experience has disclosed that the easiest and quickest way to learn to induce a trance is to be hypnotized first, thus to learn the "feel" of it. [1964]
(In Erickson, 1980, Vol. I, chap. 10, p. 279)

Anybody who has been hypnotized can employ it to hypnotize others, given cooperation and the patience to make use of it.
(Erickson, 1941b, p. 15)

R: How do you make use of their interest? You direct it to the inner parts of their own world?
E: Yes. And then I stay there with them.
(Erickson & Rossi, 1979, p. 368)

Staying with your patient is so important.
(Erickson, Rossi & Rossi, 1976, p. 103)

How does one validate another's subjective experience? By participating, if possible! [1964]
(In Erickson, 1980, Vol. I, chap. 15, p. 345)

I soon learned during the process of developing that technique [hand-levitation] that I almost invariably would find my hand lifting and my eyelids closing. Thus I learned the importance of giving my subjects suggestions in a tone of voice completely expressive of meaningfulness, expectation and of "feeling" my words and their meanings within me as a person. [1964]
(In Erickson, 1980, Vol. I, chap. 15, p. 344)

I was careful to emphasize the importance in inducing hypnosis, of speaking slowly, impressively and meaningfully, and literally to "feel" at the moment within the self the full significance of what is being said. [1964]
(In Erickson, 1980, Vol. I, chap. 15, p. 344)

Usually when a patient comes into your office and
needs advanced psychotherapy or hypnotherapy you do
not have that time for preparation. You've simply got to
rely upon your past experience and your past understandings. And I think that's the most important thing that
you ought to bear in mind, that you do have a body of
experience, a body of learning upon which you can draw.

(ASCH, 1980, Taped Lecture, 8/14/66)

You go into autohypnosis to achieve certain things or
acquire certain knowledge. When do you need knowledge? When you have a problem with a patient you
think it over. You work out in your unconscious mind
how you're going to deal with it. Then two weeks later
when the patient comes in you say the right thing at the
right movement. But you have no business knowing it
ahead of time because as surely as you know it consciously, you start to improve on it and ruin it.

(Erickson & Rossi, 1977, p. 44)

I recently shared my experiences with him and posed
my tentative new theoretical construct about how he
works: that during trance he is *in an almost continual
hypnotic trance....* I asked Milton Erickson what he
thought of my formulation. He replied with a smile,
"You're on the right track."

(Beahrs, 1977, p. 67)

At the present time if I have any doubt about my
capacity to see the important things I go into a trance.
When there is a crucial issue with a patient and I don't
want to miss any of the clues I go into trance.

(Erickson & Rossi, 1977, p. 42)

It [autohypnotic trance during therapy] happens
automatically because I start keeping close track of every

moment, sign, or behavioral manifestation that could be important....It happened automatically, the terrible intensity. The word "terrible" is wrong, it's pleasurable.

(Erickson & Rossi, 1977, p. 42)

Now and then I became aware that I had been so attentive to my patient that I had forgotten where I was, but I would comfortably and instantly reorient myself. [1966]

(In Erickson, 1980, Vol. II, chap. 34, p. 352)

Yes, I discovered I was in a trance with my subject. The next thing I wanted to learn was could I do equally good work with reality all around me or did I have to go into trance. I found I could work equally well under both conditions.

(Erickson & Rossi, 1977, p. 42)

Utilizing Autohypnosis

Entering hypnosis without the aid of a hypnotist can be a confusing business. The normal tendency, emphasized by numerous popular books on the subject, is to use the internal chatterings of the conscious mind as a sort of pseudo-hypnotist. This attempt to talk oneself into a hypnotic state is a contradiction in terms, because the whole point of entering a hypnotic trance is to relinquish conscious control of internal awareness.

It is much easier to experience autohypnosis after a successful hetero-hypnotic episode. Once you have learned what the experience is like with the aid of an effective hypnotist, it is much easier to allow yourself to re-enter the state on your own. Autohypnosis does not really differ from ordinary hypnosis in any particular way except that you must have total trust in your own unconscious to guide and direct the process instead of a hypnotist. When you enter an autohypnotic state, you must do so with no conscious effort to control or direct the process. Once you have decided what you want to accomplish within the autohypnotic condition, your unconscious knows what you have decided and it will either act or not act upon that decision after the hypnotic state has been allowed to develop.

Behavior in an autohypnotic state may be difficult to differentiate from ordinary waking behavior. [1966]
(In Erickson, 1980, Vol. IV, chap. 18, p. 206)

Autohypnosis or self-hypnosis is both possible and feasible, but is often a sterile procedure because of misconceptions of its nature and use. Usually the autohypnotist tries too hard to direct *consciously* the activities he wishes to take place at the hypnotic level of awareness, thus nullifying the effort.

Acceptance of autohypnotic processes, rather than attempted direction of them, leads to productive results.
(Erickson, 1970, p. 996)

Whenever you attempt self-hypnosis and you attempt to be consciously aware, then you're consciously aware. You ought to be aware of just one thing, that if you want to learn self-hypnosis your own unconscious mind knows it too, that your unconscious mind is aware of your desires to learn self-hypnosis. And you do not have to tell your unconscious mind what to do because it knows what to do a great deal better than you do. Because consciously you behave in accord with the conscious universe, the conscious patterns of behavior. Your unconscious behaves in accord with its own code of behavior. Therefore, if you want to learn self-hypnosis a better way of doing it is to allot yourself a given length of time and hope, just hope, that your unconscious is as interested in

learning it as you are. **Because if your unconscious is as willing to learn it, it will do so.**

(ASCH, 1980, Taped Lecture, 2/2/66)

In other words, you don't tell yourself what you are going to do in a trance state. Your unconscious mind knows an awful lot more than you do. If you *trust* your unconscious mind, it will do the autohypnosis that you want to do. And maybe it has a better idea than you have.

(Zeig, 1980, p. 192)

You don't know all the things you can do. Use autohypnosis to explore, knowing you are going to find something that you don't know about yet.

(Erickson & Rossi, 1977, p. 43)

No way you can consciously instruct the unconscious.

(Erickson & Rossi, 1977, p. 43)

You go into autohypnosis to achieve certain things or acquire certain knowledge.

(Erickson & Rossi, 1977, p. 44)

R: In using autohypnosis you can tell yourself what you want to achieve but —
E: Then you leave it to your unconscious.

(Erickson & Rossi, 1977, p. 45)

Everytime you go into trance you go in prepared for all other possibilities.

(Erickson & Rossi, 1977, p. 43)

By that time I could relegate things to my unconscious because I knew I had gone through all that before. I just go into trance saying, "Unconscious, do your stuff."

(Erickson & Rossi, 1977, p. 47)

If you want to do autohypnosis do it privately. Sit down in a quiet room and *don't decide what you are going to do*. Just go into a trance. Your unconscious will carry out the thing that needs to be done.

(Erickson & Rossi, 1977, p. 50)

You can go as deeply in the trance as you wish, the only thing is you don't know when. In teaching people autohypnosis I tell them that their unconscious mind will select the time, place, and situation. Usually it's done in a much more advantageous situation than you consciously know about.

(Erickson & Rossi, 1977, p. 43)

When you fall into those states you explore them and *enjoy it*! You can learn to prolong your hypnogogic and hypnopompic states and experiment with yourself in these states. You can awaken from a dream and then go beck to sleep to continue that dream.

(Erickson & Rossi, 1977, p. 49)

It [hypnogigic, autohypnotic state] gives you an opportunity to learn to dissociate any part of your body. If you don't get frightened, it gives you a chance to start examining the autohypnotic state.

(Erickson & Rossi, 1977, p. 48)

At least for me, physiological sleep will cause ordinary hypnosis to disappear.

(Erickson & Rossi, 1977, p. 46)

Exceptions

The final quotation presented in this book was originally used by Jay Haley to close his discussion of Erickson's work

(Haley, 1967). Lest we become too complacent or self-satisfied in our understanding of Erickson, of hypnosis, of psychotherapy or of people in general, it is best to keep in mind that no matter what rules or understandings we develop:

> **"There's always an exception."**
>
> *(In Haley, 1967, p. 549)*

Overview Summary and Conclusion

Erickson depended upon careful, objective observations of human behavior for the insights that allowed him to become one of this century's most remarkable clinicians. His most general observation was that people have both a conscious mode of functioning and an unconscious mode of functioning. The conscious mind represents a prejudiced and limited perspective on reality which can result in various distortions and behavioral anomolies. The unconscious mind, on the other hand, is a flexible system of thought and awareness which perceives and responds to the literal or objective qualities of reality. It is relatively unprejudiced, is very intelligent, and contains a vast reservoir of previously acquired, experientially based knowledge and memories. It serves the needs of the conscious mind and protects it from painful or unacceptable stimuli, even when these protections may generate serious neurotic or psychotic outcomes.

The consequences of the protective conscious/unconscious dissociative relationship expand over time and make it increasingly difficult for people to perceive, accept or respond to the external and internal events of their lives realistically or to use their unconscious potentials effectively. For most people, the distortions of reality caused by this process result in minor disruptions in personal functioning and interpersonal relationships, but for others the distortions result in major disabilities and discomfort. By the time they seek assistance from a therapist, these people have usually become unable to profit from their experiences and to face specific aspects of reality directly or they have developed such a distorted image of reality that their behavior is counterproductive and ineffectual. They cannot describe their situation accurately and may even actively resist attempts to help them.

The goal of the therapist, according to Erickson, is to help patients perceive, accept, and respond to their realities realistically. The problem of the therapist is how to motivate patients to undergo whatever transformations or reorganizations in conscious thought or awareness are necessary to allow them to utilize their potentials effectively toward that end. Rigid, self-limiting, arbitrary, delusional and self-defeating patterns of thought and behavior must be shattered and replaced. Barriers preventing an effective use of unconscious potentials must be removed.

This general goal is given limits and specificity by the unique needs and circumstances of each patient. The degree of reorganization, transformation, or release of unused potentials needed is defined by the particular problems, personality, and situational demands of each unique patient. Furthermore, therapeutic change is ultimately the responsibility of the patient. Therapists merely provide an environment conducive to change. They help patients feel comfortable, protected, and willing to cooperate by accepting and respecting whatever patients are or do. Therapists then offer events designed to help stimulate the learning experience necessary for change to occur. Change, however, occurs within the patients and is done by the patients. Therapists do not do therapy; they provide conditions that motivate and enable patients to do it.

Erickson emphasized that therapists can accomplish these

components of therapy more efficiently if they utilize the individual attitudes, interests, emotions, language, and behavior patients bring into therapy with them. Such utilization of a patient's natural interests and inclinations can speed and smooth the change process considerably. Whatever interests, motivates, or captures the attention of a patient should be examined carefully to determine how it can be redirected or used to enhance cooperation and to trigger a reorganizational learning experience. Patients can be led to violate and replace their restrictive patterns of thought and response comfortably, without a conscious recognition, if their typical or dominant interests, motives, and emotions are used to do so.

Hypnosis offers a useful tool with which to accomplish these therapeutic goals. Hypnotized patients are able to focus their attention more comfortably and fully upon the problem at hand and can even be taught to become completely unaware of or unable to remember their ensuing memories, understandings or responses. Awareness can be focused entirely through the unconscious mind which can precipitate revivification experiences, realistic projections into the future, dissociative awareness, ideomotor communications, amnesias, and other unusual and useful phenomena. By focusing a patient's attention upon internal events and away from external reality, a hypnotic trance can be precipitated wherein patients become less distracted by irrelevancies and more able to utilize their previously hidden capacities and experientially based knowledge to learn objective awareness, full use of potentials and control of emotional, physical, and psychological pain.

There is no easy way to become an effective Ericksonian hypnotherapist. It has been reiterated numerous times that there is no single theory to memorize and apply with every patient; there is no list of particular skills to master that can be used in any situation; there is no mystical alteration in consciousness that will provide universal truth overnight. Effective hypnotherapy and psychotherapy in an Ericksonian tradition are not just special techniques such as voice inflections, word games, puns, metaphors, or anecdotes. It is the recognition and acceptance of reality coupled with the willingness and ability to use whatever reality offers to accomplish the results desired. It is a total committment to being a hypnotherapist in all aspects of life and not just a feeble attempt to act like one during office hours. It is the slow painstaking accumulation of detailed and accurate observations and related skills. It is the willingness to participate in the hypnotherapeutic process oneself and to learn from direct personal experience as a hypnotic subject what hypnotherapy is all about and what the tool of hypnosis can accomplish. It is the ability to access one's own unconscious potentials via autohypnosis and the choice to use and to be guided by them. Ericksonian hypnotherapy and psychotherapy are crafts that demand practice and dedication. They may very well be the most demanding crafts there are.

There are many training seminars and books on Ericksonian hypnotherapy now available. The aspiring hypnotherapist can acquire valuable experiences, skills, and insights form these sources. Like the understandings obtained from this book, however, the information and skills acquired from them will be of value only to the extent that they are incorporated into one's daily patterns of experience and response. Becoming and effective hypnotherapist means adopting a hypnotherapeutic style of life. The words and concepts uttered by Erickson can serve as a source of motivation and as a guide, but they cannot serve as the answer. The answer lies within each one of us, in our total commitments to learning by objective observation and experiences how to use our full range of conscious and unconscious capacities and how to help others learn how to do the same.

Erickson's death forced me to search elsewhere to discover the full implication of his teachings. I turned to his writings and lectures where I found examples of his efforts to teach others professionals what they needed to learn, including the particular perspective necessary for that learning to occur. I became absorbed by his words and his message. The result of that absorption is this book which is my tribute to him and those who would understand what he tried to teach us. I certainly hope that my efforts have done no significant violence to his intended meanings and that this work will prove to be of value. The unpleasant fact of the matter is that we are now on our own. We no longer have Milton H. Erickson to redirect our attention, to correct our erroneous interpretations, or to chide us for our naive acceptance of whatever "truth" comes our way. Maybe, just maybe, therapists will fill that void with their own objectively based wisdom and experientially derived skills instead of new theoretical school or a new personality to emulate. If so, then Erickson's message and example will have gotten through. If not, then someone else must begin again the struggle to open up our eyes and our minds. One way or another, we must eventually put away our childish tendencies to seek out simple solutions and idols to imitate. We have to grow up, accept the wisdom given to us, and admit that this is a difficult business, a complex craft. We owe it to our patients to use Erickson's wisdom wisely. More importantly, we owe it to ourselves.

REFERENCES

American Society of Clinical Hypnosis (Producer) *Milton H. Erickson classic cassette series.* 1980, Audio taped lectures by Dr. Erickson from 8/8/64, 7/16/65, 7/18/65, 2/2/66 and 8/14/66.

Bandler, R. & Grinder, J. *Patterns of the hypnotic techniques of Milton H. Erickson, M.D.,* Cupertine, Cal.: Meta Publications, 1975.

Beahrs, J.O. Integrating Erickson's approach. *American Journal of Clinical Hypnosis,* 1977, *20,* 55–68.

Erickson, M.H. A brief survey of hypnotism. *Medical Record,* 1934, *140,* 609–613.

Erickson, M.H. An experimental investigation of the possible anti-social use of hypnosis. *Psychiatry,* 1939a, *2,* 391–414.

Erickson, M.H. The application of hypnosis to psychiatry. *Medical Record,* 1939b, *150,* 60–65.

Erickson, M.H. The early recognition of mental disease. *Diseases of the Nervous System,* 1941a, *2,* 99–108.

Erickson, M.H. Hypnosis: a general review. *Diseases of the Nervous System,* 1941b, *2,* 13–18.

Erickson, M.H. The therapy of a psychosomatic headache. *Journal of Clinical and Experimental Hypnosis,* 1953, *4,* 2–6.

Erickson, M.H. A clinical note on indirect hypnotic therapy. *Journal of Clinical and Experimental Hypnosis,* 1954a, *2,* 171–174.

Erickson, M.H. Hypnotism. Encyclopaedia Britannica, 14th edition, Vol. 12, 1954b, 22–24.

Erickson, M.H. Pseudo-orientation in time as on hypnotherapeutic procedure. *Journal of Clinical and Experimental Hypnosis,* 1954c, *2,* 261–283.

Erickson, M.H. Special techniques of brief hypnotherapy. *Journal of Clinical and Experimental Hypnosis*, 1954d, *2*, 109–129.

Erickson, M.H. Self-exploration in the hypnotic state. *Journal of Clinical and Experimental Hypnosis*, 1955, *3*, 49–57.

Erickson, M.H. Hypnosis. *Encyclopaedia Britannica,* 14th Edition, Vol. 11, 1970, 995–997 (also in 14th Edition, 1961, Vol. 12, 23–24A).

Erickson, M.H. A field investigation by hypnosis of sound loci importance in human behavior. *American Journal of Clinical Hypnosis*, 1973, *16*, 92–109.

Erickson, M.H. Control of physiological functions by hypnosis. *American Journal of Clinical Hypnosis*. 1977a, *20*, 8–19.

Erickson, M.H. Hypnotic approaches to therapy. *American Journal of Clinical Hypnosis*. 1977b, *20*, 20–35.

Erickson, M.H. *The collected papers of Milton H. Erickson on hypnosis* (4 vols.) (Edited by Ernest L. Rossi). New York: Irvington Publishers, 1980.

(Listed below by volume and chapter are the original references for all of Dr. Erickson's articles reprinted in this four-volume collection from which quotations were obtained for the present book.)

VOLUME I

Chapters

1. Initial experiments investigating the nature of hypnosis. *American Journal of Clinical Hypnosis,* 1964, *7*, 152–162.

2. Further experimental investigations of hypnosis: Hypnotic and nonhypnotic realities. *American Journal of Clinical Hypnosis*, 1967, *10*, 87–135.
3. A special inquiry with Aldous Huxley into the nature and character of various states of consciousness. *American Journal of Clinical Hypnosis*, 1965, *8*, 14–33.
4. Autohypnotic experiences of Milton H. Erickson. *American Journal of Clinical Hypnosis*, 1977, *20*, 1, 36–54 (with E. L. Rossi).
5. Historical note on hand levitation and other ideomotor techniques. *American Journal of Clinical Hypnosis*, 1961, *3*, 196–199.
6. Deep hypnosis and its induction. In L.M. LeCron (Ed.) *Experimental Hypnosis*. New York: MacMillan, 1952. Pp. 70–114.
7. Naturalistic techniques of hypnosis. *American Journal of Clinical Hypnosis*, 1958, *1*, 3–8.
8. Further clinical techniques of hypnosis: Utilization techniques. *American Journal of Clinical Hypnosis*, 1959, *2*, 3–21.
9. A transcript of a trance induction with commentary. *American Journal of Clinical Hypnosis*, 1959, *2*, 49–84 (with J. Haley and J.H. Weakland).
10. The confusion technique in hypnosis. *American Journal of Clinical Hypnosis*, 1964, *6*, 183–207.
11. The dynamics of visualization, levitation and confusion in trance induction. Unpublished fragment, circa 1940's.
12. Another example of confusion in trance induction. As told to Rossi in 1976.
13. An hypnotic technique for resistant patients: The patient, the technique and its rationale, and field ex-

periments. *American Journal of Clinical Hypnosis*, 1964, *7*, 8–32.

14. Pantomime techniques in hypnosis and the implications. *American Journal of Clinical Hypnosis*, 1964, *7*, 64–70.

15. The "surprise" and "my-friend-John" techniques of hypnosis: Minimal cues and natural field experimentation. *American Journal of Clinical Hypnosis*, 1964, *6*, 293–307.

16. Respiratory rhythm in trance induction: The role of minimal sensory cues in normal and trance behavior. Unpublished fragment, circa 1960's.

17. An indirect induction of trance: Simulation and the role of indirect suggestion and minimal cues. Unpublished paper written in the 1960's.

18. Notes on minimal cues in vocal dynamics and memory. Unpublished material written in 1964.

19. Concerning the nature and character of post-hypnotic behavior. *Journal of General Psychology*, 1941, *24*, 95–133 (with E. M. Erickson).

20. Varieties of double-bind. *American Journal of Clinical Hypnosis*, 1975, *17*, 144–157 (with E. L. Rossi).

21. Two level communication and the microdynamics of trance and suggestion. *American Journal of Clinical Hypnosis*, 1976, *18*, 153–171 (with E. L. Rossi).

22. Indirect forms of suggestion. Paper presented at 28th Annual Meeting of the Society for Clinical and Experimental Hypnosis, 1976 (with E. L. Rossi).

23. Indirect forms of suggestion in hand levitation. Unpublished paper with E. L. Rossi. 1976–78.

24. Possible detrimental effects from experimental hypnosis, *Journal of Abnormal and Social Psychology*, 1932, *27*, 321–327.

25. An experimental investigation of the possible anti-social use of hypnosis. *Psychiatry*, 1939, *2*, 391–414.
27. Stage hypnotist back syndrome. *American Journal of Clinical Hypnosis.* 1962, *5*, 141–142.
28. Editorial. *American Journal of Clincal Hypnosis*, 1964, *7*, 1–3.
29. Editorial. *American Journal of Clinical Hypnosis*, 1965, *8*, 1–2.

VOLUME II

Chapters
1. The hypnotic induction of hallucinatory color vision followed by pseudo-negative after-images. *Journal of Experimental Psychology*, 1938, *22*, 581–588 (with E. M. Erickson).
3. The induction of color blindedness by a technique of hypnotic suggestion. *Journal of General Psychology*, 1939, *20*, 61–89.
4. An experimental investigation of the hypnotic subject's apparent ability to become unaware of stimuli. *Journal of General Psychology*. 1944, *31*, 191–212.
8. An investigation of optokinetic nystagmus. *American Journal of Clinical Hypnosis.* 1962, *4*, 181–183.
9. Acquired control of pupillary responses. *American Journal of Clinical Hypnosis,* 1965, *7,* 207–208.
10. A study of clinical and experimental findings on hpnotic deafness: I. Clinical experimentation and findings. *Journal of General Psychology*, 1938, *19*, 127–150.
11. A study of clinical and experimental findings on hypnotic deafness: II. Experimental findings with a condition-

ed response technique. *Journal of General Psychology*, 1938, *19*, 151–167.

12. Chemo-anesthesia in relation to hearing and memory. *American Journal of Clinical Hypnosis,* 1963, *6*, 31–36.

13. A field investigation by hypnosis of sound loci importance in human behavior. *American Journal of Clinical Hypnosis*, 1973, 16, *92–109.*

14. Hypnotic investigation of psychosomatic phenomena: Psychosomatic interrelationships studied by experimental hypnosis. *Psychosomatic Medicine*, 1943, *5*, 51–58.

18. Control of physiological functions by hypnosis. *American Journal of Clinical Hypnosis,* 1977, *20*, 1, 8–19.

19. The hypotic alteration of blood flow: An experiment comparing waking and hypnotic responsiveness. Paper presented at the American Society of Clinical Hypnosis Annual Meeting, 1958.

20. A clinical experimental approach to psychogenic infertility. Paper presented at the American Society of Clinical Hypnosis Annual Meeting, 1958.

21. Breast development possibly influenced by hypnosis: Two instances and the psychotherapeutic results. *American Journal of Clinical Hypnosis*, 1960, *11*, 157–159.

23. The appearance in three generations of an atypical pattern of the sneezing reflex. *Journal of Genetic Psychology*, 1940, *56*, 455–459.

29. Clinical and experimental trance: Hypnotic training and time required for their development. Unpublished discussion, circa 1960.

30. Laboratory and clinical hypL.is: The same or different phenomena? *American Journal of Clinical Hypnosis*, 1967, *9*, 166–170.

31. Explorations in hypnosis research. Paper presented at the Seventh Annual University of Kansas Institute for Research in Clinical Psychology in Hypnosis and Clinical Psychology, May, 1960.
32. Expectancy and minimal sensory cues in hypnosis. Incomplete report written in the 1960's.
33. Basic psychological problems in hypnotic research. In Estabrooks, G., *Hypnosis: Current Problems*. New York: Harper and Row, 1962. Pp. 207-223.
34. The experience of interviewing in the presence of observers. In L. A. Gottschalk and A. H. Aeurbach (Eds.), *Methods of Research in Psychotherapy*. New York: Appleton-Century-Crofts, 1966. Pp. 61-64.

VOLUME III

Chapters

1. A brief survey of hypnotism. *Medical Record*, 1934, 140, 609-613.
2. Hypnosis: A general review. *Diseases of the Nervous System*, 1941, *2*, 13-18.
4. The basis of hypnosis. Panel discussion on hypnosis. *Northwest Medicine*, 1959, 1404-1408.
5. The investigation of a specific amnesia. *British Journal of Medical Psychology*, 1933, *13, 143-150*.
6. Development of apparent unconsciousness during hypnotic reliving of a traumatic experience. *Archives of Neurology and Psychiatry*, 1937, *38*, 1282-1288.
7. Clinical and experimental observations on hypnotic amnesia: Introduction to an unpublished paper. Circa 1950's.

8. The problem of amnesia in waking and hypnotic states. Unpublished manuscript, circa 1960's.

9. Varieties of hypnotic amnesia. *American Journal of Clinical Hypnosis*, 1974, *16*, 225–239 (with E. L. Rossi).

10. Literalness: An experimental study. Unpublished manuscript, circa 1940's.

11. Literalness and the use of trance in neurosis. Dialogue with E. L. Rossi, 1973.

13. Past weekday determination in hypnotic and waking states. Unpublished manuscript with A. Erickson, 1962.

16. The experimental demonstration of unconscious mentation by automatic writing. *Psychoanaltyic Quarterly*, 1937, *6*, 513–529.

17. The use of automatic drawing in the interpretation and relief of a state of acute obsessional depression. *Psychoanalytic Quarterly*, 1938, *7*, 443–466 (with L. S. Kubie).

18. The translation of the automatic writing of one hypnotic subject by another in a trance-like dissociated state. *Psychoanalytic Quarterly*, 1940, *9*, 51–63 (with L. S. Kubie).

19. Experimental demonstrations of the psychopathology of everyday life. *Psychoanalytic Quarterly*, 1939, *8*, 338–353.

20. Demonstration of mental mechanisms by hypnosis. *Archives of Neurology and Psychiatry*, 1939, *42*, 367–370.

21. Unconscious mental activity in hypnosis—psychoanaltyic implications. *Psychoanalytic Quarterly*, January, 1944, Vol. XIII, No. 1 (with L. B. Hill).

22. Negation or reversal of legal testimony. *Archives of Neurology and Psychiatry*, 1938, *40*, 549–555.

23. The permanent relief of an obsessional phobia by means of communication with an unsuspected dual personality. *Psychoanalytic Quarterly*, 1939, *8*, 471–509 (with L. S. Kubie).
24. The clinical discovery of a dual personality. Unpublished manuscript, circa 1940's.
28. A study of an experimental neurosis hypnotically induced in a case of ejaculatio praecox. *British Journal of Medical Psychology*, 1935, *15*, 34–50.
29. The method employed to formulate a complex story for the induction of an experimental neurosis in a hypnotic subject. *Journal of General Psychology*, 1944, *31*, 67–84.

VOLUME IV

Chapters

1. The applications of hypnosis to psychiatry. *Medical Record,* 1939, *150*, 60–65.
2. Hypnosis in medicine. *Medical Clinics of North America.* New York: W. B. Saunders Co., 1944, 639–652.
3. Hypnotic techniques for the therapy of acute psychiatric disturbances in war. *American Journal of Psychiatry*, 1945, *101*, 668–672. (copyright 1945, American Psychiatric Association)
4. Hypnotic psychotherapy. *Medical Clinics of North America.* New York: W. B. Saunders Co., 1948, 571–584.
5. Hypnosis in general practice. *State of Mind.* 1957, 1.
6. Hypnosis: Its renascence as a treatment modality. *American Journal of Clinical Hypnosis*, 1970, *13*, 71–89. (Originally published in *Trends in Psychiatry*, Merck, Sharp & Dohme, 1966, 3 (3), 3–43.

7. Hypnotic approaches to therapy. *American Journal of Clinical Hypnosis*, 1977, *20*, 1, 20–35.

10. Experimental hypnotherapy in Tourette's Disease. *American Journal of Clinical Hypnosis*, 1965, *7*, 325–331.

11. Hypnotherapy: The patient's right to both success and failure. *American Journal of Clinical Hypnosis*, 1965, *7*, 254–257.

12. Successful hypnotherapy that failed. *American Journal of Clinical Hypnosis*, 1966, *9*, 62–65.

15. Pediatric Hypnotherapy. *American Journal of Clinical Hypnosis*, 1959, *1*, 25–29.

16. The utilization of patient behavior in the hypnotherapy of obesity: three case reports. *American Journal of Clinical Hypnosis*, 1960, *3*, 112–116.

17. Hypnosis and examination panics. *American Journal of Clinical Hypnosis*, 1965, *7*, 356–358.

18. Experiential knowledge of hypnotic phenomena employed for hypnotherapy. *American Journal of Clinical Hypnosis*, 1966, *8*, 299–309.

19. The burden of responsibility in effective psychotherapy. *American Journal of Clinical Hypnosis*, 1964, *6*, 269–271.

20. The use of symptoms as an integral part of therapy. *American Journal of Clinical Hypnosis*, 1965, *8*, 57–65.

21. Hypnosis in obstetrics: Utilizing experiential learnings. Unpublished manuscript, circa 1950's.

22. A therapeutic double bind utilizing resistance. Unpublished manuscript, 1952.

23. Utilizing the patient's own personality and ideas: "Doing it his own way." Unpublished manuscript, 1954.

24. An introduction to the study and application of hypnosis for pain control. In J. Lassner (Ed.), *Hypnosis and Psychosomatic Medicine: Proceedings of the Interna-*

tional Congress for Hypnosis and Psychosomatic Medicine. Springer Verlag, 1967.

26. Migraine headache in a resistant patient. Unpublished manuscript, 1936

27. Hypnosis in painful terminal illness. *American Journal of Clinical Hypnosis*, 1959, *1*, 117–121.

28. The interspersal hypnotic technique for symptom correction and pain control. *American Journal of Clinical Hypnosis*, 1966, *8*, 198–209.

29. Hypnotic training for transforming the experience of chronic pain. Dialogue with E. L. Rossi, 1973.

30. Hypnotically oriented psychotherapy in organic brain damage. *American Journal of Clinical Hypnosis*, 1963, *6*, 92–112.

31. Hypnotically oriented psychotherapy in organic brain damage: An addendum. *American Journal of Clinical Hypnosis.* 1964, *6*, 361–362.

33. Experimental hypnotherapy in speech problems: A case report. *American Journal of Clinical Hypnosis*, 1965, *7*, 358–360.

34. Provocation as a means of motivating recovery from a cerebrovascular accident. Unpublished manuscript, circa 1965.

35. Hypnotherapy with a psychotic. Unpublished manuscript, circa 1940's with dialogue with E. L. Rossi added later.

36. Symptom prescription for expanding the psychotic's world view. Portion of a paper with J. Zeig presented to the 20th Annual Scientific Meeting of the American Society of Clinical Hypnosis, 1977.

38. Psychotherapy achieved by a reversal of the neurotic processes in a case of ejaculatio praecox. *American Journal of Clinical Hypnosis*, 1973, *15*, 217–222.

39. Modesty: An authoritarian approach permitting recon-

ditioning via fantasy. Unpublished manuscript, circa 1950's.

40. Sterility: A therapeutic reorientation to sexual satisfaction. Unpublished manuscript, circa 1950's.
41. The abortion issue: Facilitating unconscious dynamics permitting real choice. Unpublished manuscript, circa 1950's.
42. Impotence: Facilitating unconscious reconditioning. Unpublished manuscript, 1953.
44. Vasectomy: A detailed illustration of a therapeutic reorientation. Unpublished manuscript, circa 1950's.
46. Facilitating objective thinking and new frames of reference with pseudo-orientation in time. Unpublished manuscript, circa 1940's.
49. The reorganization of unconscious thinking without awareness: Two cases with intellectualized resistance against hypnosis. Unpublished manuscript, 1956.
50. Rossi, E.L. Psychological shocks and creative moments in psychotherapy. *American Journal of Clinical Hypnosis*, 1973, *16*, 1, 9–22.
51. Facilitating a new cosmetic frame of reference. Unpublished manuscript, 1927.
52. The ugly duckling: Transforming the self-image. Unpublished manuscript, 1933.
53. A shocking breakout of a mother domination. Unpublished manuscript, circa 1936.
54. Shock and surprise facilitating a new self-image. Unpublished manuscript, circa 1930's..
55. Correcting an inferiority complex. Unpublished manuscript, 1937–1938.
56. The hypnotherapy of two psychosomatic dental problems. *Journal of the American Society of Psychosomatic Dentistry and Medicine.* 1955, *1*, 6–10.

57. The identification of a secure reality. *Family Process,* 1962, *1*, 294–303.

58. The hypnotic corrective emotional experience. *American Journal of Clinical Hypnosis,* 1965, 7, 242–248.

Erickson, M.H. & Lustig, H.S. *Verbatim transcript of the "Artistry of Milton H. Erickson, M.D." (2 Parts) 1975.*

Erickson, M.H. & Rossi, E.L. Varieties of double bind. *American Journal of Clinical Hypnosis,* 1975, *17*, 143–157.

Erickson, M.H. & Rossi, E.L. Two level communication and the microdynamics of trance and suggestion. *American Journal of Clinical Hypnosis,* 1976, *18* 153–171.

INDEX

NEW FROM IRVINGTON

ERICKSONIAN HYPNOSIS: Handbook of Clinical Practice
By Lee C. Overholser

1984   ISBN 0-8290-0738-5 $29.50   325pp

LIFE REFRAMING IN HYPNOSIS: The Seminars, Workshops,
and Lectures of Milton H. Erickson, Vol. II
By Milton H. Erickson
Edited by Ernest L. Rsssi and Margaret O. Ryan
Includes 1-hour audio tape
1985   0-8290-1581-7 $39.50   332pp

HYPNOTHERAPY FOR TROUBLED CHILDREN
Includes Audio Cassette
By Robert E. Duke

1984   ISBN 0-8290-1014-9 $24.95   255pp

PREVIOUSLY PUBLISHED

HEALING IN HYPNOSIS: The Seminars, Workshops, and
Lectures of Milton H. Erickson, Vol. I
1984   ISBN 0-8290-0963-9 $38.50   311pp
By Milton H. Erickson
Edited by Ernest L. Rossi, Margaret O. Ryan, and Florence A. Sharp
Includes Audio Cassette

HYPNOTIC TECHNIQUES FOR INCREASING SELF-ESTEEM
R. A. Steffenhagen, Editor

1982   ISBN 0-8290-0775-X $26.50   268pp

TIME DISTORTION IN HYPNOSIS
By Linn F. Cooper and Milton H. Erickson
Reissue

1982   ISBN 0-8290-0650-8 $24.50   206pp